Clinical Sports
Anatomy

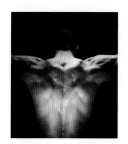

Dedication

ATM would like to dedicate his contribution to this book to his beautiful, and ever-supportive wife Shannon and children William, Noah and Sienna, who have yet to understand what daddy really does.

EF dedicates his work to Nina for her unwavering love, friendship and general hotness; to Ava, a bright light in dark days; and to Anna and Jeremiah for bestowing belief and leading by example.

PM would like dedicate his contribution to his partner, Helena, his best and most loving critic, and to his children, Rebecca and Connor, for their ongoing interest in the project.

Clinical Sports
Anatomy

Andy Franklyn-Miller
MBBS, MRCGP, MFSEM(UK)

Éanna Falvey
MB, BCh, MRCPI, FFSEM, MMedSc(Sports & Exercise Medicine)

Paul McCrory
MBBS, PhD, FRACP, FACSP, FACSM, FFSEM, FASMF, FRSM, GradDipEpidStats

Peter Brukner
OAM, MBBS, DRCOG, DipRACOG, FACSP, FACSM, FASMF, FFSEM(UK)

The **McGraw·Hill** *Companies*

Sydney New York San Francisco Auckland
Bangkok Bogotá Caracas Hong Kong
Kuala Lumpur Lisbon London Madrid
Mexico City Milan New Delhi San Juan
Seoul Singapore Taipei Toronto

The *McGraw·Hill* Companies

Notice

Medicine is an ever-changing science. As new research and clinical experience broaden our knowledge, changes in treatment and drug therapy are required. The editors and the publisher of this work have checked with sources believed to be reliable in their efforts to provide information that is complete and generally in accord with the standards accepted at the time of publication. However, in view of the possibility of human error or changes in medical sciences, neither the editors, nor the publisher, nor any other party who has been involved in the preparation or publication of this work warrants that the information contained herein is in every respect accurate or complete. Readers are encouraged to confirm the information contained herein with other sources. For example, and in particular, readers are advised to check the product information sheet included in the package of each drug they plan to administer to be certain that the information contained in this book is accurate and that changes have not been made in the recommended dose or in the contraindications for administration. This recommendation is of particular importance in connection with new or infrequently used drugs.

First published 2011

Copyright © 2011 McGraw-Hill Australia Pty Limited CHECK WITH EDITORIAL

Additional owners of copyright are acknowledged on the acknowledgments page

Every effort has been made to trace and acknowledge copyrighted material. The authors and publishers tender their apologies should any infringement have occurred.

Reproduction and communication for educational purposes

The Australian *Copyright Act 1968* (the Act) allows a maximum of one chapter or 10% of the pages of this work, whichever is the greater, to be reproduced and/or communicated by any educational institution for its educational purposes provided that the institution (or the body that administers it) has sent a Statutory Educational notice to Copyright Agency Limited (CAL) and been granted a licence. For details of statutory educational and other copyright licences contact: Copyright Agency Limited, Level 15, 233 Castlereagh Street, Sydney NSW 2000. Telephone: (02) 9394 7600. Website: www.copyright.com.au

Reproduction and communication for other purposes

Apart from any fair dealing for the purposes of study, research, criticism or review, as permitted under the Act, no part of this publication may be reproduced, distributed or transmitted in any form or by any means, or stored in a database or retrieval system, without the written permission of McGraw-Hill Australia including, but not limited to, any network or other electronic storage.

Enquiries should be made to the publisher via www.mcgraw-hill.com.au or marked for the attention of the Rights and Permissions Manager at the address below.

National Library of Australia Cataloguing-in-Publication data

Title:	Clinical sports anatomy / Andrew Franklyn-Miller [et al.].
Edition:	1ed.
ISBN:	9780070285552 (pbk.)
Series:	Clinical sports medicine.
Notes:	Includes bibliographical references and index.
Subjects:	Musculoskeletal system. Wounds and injuries. Diagnosis. Sports injuries, Diagnosis. Sports medicine.
Other authors/contributors:	Franklyn-Miller, Andrew.
Dewey Number:	617.1027

Published in Australia by
McGraw-Hill Australia Pty Ltd
Level 2, 82 Waterloo Road, North Ryde NSW 2113
Publisher: Elizabeth Walton
Art director: Astred Hicks
Production editor: Michael McGrath
Editor: Mary-Jo O'Rourke
Illustrator: Levent Efe
Proofreader: Nicole McKenzie
Indexer: Mary Coe
Internal design: David Rosemeyer
Cover design: Pier Vido
Typeset in Scala by Midland Typesetters, Australia
Printed in China by 1010 Printing International Ltd.

1 2 3 4 5 6 7 8 9 10

Foreword

The subject of clinical anatomy has undergone tremendous changes in profile over the years .

In the 1800s it provided all the novel data available—it was the MRI of its time. In more recent years the vogue has been to regard anatomy as a thing of the past, which is certainly an unfortunate trend for sport and exercise medicine. Diagnosis is the key to successful treatment, and anatomy is the key to accurate musculoskeletal injury diagnosis.

During my medical training, attention to the "clinical" part of anatomy was an aspirational goal. My recollection is of dry textbooks, reflecting the rather dry lectures that preceded dissection.

Clinical Sports Anatomy changes all that, with numerous innovations that will launch future clinicians on a much more enjoyable, and thus more productive, experience in anatomy teaching. The book is particularly timely when anatomy dissection time has been sliced and, as a result, the critical musculoskeletal anatomy curriculum has all but disappeared.

The graphics In *Clinical Sports Anatomy* are exceptional; the text is clear and clinically focused, and the idea of functional triangles is inspired. I was delighted to see clinical scenarios and jewels at the end of every chapter. This book truly represents a substantial step forward in pedagogy.

The authorship team is critical to any textbook, and here we see a terrific alliance among experts from both the Northern and Southern hemispheres. Drs Franklyn-Miller and Falvey have completed rigorous sport and exercise medicine specialization in the recent past; Drs McCrory and Brukner have been household names for several decades, but continue to represent the leading edge of sports medicine, both academically and in their active careers with individual athletes and sporting teams. This combination provides the innovation that comes with new blood, tempered with the experience of knowing how to make messages "stick". The final product is attractive, comprehensive and eminently useable.

I commend any clinician whose work includes musculoskeletal diagnosis and treatment, to examine this book carefully—it makes a wonderful addition to McGraw-Hill's Sports Medicine Series.

Karim Khan MBBS, PhD, FACSP
Sports and Exercise Physician

Professor, Department of Family Practice and Centre for Hip Health and Mobility
Faculty of Medicine, University of British Columbia

Editor, *British Journal of Sports Medicine*.

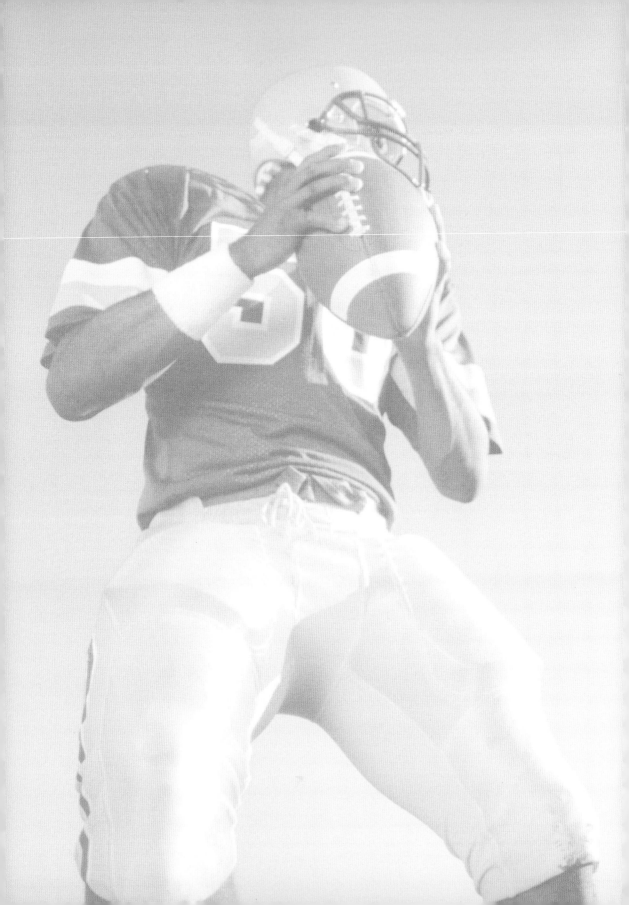

Contents

Preface

As medical students we are interested in anatomy partly because we feel we ought to be (given we are starting a career in medicine), but also out of necessity, as someone will invariably examine us on our learning every six weeks or so. In today's medical curriculum, things have changed. Often the chance to spend time dissecting a cadaver oneself with a guiding hand to prevent the unnecessary destruction of vital nerves, vessels or muscle insertions, has been reduced to the bare minimum. In the miniscule amount of time afforded to the whole of anatomy, musculoskeletal anatomy takes a back seat to the major organs. Physiotherapy students, although afforded more time, still do not have the opportunities of their predecessors as time is squeezed. To paraphrase the polymath Goethe: Eine Person hoert nur, was sie verstehen' (a person hears only what they understand); when the clinician approaches an injury, so too 'they will only see what they know'. How is the modern student/clinician to wade through the morass of information on musculoskeletal pathology and its treatment, without a firm knowledge of the basics—the anatomy?

The authors spent time teaching anatomy at the University of Melbourne, Australia, and were struck by the massive opportunity presented by a 'second chance'—the ability to approach anatomy with some clinical insight. We were uniquely afforded the opportunity as clinicians to go back into the prosection room to spend unlimited amounts of time. Not burdened by examination or learning objectives, we were able to satisfy our curiosities and really understand the clinical challenges posed, both when learning the relevant anatomy but also organising it into clinically relevant segments. This process was something of a revelation, and often, while in the process of examining a joint or the layering of muscles and fascia, we reminded ourselves how lucky a position we were in. This experience was tempered by the opportunity to experience first-hand the challenge of imparting this information to anatomy students.

The Baretto Espresso Bar in the Law Building at the University of Melbourne has a lot to answer for. We have spent hours and thousands of dollars on lattes and sandwiches while we came up with triangles, revised anatomy and generally bounced ideas between us. From this, the idea of the book arose.

This first edition includes over 60 original illustrations by Dr Levent Efe. We have attempted to deconstruct our laboratory work to aid you, the reader, and afford you something of the opportunity we had. It is not perfect—nothing outside the dissection room is—and we would encourage all of you to make the most of any time spent with cadaveric tissue. We include case histories to help apply the anatomy and, in particular, our way of orientating the reader to the anatomy in easily digestible sections. We hope it enlightens you in a small way and inspires further work.

Dr Andy Franklyn-Miller

MBBS MRCGP MFSEM (UK)

Dr Andy Franklyn-Miller is one of the first doctors in the United Kingdom to hold a substantive consultant post in sports and exercise medicine. He is Director of the Centre for Human Performance, Rehabilitation and Sports Medicine at the Defence Medical Rehabilitation Centre, Surrey, London. A clinician and academic, he holds fellowship of the Faculty of Sports and Exercise Medicine and is part of the Education Committee of the British Association of Sports and Exercise Medicine and the European Faculty of Sports and Exercise Medicine. He remains a fellow at the Centre for Health, Exercise and Sports Medicine at the University of Melbourne, Australia, and his research interests lie in the role of fascia in lower limb injury, the physiological demands of rehabilitation, and the cardiovascular risk of complex trauma.

Having been team doctor and medical and performance advisor for a variety of international organizations including the men's Great British Rowing Team, Melbourne Storm Rugby League Football Club, New Zealand Women's Rugby Football Union, UK men's Athletics and England U16 RFU among others, he maintains currency in the optimisation of athlete performance, altitude, and acclimatisation strategies, and the prevention of lower limb injuries.

Dr Éanna Falvey

MB, BCh, MRCPI, FFSEM, MMedSc(Sports & Exercise Medicine)

Dr Eanna Falvey is one of a few clinicians in Ireland to specifically train for, and gain speciality recognition in, sports and exercise medicine. He is currently Director of Sports Medicine at the Sports Surgery Clinic in Dublin, Ireland, working as a Consultant Sports Physician. As a Fellow of the Centre for Health Exercise & Sports Medicine at the University of Melbourne, Eanna is a member of the musculoskeletal research group which has produced work on groin pain and the role of fascia in lower limb injury. He is published in sports injury epidemiology and EIB, is a reviewer for the BJSM and BMJ, and enjoys post-graduate sports medicine teaching

A former international amateur super-heavyweight boxer, Eanna retains a keen interest in boxing, hurling, gaelic football, and rugby. He is team physician to the Irish Senior Rugby Team and the Irish Amateur Boxing Association's high performance unit. He has worked in professional rugby since 2003, and has team experience in hurling, football, athletics, Australian rules football, and water polo. Eanna's clinical interests include tendinopathy, groin pain, and hamstring pathology.

A/Prof Paul McCrory

MBBS PhD FRACP FACSP FACSM FFSEM FASMF FRSM GradDipEpidStats

Dr McCrory is a consultant neurologist, general physician, and a sports and exercise physician. He has extensive clinical and research experience, particularly in the area of management of sport-related neurological injury including brain, peripheral nerve, and spinal cord injury. For 15 years, he was team doctor for a professional Australian football club and he also worked at the Sydney 2000 Olympic Games, as well as in individual athlete care. He is past-president of the Australasian College of Sports Physicians and an executive board member for the Institute of Sports and Exercise Medicine in the UK, as well as serving on a variety of committees for national and international bodies. He has an extensive publication record and is the former editor-in-chief of the *British Journal of Sports Medicine*, as well as an associate editor of the *Clinical Journal of Sports Medicine*, and an editorial board member of *Physician and Sports Medicine* and *Current Sports Medicine Reports*. He is founding member and co-chair of the Concussion in Sport Consensus Group formed following the 1st International Conference of Concussion in Sport in 2001, and does ongoing consulting work for the medical commissions of The British Horseracing Authority, the International Olympic Commission, the International Rugby Board and FIFA. He has an ongoing professional interest in eHealth, and is currently involved in the design and production of medical software for general practice.

Peter Brukner

OAM, MBBS, DRCOG, DipRACOG, FACSP, FACSM, FASMF, FFSEM(UK)

Peter Brukner is a specialist sports and exercise physician and founding partner of the *Olympic Park Sports Medicine Centre* in Melbourne, Australia. Peter is a world-renowned sports medicine clinician and researcher, and is currently Associate Professor in Sports Medicine at the Centre for Health, Exercise and Sports Medicine at the University of Melbourne. He has served two terms as President of the Australian College of Sports Physicians, during which time he was instrumental in the establishment of a specialist level training program in Australia for sports medicine physicians.

Peter has published widely internationally with a number of books, book chapters, and original research articles. He is the co-author of *Clinical Sports Medicine*, a best-selling general sports medicine text now in its third edition, as well as *Stress Fractures, Food for Sport* and the *Encyclopedia of Exercise and Sport Health*. Peter has been team physician for Melbourne and Collingwood AFL clubs as well as national athletics, swimming, soccer, and men's hockey teams. He was an Australian Team Physician at the Atlanta and Sydney Olympic Games, and Socceroos Team Doctor for the 2010 World Cup. In 2010 he commenced as Head of Sports Medicine and Sports Science at Liverpool Football Club in the United Kingdom.

His contribution to sports medicine has been recognised by the award of the inaugural Citation for Distinguished Service by the Australian College of Sports Physicians, and the Citation Award of the American College of Sports Medicine. In 2006 Peter was awarded the Medal of the Order of Australia (OAM) for services to sports medicine.

Acknowledgments

The authors would like thank:

The donors and the families of the cadavers left to research at the Department of Cell Biology and Anatomy at the University of Melbourne. We will be eternally grateful for your gift.

Professor Chris Briggs and Dr Priscilla Barker from the Department of Anatomy at the University of Melbourne who sustained our endless requests and guided our embryonic dissection skills to something resembling competence, and allowed us the opportunity to teach both physiotherapy and medical students, which was essential in understanding our concepts.

Susan Kerby and Lauren Richardson from the Dissection Room at the University of Melbourne, who always would listen to our strange requests and amazingly arranged our fresh cadaver access with Ian Bouch.

Professor Michael G. Molloy, for his unparalleled help, support, and friendship.

Stuart Thyer, whose excellent medical photography was key to our original work.

Levent Efe, our medical illustrator, whose ability to interpret our scribbles and non-artistic interpretations of new orientations and the triangle concepts never ceased to amaze. Also to his steady education in the process of illustration and business.

Peter Brukner and Karim Khan for the use of the 'case history' photographs from *Clinical Sports Medicine*.

Elizabeth Walton, who believed in us, cajoled us, and never appeared flustered despite Professor Karim Khan's warning that whatever the time we believed it would take us to write, triple it and then we might be close (he was correct). Lizzie, thank you for your guidance and patience!

The staff at the Olympic Park Sports Medicine Centre in Melbourne, Australia, who welcomed us during our respective fellowships and provided unrivalled clinical experience and inspiration.

The staff of the Baretto Espresso Bar in the Law Building at the University of Melbourne for keeping us in lattes!

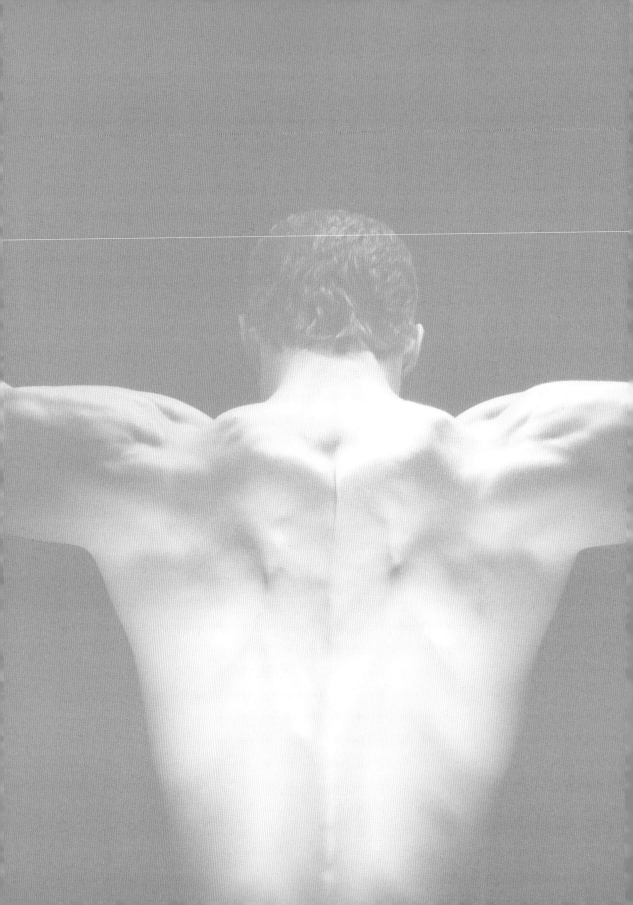

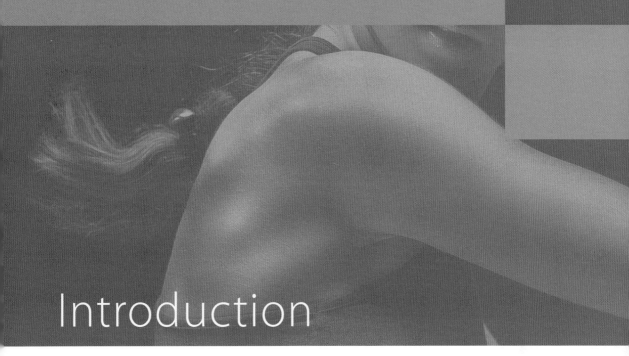

Introduction

History of anatomy teaching

Alcmaeon of Croton in the mid-5th century BC is the first person reported to have performed human dissection; this was in a misguided quest to find "intelligence" rather than from a burning desire to study anatomy. The first anatomical descriptive work came from Herophilus (335–280 BC), the so-called "father of anatomy", who publicly dissected convicted criminals, and so laid the foundation stones of the science of anatomy. The guiding ethical principle of his work, similar to that of modern anatomy, was that from the suffering of few, the many will be helped.

Claudius Galen (129–c200 AD) was arguably the first professional sports physician (Fig. 1). Given his medical training in the great center of learning of Alexandria, and his professional role as a physician for the gladiatorial contests in Permagmum in Asia Minor, he was in an ideal position to consider the anatomical aspects of the injuries he saw in his daily professional life. Perhaps driven by a quest to understand such injuries, he performed a number of documented dissections of animals, which formed the basis of his medical tracts, of which over a hundred survive. His work *On the use of the parts of the human body* was a significant step forward in anatomical knowledge. However, his use of primate, rather than human, dissection resulted in many fundamental errors which took almost 1500 years to correct, although his theory that the constituent of arteries was blood, not air, was proved accurate.

Leonardo da Vinci (1452–1519), the archetype of the Renaissance man, is renowned as a painter whose understanding of the human form was firmly based on anatomical study. Leonardo's master, Andrea del Verrocchio, had insisted that all his pupils learn anatomy. As a successful artist, he was given permission to dissect human corpses at the Hospital of Santa Maria Nuova in Florence, and later at hospitals in Milan and Rome. In 1510, he collaborated with Marcantonio della Torre on an anatomical treatise (*Treatise on painting*), for which Leonardo

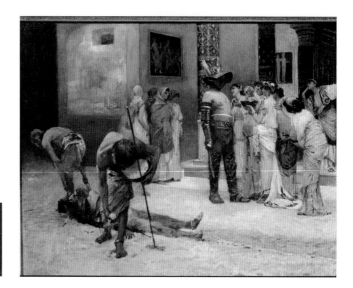

Figure 1 Claudious Galen's work on injured gladiators and animal dissection advanced anatomical knowledge

made more than 200 drawings. It was first published in 1680, some 161 years after his death. Leonardo's vivid series of anatomical drawings detailing the structure of bone, visceral organs, the brain, and musculature took medicine to the next level.

One of his most enduring anatomical images is the *Vitruvian man* (Fig. 2), which illustrates the proportions of the human body. It is perhaps the first study of anthropometrics, and has become a cultural icon in its own right. The Vitruvian man demonstrates the relationships of proportion in a way that we have borrowed for this book, in order to create a number of new anatomical points as references for the triangle concept contained here. These reference points rely on the reliable transference of proportion from one skeleton to another, regardless of body habitus or size.

Andreas Vesalius (1514–1564) was an anatomist, physician, and author of one of the most influential books on human anatomy, *De humani corporis fabrica* (*On the structure of the human body*), published in 1543. Vesalius is often referred to as the founder of modern human anatomy. His insistence on studying human, rather than animal, anatomy corrected many of the inaccuracies which had persisted since the work of Galen almost 1200 years earlier.

Change in current teaching

Modern anatomical texts largely stem from the work of the British anatomist and surgeon, Henry Gray (1827–1861). In 1858, Gray published the first edition of his book *Anatomy*, which covered 750 pages and contained 363 figures (Fig. 4). He had the good fortune of securing the help of his friend Henry Vandyke Carter, a skilled draftsman and former demonstrator of anatomy at St George's Hospital. The success of the book was undoubtedly due in no small measure to the excellence of its illustrations. Gray's death from smallpox came just three years after the publication of *Anatomy: Descriptive and surgical*, which is now in its 40th edition.

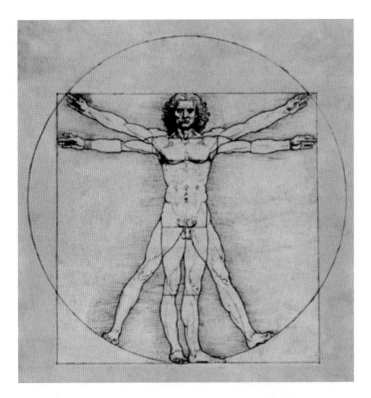

Figure 2 Leonardo da Vinci's Vitruvian man

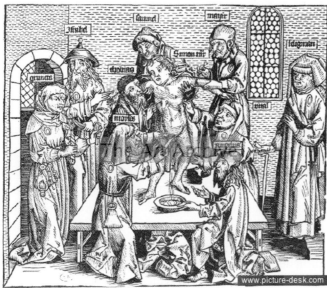

Figure 3 Anatomy class from a 15th century German engraving

Anatomy is currently of great interest to the public[1, 2], which of course includes the sporting population, whose understanding of anatomical functions is likely to be above that of the lay person. Traditional anatomical texts often do not relate the clinical pathology to the structure responsible, nor indeed concentrate on the functional aspects of musculoskeletal anatomy in

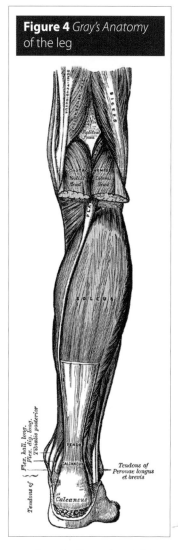

Figure 4 *Gray's Anatomy of the leg*

any great detail. Von Hagens' *BodyWorks* (Fig. 5), although it relates dramatic cadaveric images to function, does not inform in sufficient detail regarding pathology, although it is certainly a step forward.

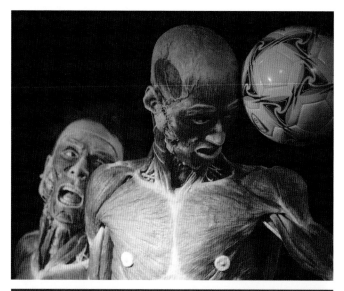

Figure 5 Professor Gunther Von Hagens' plasticized cadavers on public display.

The authors have been fortunate to spend 12 months preparing for this book by performing original anatomical prosection under the guidance of Associate Professor Christopher Briggs and Dr Priscilla Barker in the human anatomy laboratory of the University of Melbourne. As practicing clinicians, the authors have been able to relate the anatomical difficulties in complex clinical diagnosis directly to cadaveric dissection. This approach brought success in the sports medicine clinic, and thus the concept of *Clinical Sports Anatomy* was conceived.

A thorough understanding of anatomy is essential in musculoskeletal and sports medicine, in order to make accurate diagnoses. Anatomy teaching has been in steady decline over recent years in the United Kingdom, the United States, and Australia.[4, 5] Students of today's generation are exposed to significantly less anatomy teaching than their predecessors[6], and there is concern from professional medical colleges over the resultant reduction in anatomical knowledge at the graduate level[7], although this concern has unfortunately brought about little change to modern teaching methods[8] in undergraduate curricula.

The transformation in teaching strategy at many universities[9] has led to a fundamental paradigm shift, away from the absolute requirement for students to build a systematic knowledge base of anatomy, pathology, and physiology. These foundation skills were traditionally the basis for constructing a diagnosis, but have been replaced in recent graduates with a common problem-solving framework, the ability to search for online medical information, and a composite learning experience. Whether this problem-based medical curriculum will result in improved quality of medical graduates remains to be seen.

Fundamentals of the diagnostic process

Sir William Osler (1849–1919) insisted that his students learned medicine from seeing and talking to real patients, and this approach was instrumental in the establishment of medical training programs within hospitals. Osler has been quoted as saying, "He who studies medicine without books sails an uncharted sea, whereas he who studies medicine without patients does not go to sea at all".

Osler believed that the best textbooks were the patients themselves, and the application of foundation knowledge of anatomy, physiology, and pathology were crucial in the bedside understanding of patients' conditions.[10] Clinicians draw on their knowledge base to refine a possible diagnosis from triggers in a patient's illness history. Pattern recognition forms a critical part of the diagnostic process, and allows discrimination between a number of diagnostic possibilities, which in turn focuses the physical examination and future investigation.[11] Many esteemed colleagues agree[6, 12] with the need for more anatomical teaching; however, with basic science being out of vogue at present, such skills are in dangerous decline.

The 4-step approach

In order to refocus attention on such a vital area, we outline a 4-step compartmentalization of the diagnostic process[13, 14], which emphasizes history and examination, in an effort to target investigation appropriately in the final step in the process. Dividing the method into a 4-step approach is a means by which the emphasis on traditional skills can be focused by the clinician, teacher or student on the clinical problem at hand.

Step 1: Define and align

The clinician must first ascertain from where the pain emanates. Defining the joint or relevant area affected is the initial task. When the area has been identified, the clinician locates the important anatomical landmarks for that joint or area. For a patient presenting with lateral elbow pain, the obvious "define" is the elbow. We then suggest that the clinician "align" the elbow triangles with the identified landmarks. Clinicians should also focus their examination to include those structures potentially damaged within the area, such as the ulnar nerve, the common extensor origin, the radial head, and the lateral epicondyle.

The text of each chapter will familiarize the reader with the structures encountered in the particular area of interest, presented in a logical manner as they are anticipated, moving along the borders of the triangle. It can be seen that this aligns the questioning and subsequent examination to focus on particular structures which may have been injured, far more than only thinking about the elbow.

Step 2: Listen and localize

Following on from step 1, tables in this section (Fig. 4) direct the reader to targeted questioning, in order to differentiate, if possible, between various diagnoses in the region localized by the triangle. Lateral elbow pain worsened by activity such as playing golf or sweeping the floor requires specific questioning and examination to narrow the diagnosis.

Rather than pose the nebulous question, "What could this diagnosis be?" it is important to pose the question, "What is it not?" Rather than creating an exhaustive list of potential diagnoses, the clinician is better served by eliminating potential diagnoses through discriminative questioning, followed by directed examination.

The patient may have common extensor origin tendinopathy, but the diagnosis could equally well involve the radial head, the radial nerve, the articular surface of the capitellum, or in fact be referred from the cervical spine; so important negatives require attention and training in application. To exclude other sources of pathology, questioning should be targeted at relevant systems or anatomical areas. The consultation must be approached, following step 1, with a list of conditions to be excluded. This requires knowledge of the underlying anatomy and pathology.

We have attempted to package the anatomy in easily digested segments, using the triangle superimposition. By focusing on the functions of those anatomical structures in the relevant sections, it is possible to focus the discriminative questioning.

Step 3: Palpate and re-create

The next step is to focus on the most evidence-based diagnostic tests or maneuvers. The authors conducted extensive, systematic reviews in order to advise on the most evidence-based tests.

The aim of this is to examine with a specific purpose, not just doing such a test for completeness, but in order to identify or dismiss specific pathology. Too often, as students, we attempted to perform a McMurray test or elicit Trendelenberg's sign without thinking about why we were attempting this, other than it being what we were taught to do by our teachers during our training. The adage "see one, do one, teach one" is enshrined in medical teaching; however, in many cases, the reason for doing such tests in the first place is never clearly thought through.

In the example of lateral elbow pain, it is important to connect the test with the potentially damaged structure; resisted extension of the wrist is the examination of choice for extensor tendinopathy, but assessment of resisted supination or extension of the third digit are helpful in excluding radial nerve entrapment. Passive range of movement of the radial head and elbow joint also need to be cleared, in order to exclude articular involvement. Similarly, a thorough examination of the cervical spine and peripheral nervous system of the upper limb is needed in order to assess the possibility of referred pain. Without this basic understanding, an important injury may be missed. In the absence of underpinning anatomical knowledge, such an approach simply cannot be contemplated.

Step 4: Alleviate and investigate

Finally, we direct the reader to the most evidence-based final investigation, where discrimination is not possible by physical examination alone. Often this is of dual function i.e. a diagnostic and potentially pain-alleviating injection, which serves to confirm and treat simultaneously. Injection of local anesthetic into the radial tunnel distal to the lateral epicondyle may abolish symptoms, making a diagnosis of radial tunnel syndrome likely. But, more often, it relies on modern imaging techniques. In the case of ambiguity, an magnetic resonance imaging (MRI) request form with "common extensor tendinopathy" is of far more value to both the patient and the radiologist than "elbow pain". It is critical to emphasize that the most appropriate and cost-effective investigation should be the final step in the diagnostic pathway, rather than the first resort.

Decline of examination skills

Bedside teaching, the mainstay of many generations of clinical education, has been lost in favor of simulated patients, objective examination assessments, and clinical problems designed to fit the curriculum teaching modules and the standardized examination process.[3] Sadly, real-life clinical scenarios rarely fit into neat boxes, an unpalatable truth which poses a fundamental problem for any problem-based learning (PBL) curriculum. There are those who suggest that basic anatomical skills are best abandoned for more modern diagnostic techniques centered on imaging and laboratory tests. They argue that the diagnostic power of history and examination are poor, and that no single symptom or sign is sufficiently discriminative.[15, 16]

The judicious use of modern advances in investigation has improved understanding and diagnostic yield in some situations, but there have also been sharp increases in their use diagnostically, economically, and medico-legally as physicians seek to protect themselves from the threat of litigation. Iglehart looked at the use of imaging services in the US[17] and found a spiraling use of MRI which did not necessarily improve diagnostic yield.

The authors argue that focusing on a thorough clinical history and examination, using the traditional teaching model, not only has the potential to reduce the burden of unnecessary investigation, but it can also target essential investigation more accurately and appropriately.

Indeed, the benefits of improved clinical reasoning and a more refined list of differential diagnoses include not only an increase in the quality and efficacy of referral patterns for radiological investigation. The sensitivity and resolution of modern imaging modalities, particularly MRI, means that clinically insignificant findings can be observed and reported, but are only acted on if not compared with the result of a sound examination.

A chronically painful groin provides many such situations; for example, pathology of the adductor origin could be reported on an MRI of the pelvis in a patient who has pain located and clinically confirmed in and around the iliopsoas muscle. This information may be monitored, but not necessarily acted on, if it is clinically unrelated to the presenting pain.

The tables in each chapter refer to commonly used filtering questions in the history, and then the most evidence-based examination or test available in the current literature, and

Table 5.3 Patho-anatomic approach; within the greater trochanter triangle (adult), (diagnoses appear in order of frequency in an athletic population)				
Define and align	Pathology	Listen and localize	Palpate and recreate	Alleviate and investigate
Within the triangle (adult)	Femoro-acetabular impingement Labral injury	Mechanical symptoms, clicking ± locking	Impingement test[7]	Plain film x-ray, MRI ± arthrogram[17]
	Osteoarthritis	Insidious onset, night pain	Limited ROM, especially internal rotation[18]	Plain film x-ray
	Femoral stress fracture Neck	Groin pain, recent increase in activity levels	Hop test[19]	Plain film x-ray, isotope bone scans, MRI
	Shaft	Proximal thigh/knee pain, recent increase in activity levels	Fulcrum test[20]	Plain film x-ray, isotope bone scan, MRI
	Inflammatory conditions	Features of systemic inflammation	Systemic manifestations of particular condition[21]	Plain film x-ray, ultrasound-guided joint aspiration
	Septic arthritis	Systemic inflammatory response	Inability to weight bear, limited range of motion, ± sepsis[22]	Plain film x-ray, fluoroscopically/ ultrasound-guided joint aspiration
	Avascular necrosis of femoral head	Mechanical symptoms more prominent than functional limitation	Limited ROM[23]	Plain film x-ray, MRI
	Tumor	Systemic "red flags", absence of appropriate physical stressors[24]	May mimic stress fracture[24]	Plain film x-ray, computerised tomography (CT)/ MRI,[25] biopsy
	Transient osteoporosis of the hip	Women 3rd trimester of pregnancy, men 40–70, hip and groin pain, varied onset[26]	Pain on weight bearing and torsion, positive impingement test[26]	Plain film x-ray, MRI[27]

Figure 6 Sample of a table from Chapter 5

finally the most reliable investigations to confirm the diagnosis. It is hoped that these tables form an aid to diagnosis at steps 2, 3, and 4 of the diagnostic process. By focusing on the relevant anatomy, this text will help the reader to request appropriate imaging, by specifying the exact area about which more detail is required. The authors do not cover individual examination techniques, as these are comprehensively detailed in the core volume, *Clinical Sports Medicine*.

Anatomical triangles and illustrations

The authors have applied the Vitruvian man principle of Leonardo Da Vinci to overlay the relevant areas of the anatomy with triangles (Fig. 5). These triangles allow the reader to focus on clearly demarcated areas of anatomy in each region, and so exclude potential pathologies in logical sequence. These diagnostic

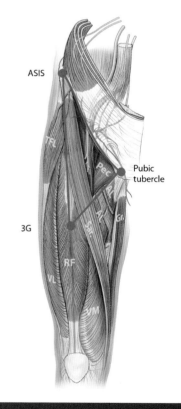

Figure 7 The groin triangle

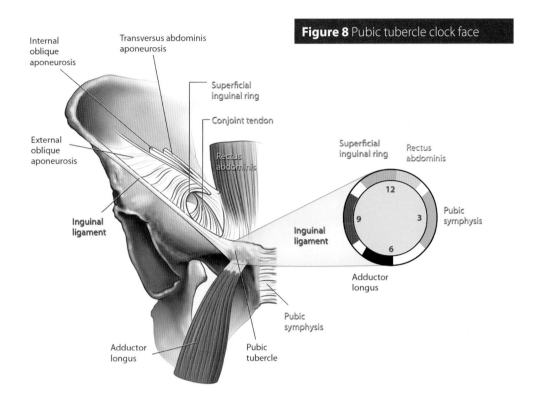

Figure 8 Pubic tubercle clock face

Internal oblique aponeurosis

Transversus abdominis aponeurosis

Superficial inguinal ring

Conjoint tendon

External oblique aponeurosis

Rectus abdominis

Inguinal ligament

Superficial inguinal ring

Rectus abdominis

Pubic symphysis

Inguinal ligament

Adductor longus

Adductor longus

Pubic symphysis

Pubic tubercle

triangles are essential to the working of the book. In some areas, we have created new anatomical reference points and carefully defined them, based on over 60 cadaveric dissections.

This book contains over 60 original anatomical illustrations, and comprehensively covers the musculosketal system. The anatomical descriptions are based on our own dissections, which have allowed us to emphasize those clinically important areas. These triangles allow the chapters to divide the pathology accordingly to the location of the presentation of pain or injury in relation to the relevant triangle. This allows the reader to immediately refine their examination and questioning. A further advantage lies in the memory aids for the anatomical structures and the clinical conditions.

In some chapters, we have used an "anatomical clock" (Fig. 6) in order to allow the reader to clearly relate what they are palpating on examination to the anatomy and to commit this to memory. We have found early feedback on this concept encouraging, and hope the reader finds it useful. For each palpable point, we have endeavored to clarify the insertions and overlapping structures. While there are always anatomical variants, we have avoided discussion of too many variants unless clinically important.

In other chapters, we have created, with our illustrator, Levent Efe, "exploded" views (Fig. 7), which again seek to clarify complex palpable anatomy in order to aid the clinical examiner in differentiating pathologies. In the wrist, for example, we highlight which structures are palpable overlying the carpal bones and where they insert. This also helps

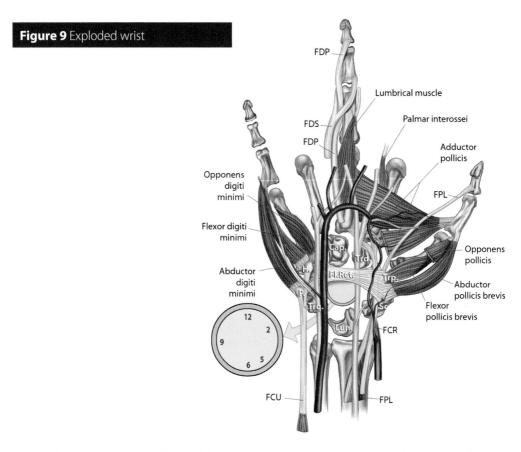

Figure 9 Exploded wrist

FDP

Lumbrical muscle

FDS

Palmar interossei

FDP

Adductor
pollicis

Opponens
digiti
minimi

FPL

Flexor digiti
minimi

Opponens
pollicis

Abductor
digiti
minimi

Abductor
pollicis brevis

Flexor
pollicis brevis

FCR

FCU

FPL

to explain the muscle functions of those structures inserting at or originating on the carpal bones, and to clarify any area of poor understanding.

We have not always included every anatomical detail in the illustrations, where we felt it was not clinically relevant. Rather than burden the reader with detail, we have sought to be both inclusive where needed, and exclusive in order to simplify certain regions. Having said this, we have thoroughly covered each region of the musculoskeletal anatomy, and nothing has been intentionally omitted.

Summary

This book aims to stimulate an understanding of clinical and functional anatomy relevant to all sports and exercise medicine, and to those involved in clinical medicine, whether in a surgery or in an emergency or minor-injury room. We hope that the anatomical descriptions and the accurate orientation which the triangle system affords will aid the reader's diagnostic skills and improve accuracy, which in turn should speed the rapid return of their patients through the rehabilitation process.

We have not aimed to provide treatment options or to explain particular examination techniques, as these are already covered in the excellent core volume, *Clinical Sports Medicine*.

Our case histories allow the reader to become familiar with the process of "Define and align", and to the layout of the diagnostic tables, which serve as a rapid reference to the patient, whether on the field or pitchside, or in the confines of the clinic, and will also prove useful to the student and the clinician involved in teaching.

Above all, we hope that this text will re-emphasize the need for accurate and comprehensive understanding of human anatomy, which is, in essence, the pathological basis for all injury in sport.

Bibliography

1. Regan de Bere S, Petersen A. Out of the dissecting room: News media portrayal of human anatomy teaching and research. *Soc Sci Med* 2006; 63(1):76–88.
2. Singh D, von Hagens G. Scientist or showman? *BMJ* (clinical research edn) 2003; 326(7387):468.
3. Christianson CE, McBride RB, Vari RC, Olson L, Wilson HD. From traditional to patient-centered learning: Curriculum change as an intervention for changing institutional culture and promoting professionalism in undergraduate medical education. *Acad Med* 2007; 82(11):1079–88.
4. Dyer GS, Thorndike ME. *Quidne mortui vivos docent?* The evolving purpose of human dissection in medical education. *Acad Med* 2000; 75(10):969–79.
5. Patel KM, Moxham BJ. Attitudes of professional anatomists to curricular change. *Clinical anatomy* New York, NY, 2006; 19(2):132–41.
6. Older J. Anatomy: A must for teaching the next generation. *Surgeon* 2004; 2(2):79–90.
7. Cottam W. Adequacy of medical school gross anatomy education as perceived by certain postgraduate residency programs and anatomy course directors. *Clinical anatomy* New York, NY, 1999; 12:55–65.
8. Winkelmann A. Anatomical dissection as a teaching method in medical school: A review of the evidence. *Medical education* 2007; 41(1):15–22.
9. Sanson–Fisher RW, Lynagh MC. Problem-based learning: A dissemination success story? *Med J Aust* 2005; 183(5):258–60.
10. Osler W. *The principles and practice of medicine*, 1892.
11. Bowen JL. Educational strategies to promote clinical diagnostic reasoning. *The New England Journal of Medicine* 2006; 355(21):2217–25.
12. Turney BW. Anatomy in a modern medical curriculum. *Ann R Coll Surg Engl* 2007; 89(2):104–07.
13. Franklyn–Miller A, Falvey E, McCrory P. Problem-based learning in sports medicine: The way forward or a backward step? *Br J Sports Med* 2007; 41(10):623–24.
14. Franklyn–Miller A, Falevy E, McCrory P. Patient-based not problem-based learning: An Oslerian approach to clinical skills, looking back to move forward. *Journal of Postgraduate Medicine* 2009; 55(3):198–203.
15. Sun T, Wang L, Zhang Y. Prognostic value of B-type natriuretic peptide in patients with chronic and advanced heart failure. *Intern Med J* 2007; 37(3):168–71.
16. Wang CS, FitzGerald JM, Schulzer M, Mak E, Ayas NT. Does this dyspneic patient in the emergency department have congestive heart failure? *JAMA* 2005; 294(15):1944–56.
17. Iglehart JK. The new era of medical imaging – progress and pitfalls. *The New England Journal of Medicine* 2006; 354(26):2822–28.

Photo Credits

Figure 1:   The Art Archive / Museo di Capodimonte, Naples / Alfredo Dagli Orti
Figure 2:   SuperStock
Figure 3.   The Art Archive / Bibliothèque des Arts Décoratifs Paris / Gianni Dagli Orti
Figure 4.   Gray, Henry. Anatomy of the Human Body. Philadelphia: Lea & Febiger, 1918; Bartleby.com, 2000. www.bartleby.com/107/. [Date of Printout]
Figure 5:   Getty Images

1

The shoulder triangle

Introduction

The human shoulder is prone to injury, through either trauma or overuse. In overhead sports such as tennis, baseball, and swimming, it is the most frequently injured joint; a recent survey of the world aquatic championships showed the shoulder was the most injured joint at 14.2%.[1] High-school athletes in the USA have an incidence of 10.9% for shoulder injury.[2] The wonderful range of motion of the shoulder provides allows us to perform many of the feats of athleticism we admire. This range of motion, however, comes at a cost.

Bone plays less of a role in joint stability of the shoulder than, for example, in the hip. Static stabilizers include the joint capsules and ligaments; the glenoid labrum acts to increase the diameter of the glenoid fossa. The muscles of the rotator cuff play a major role in joint stability. Athletic achievement requires athletes to push their bodies and their joints to the limit. Even slight gains in joint range of motion (already formidable in the shoulder) may confer an athletic advantage – a faster pitch, a wider spin in a tennis serve, or greater efficiency in a swimming stroke. This gain exposes stabilizers to even greater stresses. When static and dynamic stabilizers are disrupted, either violently and acutely, or chronically from overuse, a range of injuries may occur. The challenge for the clinician is to differentiate these, in and around a joint which is not easily palpated and which is biomechanically complex.

The joint

The shoulder is the articulation of the humerus with the scapula. Movements of the shoulder involve three joints or articulations: the glenohumeral; the acromioclavicular; and the sternoclavicular joints.

The **glenohumeral joint** is a ball-and-socket joint. The relatively large humeral head and shallow glenoid cavity mean that there is little surface contact between the two structures. The lack of congruity of the humeral head and cavity has been likened to "a seal balancing a ball on its nose": the glenoid labrum deepens the glenoid cavity, improving stability by providing negative intra-articular pressure by coaptation of the labrum and humeral head acting as a "suction cup".[3] This incongruity facilitates a much greater range of motion than in a similar joint such as the hip. Much of the stability of the shoulder joint is provided by static (joint capsule and glenohumeral ligaments) and active (muscular, particularly rotator cuff and deltoid) structures.

The ranges of movement of the glenohumeral joint are as follows:

> forward flexion: 0–180°

> extension: 0–60°

> abduction: 0–180°

> adduction: 0–30°

> internal rotation: 0–70°

> external rotation: 0–90°

The **acromioclavicular joint** (AC joint) acts as a "strut" between the thorax and shoulder around which the scapula rotates, giving us the ability to raise our arms above our heads. This is an inherently unstable articulation (gliding synovial joint) which is supported by the AC joint capsule and the robust **coracoclavicular (CC) ligaments**, which provide static stability. The dynamic stabilizers include the deltoid and trapezius muscles.[4] The **acromioclavicular ligaments**, in particular the superior and posterior ligaments, prevent excess motion in the horizontal plane,[5] while the coracoclavicular ligaments (conoid, trapezoid) prevent inferior migration of the scapulohumeral complex relative to the clavicle.[6] The **coracoacromial ligament**, the coracoid process and the acromion protect the head of the humerus.

The **sternoclavicular joint** (SC joint) is the joining of the flattened sternal end of the clavicle and the manubrium sterni, and the cartilage of the first rib. Like the AC joint, it is an atypical synovial joint, with a fibrocartilage disc. It is stabilized by the sternoclavicular ligaments (anterior and posterior), the interclavicular ligament (connecting both clavicles across the superior aspect of the sternum), and the strong costoclavicular ligament between the costal cartilage of the first rib and the clavicle.

The joint capsule
The joint capsule is a loose structure attached proximally to the labrum and glenoid rim, and distally to the articular margins of the head of humerus, except inferiorly where it extends 2 cm onto the neck of the humerus. This inferior laxity allows greater mobility, particularly abduction. Posteriorly and inferiorly, the capsular insertion is directly onto the labrum. Superiorly, the capsule is attached to the glenoid rim at the base of the labrum, and includes the origin of the long head of biceps tendon.

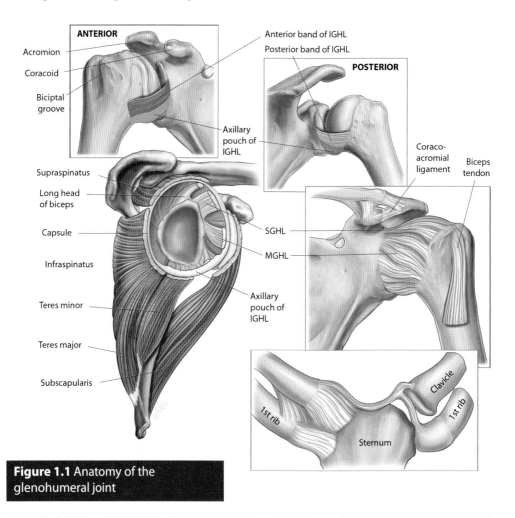

Figure 1.1 Anatomy of the glenohumeral joint

The anterior capsule has a number of condensations termed the "scapulohumeral ligaments"; these serve as the main static stabilizers of the shoulder. The tendons of the rotator cuff reinforce the capsule above, and the tendon of the long head of triceps below.

The posterior band of the inferior glenohumeral ligament and the tendon of the teres minor both strengthen the posterior capsule. The main active restraint to posterior dislocation is subscapularis.

Ligaments

The **superior glenohumeral ligament** (SGL) is the superior thickening of the capsule; it arises from the coracoid and superior labrum, and is closely related to the extra-articular **coracohumeral ligament**. The inferior border of the SGL blends with the **medial glenohumeral ligament** (MGL), which arises from the anatomic neck of the humerus and inserts into the anterior labrum. The **inferior glenohumeral ligament** (IGL) forms the thickest part of the joint capsule, and is the largest and most important of the glenohumeral ligaments. It consists of three components: the anterior band; the axillary pouch; and the posterior band, often termed the "inferior" **glenohumeral ligament complex** (IGLC), and originates from the fibrous glenoid labrum antero-inferiorly, inserting into the humeral neck at the periphery of the articular margin.

The **transverse humeral ligament** forms a tunnel of the inter-tubercular groove of the humerus, joining the greater and lesser tubercles, always above the epiphyseal line. It houses the tendon and synovial sheath of the long head of biceps.

Bursae

The **sub-acromial bursa** facilitates the smooth movement of the proximal humerus and rotator cuff under the coracoacromial arch. The bursa is a large synovial membrane that extends under the acromion and coracoacromial ligament. Laterally it is adherent to the deltoid and it lies on the rotator cuff and greater tuberosity. It is generally surrounded by peribursal fat, and in normal individuals represents a potential space only.

The **sub-scapular bursa** communicates with the glenohumeral joint between the superior and middle glenohumeral ligaments. The bursa separates the anterior neck of the scapula and subscapularis tendon, preventing friction. A large subscapular bursa may extend upwards to lie under the coracoid process. The upper part is referred to as the **subcoracoid bursa**. Similarly, there may be an isolated bursa at this site.

Landmarks of the shoulder triangle

The anatomical apex points of the triangle are as follows:

> the coracoid process

> the acromial angle of the scapula (formed where the posterior border of the spine of the scapula joins the lateral border of the acromion)

> 3G point (located at the surface markings of the joining of the anterior and posterior borders of the deltoid muscle)

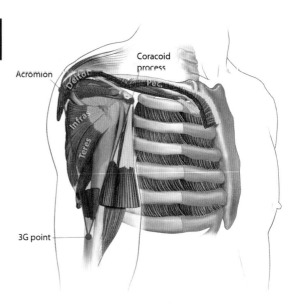

Figure 1.2 Anatomical landmarks and borders of the shoulder triangle.

Coracoid process

Acromion

Deltoid

Pec

Infra

Teres

3G point

Anatomical relations of the borders of the shoulder triangle

Depending on the muscular development of the subject, a large deltoid muscle may make palpation of the underlying structures difficult. When the shoulder is abducted to 90°, the anterior medial and posterior bundles of the deltoid may be appreciated. With the shoulder relaxed in an adducted position, the long head of biceps may be palpated in the inter-tubercular groove; this can be accentuated by gentle internal and external rotation of the arm. Flexion of the elbow, together with internal rotation (so that the hand is behind the subject's back) with the dorsum of the hand against the back, allows palpation of the superior surface of the greater tubercle of the humerus, the humeral insertion of the supraspinatus. The humeral insertion of the infraspinatus and teres minor may be palpated inferior to the postero-inferior border of the scapula when the arm is externally rotated and forward-flexed.

Superior border of the shoulder triangle

Moving from medial to lateral positions from the coracoid process of the scapula to the lateral aspect of the acromion of the scapula, although not necessarily palpable, the following structures are encountered.

The **deltoid** is the most obvious muscle of the shoulder, this arises from the anterior border of the lateral third of the clavicle, the lateral border of the acromion, and the lower lip of the scapular spine, as well as from the fascia over the infraspinatus muscle. Innervated by the radial nerve, the deltoid is a powerful abductor of the shoulder (a motion which is commenced by the supraspinatus), while the posterior bundle of the deltoid is an extensor of the shoulder. The deltoid muscle is multipennate. Tendinous septa arising from the acromion and the deltoid tuberosity interdigitate, with short muscle fibers extending between the septa. This gives the muscle a short but powerful pull.

Coracobrachialis arises from the apex of the coracoid process, in common with the short head of the biceps brachii, and from the intermuscular septum between the two muscles, and inserting as a flat tendon between the origins of the triceps brachii and brachialis on the medial aspect of the shaft of the humerus, the coracobrachialis acts to flex and adduct the shoulder.

As its name suggests, the **biceps brachii** has two heads (long and short), both of which arise in and around the shoulder. The short head arises from the coracoid process of the scapula. The long head arises from the supraglenoid tubercle, with considerable anatomical variation described in its relationship with the glenoid labrum (most often superior).[7]

The tendon is intra-articular but extra-synovial (it lies within a reflection of the synovial sheath). As the tendon passes out of the joint, through the rotator interval, and into the bicipital groove, it is stabilized proximally by the "biceps pulley" mechanism, composed of the coracohumeral ligament and superior glenohumeral ligament. Reinforcing fibers from the subscapularis and supraspinatus tendons surround the biceps tendon at its entrance to the bicipital groove.[8] Innervation is from the musculocutaneous nerve. Distally, the biceps inserts into the radial tuberosity.

Through the scapular origins of the biceps, it stabilizes the glenohumeral joint, depressing the humeral head[9] when the arm is internally rotated. The short head is a weak adductor and, when the arm is externally rotated, the long head aids in abduction, while both heads contribute to flexion. The more significant actions of the biceps are seen at the elbow and are discussed in Chapter 3.

The **supraclavicular nerve** is a sensory nerve arising from the C3 and C4 nerve roots which emerge beneath the posterior border of the sternocleidomastoid muscle, supplying the skin over the superior anterior and posterior shoulder.

The **suprascapular nerve** is a mixed motor/sensory nerve. It is formed from the C5 and C6 nerve roots (the upper trunk of the brachial plexus) with a variable contribution from the C4.[10] The nerve passes behind the middle third of the clavicle to the suprascapular notch, supplying sensory branches to the AC joint, the subacromial bursa and the coracohumeral ligaments, before passing beneath the superior transverse scapular ligament. Beyond the suprascapular notch, motor branches arise which supply the supraspinatus muscle. Approximately 1–2 cm from the posterior glenoid rim, the nerve passes through the spinoglenoid notch, first supplying the sensory branch to the posterior aspect of the glenohumeral joint; after the notch, the nerve supplies the infraspinatus nerve.

The **long thoracic nerve** arises by three roots from the fifth, sixth, and seventh cervical nerves (C5–C7). The nerve descends behind the brachial plexus and the axillary vessels, resting on the outer surface of the serratus anterior, which it supplies. It extends along the side of the thorax to the lower border of that muscle, supplying filaments to each of its digitations.

The **axillary nerve** is formed of fibers (C5, C6) from the posterior chord of the brachial plexus (which then becomes the radial nerve). It is formed at the level of the axilla, and passes posteriorly through the quadrilateral space with the posterior circumflex humeral artery. The axillary nerve supplies the deltoid (anterior and posterior) and teres minor, and supplies cutaneous branches to the skin above the lateral aspect of the shoulder.

The **quadrilateral space** is found at the posterior aspect of the shoulder. The superior border is formed by the inferior edge of the teres minor, the medial edge by the lateral border of the tendon of origin of the long head of the triceps, the inferior border by the superior margin of the teres major, and the lateral border by the humerus. The axillary nerve and posterior circumflex artery pass through the space.

The **triceps brachii** is formed of three heads of the triceps are the long head, which arises from the infraglenoid tubercle of the scapula, and the lateral and medial heads, which arise from their respective sides of the superior and inferior aspects respectively of the radial groove of the humerus. The fibers converge into a single tendon, to insert onto the olecranon process of the ulna (although this may vary).[60]

Supplied by the radial nerve, the triceps extends the elbow, also acting as an antagonist of the biceps and brachialis muscles. It can also fixate the elbow joint when the forearm and hand are used for fine movements, for example, when writing. The triceps accounts for approximately 60% of the upper arm's muscle mass.

Pectoralis major is the most prominent muscle of the chest wall arising from the anterior surface of the sternal half of the clavicle, from the anterior surface of the sternum, from the cartilages of the upper six ribs, and from the aponeurosis of the abdominal external oblique muscle. The muscle fibers are divided into superficial and deep laminae. The lower fibers of the deep lamina insert higher up on the humerus, giving the rounded appearance to the anterior border of the axilla. The upper insertions of the posterior lamina may contribute to the transverse humeral ligament. Supplied by the medial lateral pectoral nerve (C6, C7, C8), the clavicular head aids in flexion of the humerus, while the sternal head is a medial rotator of the humerus, and both aid in the adduction and accessory muscle of inspiration.

Rotator cuff

This is a collective term for the tendinous insertions of the **sub-scapularis**, **supraspinatus**, **infraspinatus**, and **teres minor** muscles. These tendons form a hood which surrounds the head of the humerus anteriorly, superiorly, and posteriorly. Co-contraction of these muscles adds to the stability of the glenohumeral joint during normal activities. This is most clearly seen in the abduction of the arm from an adducted position (the arm by the side), where the deltoid generates an almost vertical force vector; this tends to sublux the humeral heel superiorly. The force vector generated by the rotator cuff tends to be more horizontal, and their tensions combine with that of the deltoid to direct the resultant joint force vector into the superior concavity of the glenoid, improving stability.

The **infraspinatus** arises from the fossa of the same name on the posterior aspect of the scapula; it is also anchored in the overlying infraspinatus fascia which separates it from the teres minor and major. The fibers converge into a tendon, which reinforces the posterior part of the capsule of the shoulder joint, inserting into the greater tubercle of the humerus. Supplied by the suprascapular nerve, the infraspinatus externally rotates the humerus (also aiding in abduction), and provides dynamic support for the shoulder joint.

Arising from the **supraspinatus** fossa above the spine of the scapula, the tendon of this small muscle merges with the superior joint capsule, before inserting into the greater tubercle of the humerus.

Contraction of the supraspinatus muscle begins (the first 30°) abduction; beyond this point, the deltoid muscle becomes the increasingly dominant muscle of this action. When the supraspinatus is ineffective, injury studies have shown that abduction is still possible, but the deltoid tends to tire quickly.[12] Internal and external rotation of the shoulder will activate the infraspinatus and subscapularis respectively, and these muscles are capable of initiating and maintaining functional abduction.[13] The supraspinatus also helps to stabilize the shoulder joint, by keeping the head of the humerus firmly pressed medially against the glenoid fossa of the scapula, and helps to resist the inferior gravitational forces placed across the shoulder joint due to the downward pull from the weight of the upper limb.

Subscapularis, a broad triangular muscle arises from the sub-scapular fossa and most of the anterior aspect of the scapula.

The fibers pass laterally, to form a tendon which is inserted into the lesser tubercle of the humerus, and reinforces the anterior joint capsule of the shoulder joint. Innervated by the upper and lower sub-scapular muscles, it internally rotates the humerus; in abduction, it draws the humerus forward and downward. It is a powerful stabilizer (active and passive) of the front of the shoulder joint, preventing displacement of the head of the humerus.

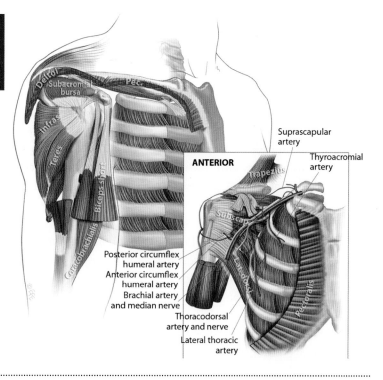

Figure 1.3 Muscles, blood vessels and nerves of the shoulder joint

The **teres minor** arises from the lateral border of the scapula (upper two-thirds), and inserts into the inferior aspect of the greater tuberosity of the humerus. It lies in close proximity to the infraspinatus, and acts with it to externally rotate the humerus. It is supplied by the axillary nerve.

The **rotator cuff interval** is located between the superior aspect of the sub-scapularis tendon and the inferior aspect of the supraspinatus tendon. This interval contains the coracohumeral ligament and the superior glenohumeral ligament.

Teres major is a flattened scapulohumeral muscle arising from the inferior angle of the scapula, and from the fibrous septa found between the muscle and the teres minor and infraspinatus. It is innervated by the lower sub-scapular nerve, and inserts into the medial lip of the bicipital groove of the humerus. This relatively anterior insertion means the teres major aids in the internal rotation of the humerus; it accentuates the action of the latissimus dorsi in adducting the humerus.

Latissimus dorsi is a broad flat muscle arising from the spines and supraspinous ligaments of the T6–12 vertebrae deep to the trapezius, and from the thoracolumbar fascia, by which it is attached to the spines of all lumbar and sacral vertebrae. Fibers also arise from the posterior iliac crest and the four ribs. It passes upward and laterally, gaining a small slip from the inferior angle of scapula. The muscle inserts to the floor of the intertubercular groove of the humerus, in a flat tendon which wraps around and, for a short distance, unites with the tendon of the teres major. A bursa lies between the two. Innervated by the thoracodorsal nerve, latissimus dorsi is a powerful adductor and extensor of the shoulder; like the teres major, the position of its tendon means that it also internally rotates the humerus.

The **subclavius** is a small triangular muscle arising from the first rib and its costal cartilage. It inserts into the inferior aspect of the middle third of the clavicle, acting to depress the clavicle and stabilize the sternoclavicular (SC) joint. It is supplied by the nerve to the subclavius, and also serves to protect the underlying brachial plexus and subclavian vessels in the case of a fractured clavicle (the most frequently broken long bone).

The **serratus anterior** arises as muscular slips from the upper eight ribs and fascia. There is inter-digitation with the external oblique origin in the lower slips. Innervated by the long thoracic nerve, it inserts into the entire length of the anterior aspect of the medial border of the scapula (passing between the sub-scapularis and the thoracic wall), and serves to protract the scapula (pull it forward around the chest wall).

The **pectoralis minor** lies beneath its larger cousin the pectoralis major, arising from the upper margins and outer surfaces of the third, forth, and fifth ribs, and from the intercostal muscle aponeurosis. The fibers form a flat tendon, passing superolaterally to insert into the medial border and upper surface of the coracoid process of the scapula. Supplied by the medial and lateral pectoral nerves, the pectoralis minor moves the scapula around the fulcrum of the AC joint, to move the shoulder girdle forward and inferiorly.

The **cephalic vein** is located in the superficial fascia of the biceps brachii muscle. In the shoulder, the vein passes through the groove between the deltoid and pectoralis major muscles (deltopectoral groove), where it empties into the axillary vein.

The **axillary vein** is formed by the basilic vein and the cephalic vein, when it crosses the teres major. It terminates at the lateral margin of the first rib, where it becomes the subclavian vein.

The **axillary artery** is formed when the subclavian artery crosses the first rib. It gives rise to branches which supply the axilla and lateral aspect of the thorax, before crossing the teres major to become the brachial artery.

Nomenclature

Instability

Just as the shoulder joint trades stability for range of motion, so the overhead athlete requires a delicate balance of mobility and stability.[14] The glenoid labrum and glenohumeral ligaments provide static stability.

The anterior and posterior bands of the **IGL**, with an interposed axillary, support the humeral head. Lying below the sub-scapularis tendon, the **IGL** prevents anterior, inferior, and posterior translation in the abducted arm, with alternating tensions in the anterior and posterior bands. The more superior **MGL** is effective primarily in the 45° abducted range; it helps to limit external rotation, and inferior translation, and prevents anterior translation of the humeral head. The **SGL** blends with the superior labrum and biceps tendon medially, and primarily limits inferior translation and external rotation of the adducted arm; it also plays a minor role in preventing anterior instability. The **coracohumeral ligament** reinforces the **SGL**.

The **rotator interval** is that part of the capsule located between the supraspinatus and subscapularis tendons. Reinforced by the **SGL** and coracohumeral ligament, the interval plays a role in inferior and posterior stability, particularly when the arm is adducted and externally rotated.

At the mid-range of abductions, the static stabilizers (capsulo-ligamentous complex) are less effective, and the burden of stability is borne by the dynamic stabilizing structures of the rotator cuff muscles, biceps tendon complex, and scapular rotators, which work optimally at mid-range positions. The synergistic tensions of the supraspinatus, infraspinatus, subscapularis, and teres minor increase the contact pressure between the humeral head and glenoid fossa.

In the early stages of abduction, the teres minor is more active, forming a force couple; a contraction of equal and opposite strength to the deltoid's action. As the arm abducts further, the sub-scapularis and infraspinatus are activated. An eccentric contraction of the latissimus dorsi provides control and fluidity to the abduction moment, while muscle activity is seen to increase as the angle of abduction increases. Beyond 90° abduction, the joint is made less stable by a diminution of rotator cuff activity, and only the sub-scapularis remains active. Further abduction is facilitated by scapular rotation, and controlled by the serratus anterior and trapezius.

Multidirectional glenohumeral instability encompasses symptomatic involuntary subluxation or dislocation of the glenohumeral joint in more than one direction, including

Table 1.1 Origins, insertions, and nerve supply to the main movers of the shoulder joint				
Muscle	Origin	Insertion	Nerve	Root
coracobrachialis	humerus, lower half, intermuscular septum	ulna; coronoid process and tuberosity	musculo-cutaneous n.	C5, C6
biceps brachii	long head – scapula; supraglenoid tubercle short head – scapula; coracoid process	radius; bicipital tuberosity, bicipital aponeurosis, deep fascia, subcutaneous ulna	musculo-cutaneous n.	C5, C6
triceps brachii	long head; scapula infraglenoid tubercle lateral head; posterior humerus lower ½ medial head; humerus, dorsal surface	olecranon of ulna	radial n.	C6–8
deltoid	clavicle: lateral third (anterior head) acromion scapula: spine, posterior border, lower lip	humerus; deltoid tuberosity, middle of lateral surface.	axillary n.	C5, C6
trapezius	occipital bone; superior nuchal line ligamentum nuchae and supraspinous ligaments to T12	clavicle; posterior border lateral 1/3 scapula; acromion, lateral spine, spine of scapula medial end	accessory n. (spinal root)	C1–5
pectoralis major	clavicle: medial half sternocostal: manubrium, sternum, upper 6 costal cartilages, rectus sheath	humerus; bicipital groove lateral lip, deltoid tuberosity anterior lip	medial pectoral n. lateral pectoral n.	C6–8
pectoralis minor	costal; ribs 3–5	scapula; coracoid process, medial and upper surface	medial pectoral n. lateral pectoral n.	C6–8
subclavius	costal; osteochondral junction 1st rib	clavicle; subclavian groove	nerve to subclavius	C5, C6
supraspinatus	scapula (bipennate); supraspinous fossa and upper surface of spine	humerus; greater tuberosity shoulder capsule; superior aspect	suprascapular n.	C5, C6
infraspinatus	scapula; medial ¾ infraspinous fossa	humerus; greater tuberosity, middle facet shoulder capsule; posterior aspect	suprascapular n.	C5, C6

Table 1.1 *(continued)*				
Muscle	**Origin**	**Insertion**	**Nerve**	**Root**
subscapularis	scapula; middle ⅔ sub-scapular fossa	humerus; lesser tuberosity, medial lip of bicipital groove shoulder capsule: anterior aspect	upper and lower subscapular n.	C5, C6
teres minor	scapula; lat border, middle ⅓	humerus; greater tuberosity (below) infraspinatus, shoulder capsule; postero-inferior aspect	axillary n.	C5, C6
teres major	scapula; lat border, lower ⅓	humerus; bicipital groove medial lip	lower sub-scapular nerve	C5–7
latissimus dorsi	thoracic spine; spinous processes and supraspinous ligaments T7–12 lumbar fascia, costal; ribs 8–12, scapula; inferior angle	humerus; bicipital groove, spirals around teres minor	thoracodorsal n.	C6–8
serratus anterior	costal: upper 8 ribs and intercostal membranes midclavicular line	scapula: 8 slips inserting form superior to inferior on medial aspect of costal surface of scapula	long thoracic nerve	C5–7

Table 1.2 Muscles responsible for the movements of the shoulder					
Flexion	**Extension**	**Abduction**	**Adduction**	**Internal rotation**	**External rotation**
pectoralis major	latissimus dorsi	deltoid	sub-scapularis	sub-scapularis	infraspinatus
deltoid (anterior fibers)	teres major	supraspinatus	pectoralis major	latissimus dorsi	teres minor
coracobrachialis	deltoid (posterior fibers)		latissimus dorsi	teres major	
biceps brachii (when elbow flexed)	triceps brachii (when elbow extended)		teres major	pectoralis major	
			gravity!	deltoid (anterior fibers)	

the inferior, anterior, or posterior directions.[15] First decribed by Neer, it is often bilateral, atraumatic, and seen in the setting of generalized ligamentous laxity.[16]

Referred pain

The term "referred pain" is used in this book to describe pain appreciated not at its site of origin but elsewhere. In the shoulder and arm, this is particularly important. Procacci et al. have described deep referred pain and superficial referred pain.[17] Deep referred pain is poorly localized and may be felt in the chest shoulder and arm, while superficial referred pain is almost exclusively appreciated in the C8–T1 dermatome.[18]

Within the triangle

Rotator cuff pathology is one of the most common causes of shoulder pain and functional impairment.[19] More common in later life (5th–7th decades), and in female patients, it is also seen frequently in both athletes and manual workers. Acute trauma and irritation secondary to other pathologies aside, the cause is often not known.[20] The terms "tendinosis" or "tendinopathy" are used to describe the pathology as seen elsewhere,[21] but "tenosynovitis" or "paratendonitis" have also been proposed.[22] Patients complain of pain on abduction, when working overhead, and difficulty in sleeping on the affected shoulder. The individual presentations of the rotator cuff muscle are discussed later, as are the pathologies associated with secondary rotator cuff pathology.

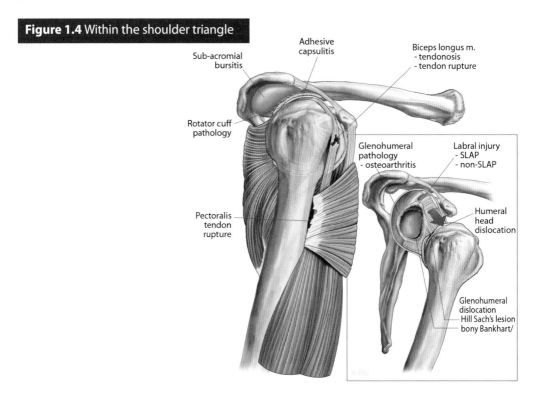

Figure 1.4 Within the shoulder triangle

Sub-acromial bursitis

Adhesive capsulitis

Biceps longus m.
- tendonosis
- tendon rupture

Rotator cuff pathology

Glenohumeral pathology
- osteoarthritis

Labral injury
- SLAP
- non-SLAP

Pectoralis tendon rupture

Humeral head dislocation

Glenohumeral dislocation
- Hill Sach's lesion
- bony Bankhart/

The **sub-acromial bursa** lies between the rotator cuff and the coracoacromial arch. When this space is decreased, irritation of the bursa may occur, causing pain and a movement deficit similar to those seen in rotator cuff pathology. Internal rotation is often limited, and pain on sleeping on the affected side is also common. Poor scapular control, AC joint pathology, and anatomical variations of acromial morphology are all associated with sub-acromial bursitis.[19] Differentiation of bursal pathology from rotator cuff pathology is clinically difficult, as often both co-exist; hence clinical examination for both pathologies is similar, and radiological investigation helps to make this distinction and to guide treatment options.

Inflammation of the long head of the biceps brachii tendon may be primary or secondary. A tenosynovitis of the tendon sheath is the classic "tendonitis", which accounts for less than 5% of pathology;[23] damage to the biceps pulley system may lead to subluxation or inflammation. Primary tendinosis is thought to be due to anatomical restraints in the area, leading to degenerative change.[24] Secondary biceps tendinopathy occurs due to pathology in other structures within the shoulder; there is often concomitant rotator cuff pathology (85% in one series[25]).

Rupture of the long head of the biceps is believed to occur most often in patients over 40 years of age. In the athletic population, however, it is of course seen earlier, usually after a violent contraction of the biceps against resistance or arm traction. Although retraction of the tendon resulting in the "Popeye" deformity is most common, occasionally partial retraction occurs, making the diagnosis more difficult.[26] A history of shoulder pain prior to the injury may denote concomitant rotator cuff pathology, with sub-acromial irritation of the tendons. Elbow flexion is usually unaffected, with a 10% decrease in supination strength.[27]

Adhesive capsulitis is a condition of unknown etiology affecting 2–5% of the general population.[28] It is more common in diabetics (10–35%).[29] The natural history of this process is up to 24 months, and four stages are described;[30] these are critical and require direct patient management[31] as shown in Table 1.3.

Glenohumeral dislocation, although common in the athletic setting, is a dramatic and painful event. The clinician must deal not only with the acute pain and the potential for fracture, but also potential sequelae such as labral injury, rotator cuff injury, and instability. Early recognition is essential. Though x-ray prior to relocation (in order to exclude fracture) is ideal; early correct relocation by the pitch-side clinician avoids muscle spasm and prolonged capsular stretching. This makes reduction easier in the longer term and potentially limits sequelae. Post-reduction films should be arranged at the emergency department (ED).[32] The clinician should be mindful of neuropathy resulting from injury or compression of neural structures around the joint, or more proximally in the brachial plexus.

The incidence of **post-traumatic shoulder instability** in the general population is approximately 1.7%.[33] Age at the time of dislocation is a reliable indicator of the risk of subsequent instability. Younger patients suffer a significantly higher rate of recurrent anterior instability after dislocation. Most instability episodes occur in the two years after the first episode.[33] One study found a 90% recurrence rate for shoulder dislocation in patients under the age of 20 years, 60% in patients aged 20–40 years, and 10% in patients over 40 years.[35]

	Pain	Movement	Timeline	Histology
Table 1.3 Stages of adhesive capsulitis[34]				
Stage 1 – early	Mild, ache at rest, sharp on activity, night pain	Progressive limitation; forward flexion, abduction, internal rotation, and external rotation Normalized examination after LA injection or EUA	0–3 months	Rare inflammatory cells Synovitis Normal underlying capsule
Stage 2 – freezing	Chronic pain and progressive loss of range of motion Rest pain, night pain, significant sleep disturbances may exist	Significant limitation; forward flexion, abduction, internal rotation, and external rotation Partial improvement after LA injection or EUA	3–9 months	No inflammatory cells Synovitis Fibroplasia and scarring of capsule
Stage 3 – frozen	Minimal pain at rest or at night, end of range of motion pain Progressive stiffness	Marked global loss of movement No improvement after LA injection or EUA	9–15 months	No inflammatory cells No synovitis, synovium "thinned" Dense fibroplasia and scarring of capsule
Stage 4 – thawing	Minimal pain, progressive decrease in stiffness	Global progressive improvement	15–24 months	No inflammatory cells No synovitis, synovium "thinned" Dense fibroplasia and scarring of capsule

Anterior dislocation often results in a Bankart lesion. This is an avulsion of the antero-inferior labrum at its attachment to the IGL complex. If a Bankart lesion has occurred, there is by definition damage to the IGL. It should be noted that in 30% of patients this will heal in a redundant position, exposing the athlete to instability. Where a fracture of the anterior inferior glenoid occurs, this is termed a "bony Bankart". The impact to create the Bankart lesion may also be seen on the humeral head. This resembles an indentation and is termed a Hill Sachs lesion.

Damage to the superior glenoid labrum is termed a **"superior labral anterior-posterior"** (SLAP) lesion of the shoulder. These are of significance, particularly in overhead athletes, and particularly in throwing sports. Despite the widespread recognition and coverage of this injury, the true incidence of symptomatic SLAP lesions is low, SLAP pathology is thought to cause approximately 6% of symptomatic shoulder pain.[36] Clinical diagnosis may be unreliable, and anatomical and age-related variance may add to the difficulties surrounding diagnosis.[37] Snyder and colleagues[38] categorized labral injuries into types I–IV, based on the involvement of the biceps anchor and the degree of superior labral injury. This is summarized in Table 1.4.

Table 1.4 Classification of SLAP lesions[39]	
Classification of SLAP lesions	
Type I	Fraying of the edge of the superior labrum
Type II	Detached biceps anchor
Type III	Bucket handle tear of the superior labrum
Type IV	Splitting of the superior labrum that continues into the biceps tendon

Osteoarthritis of the shoulder is less common than in weightbearing joints, but is similarly seen as a primary or secondary process.[34] In the athlete, degenerative arthritis appears to result from trauma. This may have many forms: instability; sport-specific loading; rotator cuff deficiency (where a large rotator cuff defect exposes the humeral head to abrasion by the acromion); or iatrogenic (excessive tightness post-capsulorrhaphy for treatment of instability).[84] Typically the area of degenerative change seen in degenerative osteoarthritis is posterior with anterior sparing, the so-called "Friar Tuck" pattern.[39]

Pectoralis major rupture is rare, occurring at either the tendon insertion into the humerus, or at the musculotendinous junction. It usually occurs in males, often in their third decade, when an extreme contraction against a heavy, eccentric load is performed. This is particularly true when the pectoral muscle is biomechanically disadvantaged, such as when bench pressing.[51] The clinician should have an index of suspicion for the injury, but be aware that persistence of the clavi-pectoral fascia may not allow palpation of a defect in the muscle where rupture is incomplete, and repeat examination is recommended when the swelling and pain have settled.[51]

Factors associated with rotator cuff pathology

In a break from the convention of the triangle process, we here devote a section to the differentiation of the pathologies responsible for rotator cuff pathology in the athletic shoulder. When the clinicians has satisfied themselves that rotator cuff pathology exists, treatment and rehabilitation may be slowed or limited if the underlying etiology remains untreated. We suggest an evidence-based means of differentiation between pathologies.

Primary rotator cuff pathology

The clinician must be adept in the examination of the rotator cuff, as pathology is often masked by other structures compensating. Clinical examination is not precise;[53] we have attempted to list the most efficient means of examination. Large tears are easily diagnosed; however, partial tears or tendinopathy are more difficult. When examining the rotator cuff, it is also important to recognize that strength testing does not necessarily reflect cuff integrity, because a torn cuff may be masked by normal manual strength, and a weak cuff may be intact but painful.[53]

The position of the supraspinatus as the most superior of the rotator cuff muscles means that, as its tendon and that of the infraspinatus pass beneath the coraco-acromial arch, they are prone to impingement. This diminution of the supraspinatus outlet is thought to be a factor in the generation of bursal-surface rotator cuff tears. The rotator cuff is responsible not only for abduction of the shoulder, but for the stabilization of the humeral head in the glenoid, but is also subjected to significant deceleration of eccentric loads in the throwing athlete.[54]

Table 1.5 Within the shoulder triangle				
Define and align	Pathology	Listen and localize	Palpate and recreate	Alleviate and investgate
Within the triangle	Rotator cuff pathology	Painful arc (60°–120°), pain working overhead, pain radiating to lateral arm, pain on sleeping	Hawkin's test, Neer's sign test[42]	Ultrasound, MRI
	Sub-acromial bursitis	Pain sleeping on affected side, limited ROM	Hawkin's test, Neer's sign test[42]	X-ray, ultrasound, MRI, Neer's impingement test[43]
	Adhesive capsulitis	Painful global limited range of motion, F:M = 2:1, Bilateral 20–30%[31] Idiopathic, post-trauma, DM or autoimmune disease	Active vs passive range of motion[31]	LA injection to stage (table x)[31] Plain film x-ray, MRI to exclude other possible causes[31]
	M biceps brachii > tendonosis > tendon rupture	Anterior shoulder pain, worse at night, clunking Rupture, ecchymosis, acute worsening of pain	Pain on palpation of bicipital groove, "Popeye" sign[8] > Yergason's test* sensitivity: 37% specificity: 86%[41] > Speed's test sensitivity: 90% specificity: 14%[41]	Ultrasound,[44] MRI[8]
	Glenohumeral dislocation	Acute trauma, fall on/blow to abducted externally rotated arm Arm held internally rotated supported by contralateral arm	Assymetry of deltoid contor, limited ROM, fullness below coracoid into axilla	Plain film x-ray, AP and West Point view[45] MRI[46]

		Table 1.5 (continued)		
Define and align	**Pathology**	**Listen and localize**	**Palpate and recreate**	**Alleviate and investgate**
	Labral injury SLAP lesion	Poorly localized anterior pain, impaired performance (worsened by overhead activity),[36] mechanical symptoms[35]	> Biceps load test, sensitivity: 89.7% specificity: 96.6%[47] > New pain provocation test sensitivity: 100% specificity: 90%[48]	MR Athrography[50]
	Bankart lesion	History anterior dislocation with subsequent instability, pain in abduction and external rotation[15]	> Crank test combined with sulcus sign and apprehension relocation tests sensitivity: 90% specificity: 85%[49] > Anterior slide test sensitivity: 78% specificity: 91%[50]	
	Glenohumeral pathology > osteoarthritis	Night pain, limitation of movement, history of trauma or surgery	Limited range of motion	Plain film x-ray, CT
	Pectoralis tendon rupture	Male, third decade, maximal contraction against heavy eccentric load, audible "pop"[51]	Weakness of adduction 'Webbing' of the anterior axillary fold[51]	X-ray to exclude bone pathology, MRI[52]

*Negative in the presence of a complete biceps tendon rupture

Electromyographic studies have failed to differentiate the functions of the infraspinatus and teres minor;[55] as such, we have considered them as a single entity for the purposes of examination. In biomechanical terms, the teres minor is responsible for up to 45% of the power of external rotation.[56] Bencardino has suggested that isolated teres minor injury due to axillary nerve injury following dislocation of the shoulder is under-reported.[57]

Electromyographic studies have shown that sub-scapularis activity dominates other muscles in the golf swing,[58] and in tennis during the serve and forehand.[59] In swimmers, the butterfly stoke has been seen to place particularly high demands on the sub-scapularis.[60] It is felt that the sub-scapularis tendon is prone to overuse microtrauma, with tendon degeneration.[61] This is thought to be due to mechanical compression between the lesser tuberosity and coracoid process, the so-called "roller wringer" effect,[62] and also potentially anterosuperior impingement, in which articular-sided abrasion may occur at the lesser tuberosity and glenoid rim interface, especially in the resisted flexed and internally rotated positions (e.g. the tennis follow-through).[63] Isolated sub-scapularis tears are rare in younger patients (> 40 years), where particular velocity or violence are required, such as glenohumeral dislocation. In the older patient, it may be an acute or chronic injury

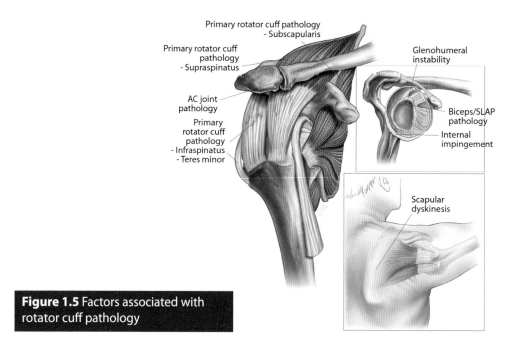

Figure 1.5 Factors associated with rotator cuff pathology

following ongoing degeneration, with patients reporting pre-existing mild pain in the anterior aspect of the shoulder.

Scapular dyskinesis has a profound effect on the caliber of the sub-acromial space. A particular pattern of scapular dyskinesis has been called the SICK scapula syndrome (Scapular malposition, Inferior medial border prominence, Coracoid pain, and dysKinesis of scapular movement).[64] Protraction of the scapula causes the coracoid to move laterally, causing adaptive tightness of the pec minor and the short head of the biceps. This further worsens the abnormal movement, causing antero-inferior angulation of the acromion and impingement-like symptoms.[64]

Shoulder instability can be due to a traumatic event, generalized joint laxity, or repeated episodes of microtrauma.[65] Anterior instability is the most common form, often resulting from frank anterior dislocation, damage to the anterior band of the inferior glenohumeral ligament, or a Bankart lesion. Generalized joint laxity, as mentioned previously, is most often seen in the setting of generalized joint laxity. The rotator cuff may be partly or fully torn in acute dislocation. In the throwing athlete, symptomatic laxity of the shoulder joint (beyond the varying degrees of laxity of the normal shoulder[66]) may lead to an exacerbation of internal impingement; the supraspinatus tendon is impinged between the humerus and glenoid.

Damage to the **biceps/SLAP complex** with labral tears may cause entrapment of the suprascapular nerve, causing weakness of the superspinatus or infraspinatus. Supraspinatus neuropathy can occur due to compression of the nerve at the suprascapular notch by a ganglion cyst (thought to result from labral injury[67]); paralabral cyst formation, due to superior labral injury with entrapment of the suprascapular nerve in the spinoglenoid notch, may result in isolated infraspinatus pathology.[68]

Internal impingement is a process seen primarily in overhead athletes; first described by Walch[69], it differs from classical impingement as the articular, rather than bursal, surface of the tendon (supraspinatus and/or infraspinatus) is affected. The tendon is pinched between the humeral head and the postero-superior glenoid rim.[70] Debate exists as to the causes of this pathology; theories include anterior joint laxity, posterior joint tightness, or a combination of both, or microinstability with over-rotation.[71]

AC joint pathology is discussed in the section Superior to the shoulder triangle. Damage to the AC joint may cause inferior osteophyte formation, which in turn may cause irritation or damage to the rotator cuff as it passes through the coracoacromial arch. When rotator cuff pathology is suspected, the AC joint must always be examined carefully.

Posterior to the triangle

Pain posterior to the triangle is often referred from elsewhere. Cervical pathology may refer pain to the shoulder, but so too can scapular dyskinesis activate the levator scapulae, trapezius, and rotator cuff, causing neck pain. Discogenic and facet-related thoracic spine pain may be felt in the peri-scapular area.

Myalgia and pain of the trapezius muscle are extremely common causes of shoulder and neck pain in the non-sporting population, being linked to office work and computer use.[91] Myofascial tightness is common in the trapezius muscle in overhead athletes.

The posterior shoulder is a common site of referred pain; the cervical spine nerve roots of C6, C7 and C8 all supply the skin over the area posterior to the shoulder triangle. Deep visceral pain may be felt in the posterior shoulder, as a diffuse pain or crushing discomfort.[18] Periscapular pain may result from facet joint pathology in the thoracic spine. Myofascial pain from the trapezius muscle, supraspinatus, and infraspinatus may also refer to the shoulder.

Scapular fractures are rare, representing 3–5% of fractures involving the shoulder girdle and 1% of all fractures.[92] They usually result from high-energy trauma, and so are seen in the sporting population. Fracture should be suspected where there is exquisite point tenderness, although it has been noted that less swelling and ecchymosis than might be expected have been seen.[93] Swelling in the rotator cuff (particularly in spinous process fracture) may lead to muscular inhibition and a so-called "pseudo-cuff rupture" picture.[94] A careful history, focusing on the mechanism of injury, may aid diagnosis. A fall on the outstretched arm, or dislocation of the glenohumeral joint can result in glenoid rim fractures. Blunt trauma over the scapula may be associated with fractures of the scapular body or glenoid neck, with possible extension into the glenoid fossa. Forces from above, such as in a football tackle, may lead to fractures of the scapular spine or acromion.[93]

Scapular dyskinesis often manifests as compression of space beneath the coraco-acromial arch, and subsequent impingement of the tendons of the rotator cuff. In the throwing athlete, however, it may present as posterior pain, or the sensation of a "dead arm".[64] It is discussed in more detail in the section Factors associated with rotator cuff impingement.

Internal impingement is also described in that section, but is a significant cause of posterior shoulder pain in throwing athletes, especially in the late cocking phase. Entrapment of the articular surface of the supraspinatus and/or infraspinatus between the humeral head and glenoid is thought to be the cause.[70]

Chronic pain at the supero-medial angle of the scapula may relate to the insertion of the levator scapulae muscle and is termed "**levator scapulae syndrome**". It is related to poor

Table 1.6 Factors associated with rotator cuff pathology				
Define and align	**Pathology**	**Listen and localize**	**Palpate and recreate**	**Alleviate and investgate**

Factors associated with rotator cuff pathology	Primary rotator cuff pathology
	
	> supraspinatous
		Night pain, insidious or acute onset, anterolateral shoulder pain, pain lying on affected limb[28]	> Jobe's (empty can) test[72, 73]
			   sensitivity: 79%
			   specificity: 50%
				MRI[74]

	Primary rotator cuff pathology
	
	> infraspinatous
	> teres minor
		Night pain, history of trauma, difficulty working overhead,[75] Posterior shoulder pain in deceleration phase of throwing[76]	> Positive Patte's dropping test[73]
			   sensitivity: 60%
			   specificity: 91.7%
				MRI[74]

	Primary rotator cuff pathology
	
	> subscapularis
		< 40 yrs, forced hyperextension and/or external rotation
		
		>40 yrs preceding symptoms, lower energy acute event
		
		Anterior shoulder pain on overhead activity and at night
		
		Report weakness on IR and instability[61]
			Lesser tuberosity tenderness
			
			Weakened IR
			
			Increased passive ER
			
			Positive bear-hug test[77]
			   sensitivity: 60%
			   specificity: 91.7%
				Plain film x-ray
				
				MRI[78]

	Scapular dyskinesis – SICK scapula syndrome	Insidious onset "dead arm", affected shoulder appears lower than unaffected side, anterior shoulder pain or signs of impingement in throwing athlete[64]	Protracted scapula, pain to palpate the coracoid process, Scapula retraction test[64]	Clinical diagnosis, MRI to exclude intra-articular complication

	AC joint pathology	Antero-superior shoulder pain, crepitus over joint	Apley scarf test
			   sensitivity: 77%[79]
			Active compression test[79]
			
			   sensitivity: 41%
			   specificity: 95%[79]
			
			Paxinos test[80]
				Plain film x-ray; Zanca view[81], cross arm view, stress x-ray
				
				Diagnostic LA injection[4]

Table 1.6 *(continued)*				
Define and align	**Pathology**	**Listen and localize**	**Palpate and recreate**	**Alleviate and investgate**
	Glenohumeral instability	Anterior: pain on overhead activity (throwing), dead arm, weakness[65] Posterior: post traumatic, pain on posterior loading of the shoulder (humerus fixed and internally rotated) – bench press, blocking in football[15] Inferior: pain and dysesthesia on carrying heavy objects[15]	No one test is sensitive or specific to diagnose individual directions of instability[41] Combination of apprehension test, relocation load and shift, inferior sulcus sign and crank tests[82]: sensitivity: 90% specificity: 85%	Plain radiology[83] MRI[84] CT for glenoid pathology
	Biceps/SLAP pathology	Burning crushing shoulder pain, weakness[85] Poorly localized anterior pain, impaired performance (worsened by overhead activity),[36] mechanical symptoms[35]	Wasting of infraspinatus or supraspinatus, tenderness in the spinoglenoid notch[86, 87]	MRI for labral abnormality,[88] EMG/NCS[89]
	Internal Impingement	Pain on overhead activity – throwing, difficulty "warming-up", pain during late cocking phase of throw	Pain on palpation of posterior joint line, internal impingement sign[70]	MRI, MR arthrogram, MRA with ABER view[90]

posture, poor work/office equipment ergonomics, and myofascial contracture in the area.[32] It may also be seen as part of the constellation of "whiplash syndrome".[95]

Neuropathy

Suprascapular nerve entrapment may cause pain and/or weakness in the shoulder. Damage or entrapment of the nerve may lead to impaired function of the supraspinatus or infraspinatus. The site of entrapment dictates the clinical presentation, but a general rule is that a proximal lesion causes pain, and a distal lesion weakness and no pain.[87] Nerve entrapment may occur due to forced depression of the shoulder due to a fall or repeated episodes such as in tackles, clavicular fracture, tumor, and paralabral cysts seen in glenohumeral labral injury[86] (Fig. 1.6).

The axillary nerve is the most commonly injured nerve when the shoulder is dislocated;[96] nerve injury of any kind is seen in up to 45% of cases of shoulder dislocation, and the risk of this is increased if the shoulder remains dislocated for >12 hours.[96] Compression by the displaced

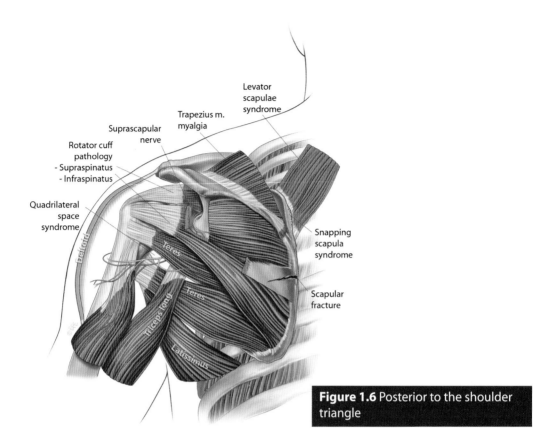

Suprascapular
nerve

Rotator cuff
pathology
- Supraspinatus
- Infraspinatus

Trapezius m.
myalgia

Levator
scapulae
syndrome

Quadrilateral
space
syndrome

Deltoid

Teres

Teres

Triceps long

Latissimus

Snapping
scapula
syndrome

Scapular
fracture

Figure 1.6 Posterior to the shoulder triangle

humeral head and/or traction of the nerve on relocation may be responsible, but it is also seen in proximal humeral fracture.[57] Injury to the nerve results in loss of sensation over a small part of the lateral upper arm; as cutaneous branches and supply to the teres minor are closest to the glenoid rim, they are most commonly injured.[97] Damage to the motor branches of the nerve causes paralysis of the teres minor and deltoid muscles. Abduction of the shoulder is impaired (Fig. 1.6).

Long thoracic nerve palsy (Fig. 1.6) leads to weakness of the serratus anterior, which has implications for scapular stability. The mechanism of injury is usually traction, either by forced depression of the shoulder, with simultaneous lateral flexion of the cervical spine in the contralateral direction (seen in tackling), or may result from prolonged aggressive stretching.[98] The clinician must exclude other, more serious causes, and counsel the patient that, despite symptoms, resolution is generally expected in 12 months.[99]

Quadrilateral space syndrome is rare, and most often seen in younger (third decade) athletes. It is rarely associated with a prior injury; the athlete complains of weakness or early fatigue, and "deadness" of the arm.[100] Thought to be caused by tethering of the neurovascular bundle passing through the space, it was first reported by Cahill et al.;[101] in 70% of cases, athletes managed well with alteration of their pitching technique and did not require surgery (Fig. 1.6).

Snapping scapula syndrome is uncommonly diagnosed, but may be overlooked as a diagnosis and mistaken for myofascial pain. Etiological factors include an altered superomedial scapular angle, fibrotic change in underlying musculature, and even osteochondroma. All of these conditions are associated with pain and crepitus on overhead rotation of the arms (which compresses the scapula against the posterior thoracic wall).[102]

Anterior to the triangle

Pectoralis major pathology usually occurs from a fall, violent contraction of the muscle, or direct trauma to the tendon. Partial tears at the musculotendinous junction are as common as complete tears, which usually occur at the tendinous insertion.[86] Given the superficial nature of the muscle, defects may be palpable, but the fascial covering may camouflage the injury.[113] Pectoralis tendinopathy, either tenosynovitis or calcific[114], or of the pectoralis minor,[115] are more common, but tend to resolve spontaneously and have featured little in the literature.

Clavicular fracture is one of the most common traumatic fractures in sport.[32] The middle third is most often fractured (80%); the medial fragment is usually displaced superiorly by traction from the sternocleidomastoid muscle. This is usually managed conservatively (operative management is indicated where the skin is compromized by bone fragments or where there is clavicular shortening > 1–2 cm), with good clinical recovery.[32] Distal clavicular fractures are more unstable, and may involve injury to the ligaments supporting the AC joint (AC and coracoclavicular ligaments).[116] Those fractures medial to the ligamentous attachment are associated with a greater risk of non-union.[116] Classification of these injuries, as per the American Shoulder and Elbow Society, is shown in Table 1.8.

Referred pain from the diaphragm may be anticipated at the shoulder, due to the phrenic nerve supplyiong the diaphragm, and the shoulder sharing a common innervation from C3–C5.[117] Pathology of the gallbladder and spleen may be anticipated at the shoulder. Post-laparoscopy, gas collects beneath the diaphragm, and may result in discomfort as it dissipates over a number of days in the postoperative period. Cardiac pain may be felt around the shoulder, neck, and arm; despite a number of theories, it is unclear why this is the case.[118]

Axillary vein thrombosis was first described by Paget and Van Schroetter and may be termed "Paget-Schroetter syndrome" or "effort thrombosis". It is theorized that chronic compression of the axillary vein between the scalenous muscle and first rib causes intimal damage, inflammation, and thrombosis.[121] It is seen in many overhead sports and, although it accounts for only 2% of all deep vein thrombosis, it has been described as the most common vascular problem in athletes.[125]

Axillary artery occlusion is a rare complication seen in elite overhead athletes such as baseball pitchers.[124] It is postulated that the cocking phase of pitching, where abduction, extension, and extreme external rotation are combined, make the axillary artery prone to compression under the pectoralis minor muscle.[122] Prolonged repetition is thought to lead to intimal damage, and endofibrosis. In severe cases, aneurysm formation has further complicated the presentation.[126] Although a rare diagnosis, loss of form and power in an

Table 1.7 Posterior to the triangle				
Define and align	**Pathology**	**Listen and localize**	**Palpate and recreate**	**Alleviate and investigate**
Posterior to the triangle	M trapezius myalgia	Pain in the descending part of the trapezius muscle, neck and posterior shoulder pain, disturbed sleep[103]	Tenderness on palpation, limited range of motion of cervical spine[103]	Investigation to exclude cervical pathology

	Rotator cuff pathology
	
	> suprasinatus
		Night pain, insidious or acute onset, antero-lateral shoulder pain, pain lying on affected limb,[28] difficulty working overhead[75]	Jobe's (empty can) test
			    sensitivity: 79%
			    specificity: 50%
				MRI[74]

	> infraspinatus	Posterior shoulder pain in deceleration phase of throwing[76]	Positive Patte's dropping test[73]
			    sensitivity: 60%
			    specificity: 91.7%	

	Referred pain > thoracic spine	Periscapular pain[104] +/− paresthesia, radiation around chest Atypical pain	Recreation of symptoms on passive thoracic rotation	Plain film x-ray, diagnostic guide injection,[107] MRI
	> neuro-myofascial	Tender muscular structures	Trigger points: supraspinatus, levator scapulae, trapezius	Response to dry-needling/deep tissue massage

	> cervical spine	Pain and paresthesias distal to the neck in the distribution of cervical spinal nerve root[105]	Spurling's compression test[105]
			    sensitivity: 40–60%
			    specificity: 92–100%[106]
				Plain film x-ray, MRI[108]

	Internal impingement	Pain on overhead activity – throwing, difficulty "warming up", pain during late cocking phase of throw	Pain on palpation of posterior joint line, internal impingement sign[70]	MRI, MR arthrogram, MRA with ABER view[90]
	Scapular dyskinesis – SICK scapula syndrome	Insidious onset "dead arm", affected shoulder appears lower than unaffected side, anterior shoulder pain or signs of impingement in throwing athlete[64]	Protracted scapula, pain to palpate the coracoid process, Scapula retraction test[64]	Clinical diagnosis, MRI to exclude intra-articular complication

	Table 1.7 *(continued)*			
Define and align	**Pathology**	**Listen and localize**	**Palpate and recreate**	**Alleviate and investigate**
	Levator scapulae syndrome	Shoulder and neck pain related to superior aspect of scapula[32]	Myofascial trigger points over levator scapulae at the superomedial angle of the scapula[95]	Soft tissue therapy, dry needling – monitor response[32]
	Neuropathy > suprascapular nerve palsy	Burning crushing shoulder pain, weakness[87]	Wasting of infraspinatus or supraspinatus, tenderness in the spinoglenoid notch[86, 87]	MRI for labral abnormality,[88] EMG/NCS[89]
	> axillary nerve compression	Post-traumatic/ shoulder dislocation, weakness on shoulder, upper arm numbness	Weakness of shoulder elevation and abduction, "regimental patch" numbness[109]	EMG, MRI for muscle changes[57]
	> long thoracic nerve palsy	Combined shoulder depression and neck bending, shoulder discomfort, weakness overhead[98]	Winging (medial) of the scapula, pain in neck and shoulder, weakness in overhead activity[99]	Clinical diagnosis, EMG[98]
	Scapular fracture	High energy trauma, painful shoulder movement	Adducted arm, flattening of scapular spine, point tenderness, "pseudo-cuff rupture"[93]	Plain film x-ray, CT[110]
	Quadrilateral space syndrome	3rd decade, insidious onset pain, non-dermatomal, non-radiating paresthesia[101]	Tenderness over quadrilateral space, reproduction of symptoms on abduction and internal rotation[101]	Clinical diagnosis, arteriography[100]
	Snapping scapula syndrome	Neck and shoulder pain, localizing at scapular insertion of rhomboid, pain on overhead movement of arms[111]	Reproduction of sound and pain on compression of superior border of scapula against chest wall while patient abducts arms[86]	Diagnostic injection of LA,[86] CT scan to exclude bony lesion[112]

Table 1.8 Classification of distal clavicle fractures	
Type	**Pathology**
I	Fracture distal to coracoclavicular ligaments with little displacement
IIa	Fracture medial to coracoclavicular ligaments
IIb	Fracture between the coracoclavicular ligaments
III	Intra-articular fracture without ligament disruption

Table 1.9 Anterior to the shoulder triangle				
Define and align	**Pathology**	**Listen and localize**	**Palpate and recreate**	**Alleviate and investigate**
Anterior to the triangle	Pectoralis pathology	Sudden onset shoulder or upper arm pain during exertion or fall, "pop" heard[86]	Pain on resisted contraction of pectoralis contraction[32] Defect visible when hands placed on the iliac crest and pectoralis contracted[86]	Plain x-ray,[113] ultrasound,[119] MRI[114]
	Clavicular fracture	Pain, crepitus, loss of motion, deformity of clavicle	Exclude concomitant injuries; AC joint, brachial plexus[120]	Plain film x-ray[120]
	Rotator cuff pathology > sub-scapularis	< 40 yrs forced hyperextension and/or external rotation > 40 yrs preceding symptoms, lower energy acute event > anterior shoulder pain on overhead activity and at night > report weakness on IR and instability[61]	> Lesser tuberosity tenderness > Weakened IR > Increased passive ER > Positive bear-hug test[77] sensitivity: 60% specificity: 91.7%	Plain film x-ray MRI[78]
	Referred pain > cardiac, diaphragm	History of recent abdominal surgery, vague ache, unrelated to movement of shoulder, cardiac pain related to exertion[117]	Normal physical examination of shoulder, manifestation of diaphragmatic irritation	ECG, CT abdomen

Define and align	Pathology	Listen and localize	Palpate and recreate	Alleviate and investigate
Table 1.9 (continued)				
	Axillary vein thrombosis	Repetitive overhead activity, dull ache, easy fatigability, heaviness and paresthesia on activity[121]	Swelling of entire upper limb, mottled cool skin, dilated veins, normal pulses, normal neurological examination[122]	Clinical diagnosis, venography
	Axillary artery occlusion	Arm pain (vague), paresthesia, cold intolerance, digital pain, fatigueability, loss of pitching speed[122]	Coolness of skin, bruit or pulse disturbance in functional position (forced hyperabduction and external rotation)[123]	Doppler US, angiography[124]

overhead athlete should lead the clinician to perform a thorough examination of the vascular supply to the upper limb.

Superior to the shoulder triangle

Acromioclavicular joint pathology may cause superior shoulder pain; acute injury most often results from direct trauma to the superior shoulder with the arm adducted. Falls on an outstretched hand or elbow may also cause AC disruption; here, coraco-clavicular ligament injury is uncommon. High-velocity displacement of the superior humeral head may result in either fracture of the acromion, or rotator cuff tear. AC joint arthrosis, or degenerative change,

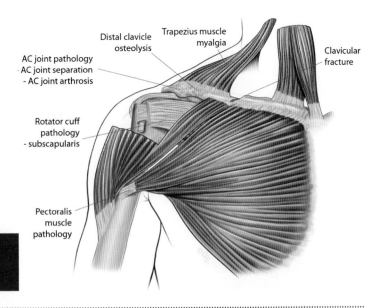

Figure 1.7 Anterior and superior to the shoulder triangle

usually has an insidious onset and may be localized or radiate to the trapezius or down the arm. Distal clavicular osteolysis is seen in athletes with a history of heavy weightlifting and, like AC joint arthrosis, has an insidious onset.

Trapezius myalgia is often seen after traumatic, high-velocity injury (often seen post-motor vehicle accident). The majority of cases settle quickly, but 10–15% may become chronic[103]. Pain is diffuse, and tends to be associated with fatigue and lack of function. Although a clinical diagnosis, the validity and reliability of a number of published diagnostic criteria have been questioned. The clinician should also bear in mind that this is a diagnosis of exclusion, and other, more serious pathologies, such as cervical spine pathology, must be excluded if suspected.

Referred pain

Superior shoulder pain should be differentiated from pain radiating from the cervical spine, neuro-myofascial pain, and neoplastic process of the upper lobe of the lung or diaphragm. The clinician must take a complete history to exclude cervical radiculopathy, and the systemic symptoms of neoplasm.

Summary

Pathology of the shoulder is truly three-dimensional; pathology within the joint may be felt anterior, posterior or superior. As with other parts of the body, and perhaps even more so in the

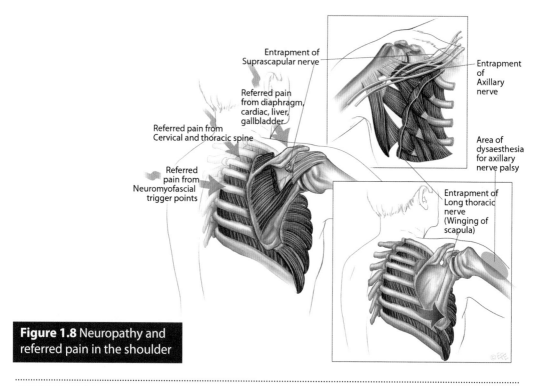

Figure 1.8 Neuropathy and referred pain in the shoulder

Table 1.10 Superior to the shoulder triangle				
Define and align	Pathology	Listen and localize	Palpate and recreate	Alleviate and investigate
Superior to the triangle	AC joint pathology	Antero-superior shoulder pain	Swelling, tenderness, visible deformity	Plain film x-ray; Zanca view[81], cross-arm view, stress x-ray
	> AC joint separation	Fall on shoulder with direct force to superior aspect and arm adducted	Apley scarf test sensitivity 77%[79]	
	> AC joint arthrosis	Older patient, idiopathic[4] or related to local injury[127]	Active compression test[129] sensitivity: 41% specificity: 95%[74]	Diagnostic LA injection[4]
	> Distal clavicle osteolysis	History of heavy weightlifting,[128] insidious onset	Paxinos test[80]	
	trapezius myalgia	Pain in the descending part of the trapezius muscle, neck and posterior shoulder pain, disturbed sleep[103]	Tenderness on palpation, limited range of motion of cervical spine, absence[103]	Investigation to exclude cervical pathology
	Referred pain neuro-myofascial	Atypical pain Tender muscular structures	Trigger points: supraspinatus, levator scapulae, trapezius	Response to dry-needling/ deep tissue massage
	cervical spine	Pain and paresthesias distal to the neck in the distribution of cervical spinal nerve root[105]	Spurling's compression test[105] sensitivity: 40–60% specificity: 92–100%[106]	Plain film x-ray, MRI[108]
	apex of lung, diaphragm	Systemic symptoms of malignancy; malaise, fever, weight loss, and fatigue[129]	Dullness to percussion and altered auscultation at lung apex	Plain x-ray, CT thorax[131] Cocaine test[132] Plain x-ray, CT thorax[131]
		Horner's syndrome[130]	Ipsilateral miosis of pupil, anhidrosis of face, ptosis of eyelid	
		Pancoast syndrome[131]	Shoulder pain, thoracic outlet obstruction	

shoulder, one pathology may in fact cause another, so shoulder instability may lead to rotator cuff pathology, which will in turn reduce stability further. The triangle method is a means of categorizing pathologies according to positions, but also allows the clinician to move from one set of differential diagnoses to another, as you will see in Case 1 below.

Case histories

Case 1

A 29-year-old former professional rugby player attends with right shoulder pain while playing tennis, particularly when serving. He has a history of intermittent shoulder trauma from his playing days, but denies ever having dislocated the joint or had any surgical procedures. When he plays a tennis match, he is quite sore afterwards, and has trouble sleeping that night. He volunteers that abducting his shoulder is painful, as is working overhead.

This is a presentation of shoulder pain. As such, proceed to step 1, define and align the shoulder triangle.

Step 1: Define and align
Expose the patient properly; a singlet will allow physical access and aid visibility.

Define the triangle: locate the coracoid process; the acromial angle of the scapula (formed where the posterior border of the spine of the scapula joins the lateral border of the acromion), and the 3G point (located at the surface markings of the joining of the anterior and posterior borders of the deltoid muscle).

Align the patient's pain on the triangle. The patient locates the pain to the lateral aspect of the shoulder, within the shoulder triangle.

From this point, we recommend that the reader attempt to exclude the potential pathologies. From Table 1.5, the potential causal structures are:

Differential diagnosis
> rotator cuff pathology
> sub-acromial bursitis
> adhesive capsulitis
> biceps brachii:
– tendonosis

>   – tendon rupture
> glenohumeral dislocation
> labral injury:
>   – SLAP lesion
>   – Bankart lesion
> glenohumeral osteoarthritis
> pectoralis tendon rupture

We proceed to differentiate between these structures (step 2).

Step 2: Listen and localize

Addressing the rotator cuff pathology we ask:

Q *Is the pain worse when working overhead, does it radiate to the lateral arm, do you have pain on sleeping?*
A Yes, it is difficult to take objects from overhead shelves and very sore to sleep at night time.

Addressing an sub-acromial bursitis we ask:

Q *Is there difficulty raising the arm from your side?*
A Yes.

Addressing an adhesive capsulitis we ask:

Q *Do you have difficulty putting your coat on? Have you noticed the range of movement in the shoulder worsening?*
A No, not always, but when it is very sore it can be painful to do anything.
Q *Do you or any of your family have diabetes mellitus?*
A No, not that I am aware.

Addressing biceps brachii pathology we ask:

Q *Is it painful to flex your bicep (demonstrate)?*
A No.

Addressing glenohumeral dislocation we ask:

Q *Have you ever dislocated your shoulder when playing rugby?*
A No, never.

Addressing labral injury we ask:

Q *Have you noticed any clicking or grinding in the shoulder?*
A No.
Q *Have you had any episodes of instability (feeling the shoulder roll or pop)?*
A No.

Addressing glenohumeral osteoarthritis we ask:

Q *Did you damage your shoulder during your rugby career?*

A I would have had your average contact but nothing exceptional.

Addressing pectoralis tendon rupture we ask:

Q *Did you have a large pop in the shoulder with bruising after trying to contract your pectoralis muscle against a heavy weight (demonstrate movement)?*

A No.

This will narrow or differential diagnosis somewhat, and we proceed to examination to narrow it further. By palpating painful structures, and recreating the pain through diagnostic maneuvers, we move toward a diagnosis (step 3).

Differential diagnosis

More likely
> rotator cuff pathology
> sub-acromial bursitis
> adhesive capsulitis
> labral injury:
>> – SLAP lesion
>> – Bankart lesion

Less likely
> m biceps brachii:
>> – tendonosis
>> – tendon rupture
> glenohumeral dislocation
> glenohumeral osteoarthritis
> pectoralis tendon rupture

Step 3: Palpate and re-create

The examination results of rotator cuff pathology and sub-acromial bursitis are similar, meaning that differentiation may be challenging. Co-existence of the problems is common. Both Hawkin's and Neer's tests are recommended.

Hawkin's test: The arm is forward-flexed to 90° and the shoulder is forcibly internally rotated. This maneuver drives the greater tuberosity further under the coracoacromial ligament, reproducing the impingement sign.[42]

Neer's test: The shoulder is moved through maximal forward flexion with internal rotation; re-creation of the pain is deemed a positive test.[42]

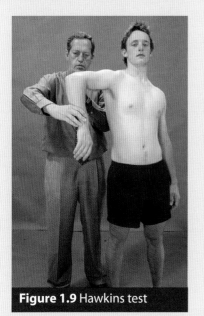

Figure 1.9 Hawkins test

A surgical study indicates that the impingement test can be used as a predictor of outcome for patients with impingement syndrome treated by arthroscopic sub-acromial decompression;[43] this is used in clinical practise regularly. Where Neer's test is positive, local anesthetic is inserted onto the sub-acromial space and testing is repeated; reduction in pain is diagnostic.

Both Neer's test and Hawkin's test are painful.

Comparison of active versus passive ranges of motion is vital in the assessment of adhesive capsulitis. The clinician should note that stage 1 adhesive capsulitis may be similar, in both presentation and examination, to rotator cuff pathology. Later in progression of the pathology, marked loss of passive range of motion is the hallmark of this pathology.

Although active range of motion is limited, passive motion is normal.

Labral pathology is assessed in this text according to position. Superior labral injury (SLAP) is best assessed with the biceps load test and/or new pain provocation test.

The biceps load test, as described by Kim, was first described with the patient sitting, but the biceps load test II[51] is used in practise by the authors. The clinician sits on the side of the shoulder being examined, grasping the wrist and elbow. The arm is elevated to 120° and maximally externally rotated; the elbow is flexed to 90° with the forearm supinated. The patient is then asked to flex the elbow against resistance. The test is positive for superior labral pathology if pain is worsened by this maneuver.

The new pain provocation test is similar to the apprehension test. The patient sits with the arm in 90° of abduction, and the examiner externally rotates the shoulder. This is repeated with the forearm supinated and pronated. The test is positive if the pain provoked is worse when the forearm is supinated.[48]

Testing for SLAP lesion is negative.

Inferior labral pathology is closely related to instability. Many of the tests we use to test for inferior labral pathology also test for instability. A pain or instability with the combination of the crank test, sulcus test, and apprehension/relocation test has excellent sensitivity and specificity.

Crank test: the shoulder is elevated to 160° in the neutral plane, and loaded axially while the humerus is rotated. Pain or a sensation of clicking are deemed positive.

Sulcus sign: the patient sits with their arm relaxed by their side. The examiner grasps the upper arm and applies an inferior load; a sulcus may be observed inferior to the tip of the acromion. This is generally indicative of complex or inferior instability.

Apprehension/relocation test: the anterior apprehension test is performed with the patient supine or seated, and the shoulder in a neutral position at 90° of abduction. The examiner applies slight anterior pressure to the humerus, and externally rotates the arm. Pain or apprehension about the feeling of impending subluxation or dislocation indicates anterior glenohumeral instability (care should be taken not to dislocate the shoulder in this maneuver). Pressure on the proximal humerus, to relocate the head of the humerus, may alleviate these symptoms.

Instability testing is negative.

Palpation of the biceps brachii tendon in the bicipital groove, and having the patient flex the bicep against resistance, should be performed to test for biceps tendinosis. Where a rupture has occurred, ecchymosis is seen and there is weakness of supination.

Palpation of the pectoralis major tendon at its insertion to the humerus should be performed; this forms the anterior fold of the axilla.

No pathology of either the biceps brachii or pectoralis major tendon are noted.

Differential diagnosis

More likely
> rotator cuff pathology
> sub-acromial bursitis

Less likely
> adhesive capsulitis
> labral injury:
  – SLAP lesion
  – Bankart lesion
> biceps brachii:
  – tendonosis
  – tendon rupture
> glenohumeral dislocation
> glenohumeral osteoarthritis
> pectoralis tendon rupture

Our clinical examination makes either rotator cuff pathology or sub-acromial bursitis likely. As the etiology of rotator cuff pathology is multifactorial, we proceed to the section Factors associated with rotator cuff pathology in order to clarify potential causes:

Differential diagnosis

> supraspinatous pathology
> infraspinatous/teres minor pathology
> sub-scapularis pathology
> scapular dyskinesis – SICK scapula syndrome
> AC joint pathology

> glenohumeral instability
> biceps/SLAP pathology
> internal impingement

Clinical evaluation of the individual muscles of the rotator cuff may be clarified.

To assess the supraspinatus, the most evidence-based test is Jobe's test: measuring strength at 90° of abduction, and neutral rotation first assesses the deltoid. The shoulder is then internally rotated, and angled forward 30°: the thumb should be pointing toward the floor. Muscle testing against resistance is then performed.[72]

Jobe's test is positive.

To assess the infraspinatus, Patte's dropping test is recommended: the examiner supports the patient's elbow in 90° of forward elevation, in the plane of the scapula (abducted from the body to 90°), and the patient is asked to externally rotate the shoulder against resistance. Pain and/or weakness indicate tendinopathy or a partial tear; a gradual dropping of the shoulder or the inability to maintain elevation indicates tendon rupture.[73]

Patte's test is negative.

To assess the sub-scapularis, the weakness of internal rotation is noted; passive external rotation is increased. The bear-hug test is the most evidence-based test;[77] the patient is standing or sitting, and is asked to place the hand of the affected side on the opposite shoulder. The examiner then holds the patient's elbow, and asks him or her to resist an external rotation force to the forearm, as the examiner tries to lift the patient's hand off the shoulder. As a result, the patient internally rotates the shoulder as the examiner attempts to externally rotate the arm and to raise the hand off the shoulder in this external rotation. If the patient cannot prevent the examiner from removing the hand from the shoulder, the test is considered positive.

Internal rotation power is good and the bear-hug test is negative.

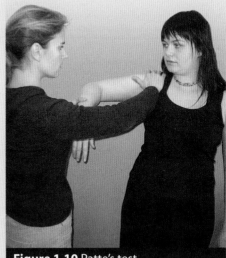

Figure 1.10 Patte's test

To assess for the SICK scapula syndrome, the patient will have a shoulder that appears lower than the unaffected side, a protracted scapula, and a positive scapula retraction test. The examiner should mark the inferior pole of the scapula, the superomedial angle, and, if necessary, the medial border on both sides. To perform the scapula retraction test, the patient is positioned supine; forward flexion in the affected shoulder is limited when compared to the contralateral side. The patient feels pain over the coracoid due to tightness of the pectoralis minor (due to coracoid malposition). The scapula is retracted (repositioned from a protracted to neutral position), and full forward flexion gives resolution of coracoid pain.[64]

Scapular positioning is normal and the scapular retraction test is negative.

To assess the AC joint, the examiner must palpate the area well, feeling for crepitus over the area when the shoulder is moved. The Apley scarf test is sensitive, while the active compression test is specific; a combination is recommended. For the scarf test, the examiner passively adducts the arm across the body horizontally, so that the elbow approximates the contralateral shoulder; the test is positive if this is painful. The active compression test has the standing patient forward-flex the arm to 90° with the elbow in full extension, and then adduct the arm 10° to 15° medial to the sagittal plane of the body, and internally rotate it so that the thumb is pointed downward. The examiner, standing behind the patient, applies a uniform downward force to the arm. With the arm in the same position, the palm is then fully supinated and the maneuver is repeated. The test is considered positive if pain is elicited during the first maneuver, and is reduced or eliminated with the second.

Crepitus is palpated, and the Apley scarf test and the active compression test are both painful.

Glenohumeral instability has already been assessed earlier in the case and is normal.

Assessment for internal impingement is best done using the internal impingement test: the patient lies supine and positions the arm into external rotation; reproduction of postero-superior pain experienced on throwing indicates a positive test. The examiner may then exert a force on the anterior shoulder to relocate the humeral head into the glenoid, then symptoms are diminished.[70]

The internal impingement test was negative.

Here the diagnosis of supraspinatus pathology is likely, and this may be secondary to impingement into the sub-acromial space by an inferior osteophyte from a degenerative AC joint. An x-ray of the shoulder (AP, cross-arm, and Zanca view[81]) will assess the AC joint and an MRI of the shoulder will assess the AC joint, sub-acromial bursa, and supraspinatus tendon.

Case 2

A 21-year-old college soccer goalkeeper presents with right-sided anterior shoulder pain. She remembers no specific trauma, but has begun to notice intermittent sharp jolts on shot-stopping powerful shots since practice one day about a month earlier. She responded well to non-steroidal anti-inflammatories initially, but this is now sore even when she has taken them. She has no history of trauma or dislocation.

This is a presentation of shoulder pain. As such, proceed to step 1, define and align the shoulder triangle.

Step 1: Define and align

Expose the patient properly; a singlet will allow physical access and aid visibility.

Define the triangle: locate the coracoid process, the acromial angle of the scapula (formed where the posterior border of the spine of scapula joins the lateral border of the acromion); and the 3G point (located at the surface markings of the joining of the anterior and posterior borders of the deltoid muscle).

Align the patient's pain on the triangle. The patient locates the pain to the anterior aspect of the shoulder, anterior to the shoulder triangle.

From this point, we recommend that the reader attempt to exclude the potential pathologies. From Table 1.9, the potential causal structures are:

Differential diagnosis

> m pectoralis pathology
> clavicular fracture
> sub-scapularis pathology
> referred pain:
  – cardiac, diaphragm
> axillary vein thrombosis
> axillary artery occlusion

Step 2: Listen and localize
Addressing pectoralis major pathology we ask:
Q *Have you felt a sharp pop at any stage followed by swelling and bruising?*
A No.
Q *Have you noticed difficulty with action such as the bench press?*
A Yes, occasionally sore, particularly when I'm tired.

Addressing clavicular fracture we ask:
Q *Have you received a kick or blow directly to the collarbone?*
A No.

Addressing subscapularis pathology we ask:
Q *Did you feel the shoulder pain first after any particular activity?*
A Yes, it was definitely during a training session when I had to get up from a press-up position and immediately save point-blank shots. This was repeated for 60 seconds 5 times; I was sore and had an ache afterwards.

Addressing referred pain from cardiac muscle or diaphragm we ask:
Q *Do you ever get the pain on activity like running without having moved your arm?*
A No, it is related to when I put my arms out and up (demonstrates a position of abduction and external rotation).
Q *Have you had any abdominal surgery recently, or any medical procedures involving your gastrointestinal or genitorinary system in the recent past?*
A No.

Q *Have you had any trauma to your abdomen in games recently?*
A No.

Addressing axillary vein thrombosis we ask:
Q *Have you noticed a feeling of heaviness or dullness in the arm after exercise?*
A Yes, when it's tired and sore, that's how it feels.

Addressing axillary artery occlusion we ask:
Q *Have you noticed any odd sensations like your arm being colder than the other side?*
A No.
Q *Is your arm easily tired?*
A Yes, when it is tired.

This will narrow or differential diagnosis somewhat, and we proceed to examination to narrow it further. By palpating painful structures, and recreating the pain through diagnostic maneuvers, we move toward a diagnosis (step 3).

Differential diagnosis

More likely
> m pectoralis pathology
> sub-scapularis pathology

Less likely
> clavicular fracture
> referred pain:
  - cardiac, diaphragm
> axillary vein thrombosis
> axillary artery occlusion

Step 3: Palpate and re-create

The diagnoses of axillary vein thrombosis and axillary artery occlusion are unlikely; as they are seen predominantly in throwing sports such as baseball, they are unlikely from this history, but we will still examine for them.

To assess the pectoralis muscle, the athlete should be asked to contract the pectoralis major against resistance. Any obvious deficit may be visualized by having the patient place their hands on the iliac crest and contract the pectoralis muscle.

No defect is visible or palpable, but there is some pain on resisted contraction of the pectoralis.

To assess the sub-scapularis, weakness of internal rotation is noted; passive external rotation is increased. The bear-hug test is the most evidence-based test;[77] the patient is standing or sitting, and is asked to place the hand of the affected side on the opposite shoulder. The examiner then holds the patient's elbow, and asks him or her to resist an external rotation force to the forearm, as the examiner tries to lift the patient's hand off the shoulder. As a result, the patient internally rotates the shoulder, as the examiner attempts to externally rotate the arm and to raise the hand off the shoulder in external rotation. If the patient cannot prevent the examiner from removing the hand from the shoulder, the test is considered positive.

Internal rotation power is limited compared to the contralateral side, and the bear-hug test is positive for pain.

The clavicle is examined and palpated for any obvious deformity.

No defect is visible or palpable.

If there is any suggestion of cardiac pain, the patient should have a resting and stress ECG. A thorough examintion of the abdomen should be performed, in order to exclude any abdominal trauma to the liver or spleen.

There is no suggestion of cardiac pain, and abdominal examination is normal.

To assess for pathology of the axillary artery or vein, the affected limb should be examined for dilated superficial veins, compared to the other side, or for mottling of the skin. The skin should be palpated for coolness, and pulses should be palpated. The patient should then hyperabduct, and observation and palpation of pulses should be repeated.

There is no obvious disturbance of arterial supply or venous drainage to the affected limb.

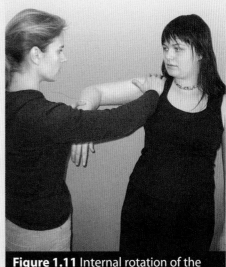

Figure 1.11 Internal rotation of the shoulder

Step 4: Alleviate and investigate

Pathology of the sub-scapularis muscle tendon is likely, although tendinosis of the pectoralis muscle may be the causal agent. It may be possible to rehabilitate this injury without investigation, but, where it is required, ultrasound or MRI would confirm the diagnosis.

Case 3

A 40-year-old recreational baseball pitcher attends complaining of posterior shoulder pain. He has played baseball in season for more than 30 years, and has had shoulder pain before, but within the joint, rather than at the back as he now feels it. His pain has come on gradually over the previous six weeks. It is particularly sore when pitching. It had tended to warm up pretty well in the beginning, but is now constantly sore, and he has difficulty sleeping with the pain.

This is a presentation of shoulder pain. Proceed to step 1, define and align the shoulder triangle.

Step 1: Define and align

Expose the patient properly; a singlet will allow physical access and aid visibility.

Define the triangle: locate the coracoid process; the acromial angle of the scapula (formed where the posterior border of the spine of scapula joins the lateral border of the acromion); and the 3G point (located at the surface markings of the joining of the anterior and posterior borders of the deltoid muscle).

Align the patient's pain on the triangle. Here the pain is located posterior to the shoulder triangle.

The patient has localized the pain to the area "posterior to the triangle". From this point, we recommend that the reader attempt to exclude the potential pathologies. From Table 1.7, the potential causal structures are:

Differential diagnosis

> m trapezius myalgia

> rotator cuff pathology:
  - m supraspinatus
  - m infraspinatus

> referred pain

> thoracic spine

> neuro-myofascial

> cervical spine

> internal impingement

> SICK scapula syndrome

> levator scapulae syndrome

> neuropathy:
  - suprascapular nerve palsy
  - axillary nerve compression
  - long thoracic nerve palsy

> quadrilateral space syndrome

> snapping scapula syndrome

> scapular

We proceed to differentiate between these structures (step 2).

Step 2: Listen and localize

Addressing trapezius myalgia we ask:

Q *Does the pain also travel up into the neck?*

A Sometimes, when it is very bad.

Addressing rotator cuff pathology we ask:

Q *Do you have difficulty raising your arms from your side?*

A Yes.

Q *Do you have pain sleeping on the affected shoulder at night time?*

A Yes.

Addressing supraspinatus pathology we ask:

Q *Do you have difficulty working overhead (taking something out of an overhead cupboard)?*

A Sometimes, only when it is bad.

Addressing infraspinatus we ask:

Q *Do you have pain after you have released the ball (deceleration pain) when pitching?*

A Yes, particularly when I pitch in competition.

Addressing referred pain from the thoracic spine we ask:

Q *Does your pain locate at the medial border of the scapula?*

A No.

Addressing neuro-myofascial referred pain we ask:

Q *Are the muscles of your neck painful?*

A No.

Addressing referred pain from the cervical spine we ask:

Q *Do you have any abnormal sensation or tingling in the arm?*

A No, I have not noticed.

Addressing internal impingement we ask:

Q *Do you have pain in the shoulder during the "cocking phase" of your swing?*

A No, it's when I release.

Addressing SICK scapula syndrome we ask:

Q *Have you had the sensation of a dead arm?*

A No.

Addressing levator scapulae syndrome we ask:

Q *Are the muscles around the shoulder sore, particularly at the supero-medial border of the scapula?*

A No, it is sore at the back of my shoulder.

Addressing suprascapular nerve palsy we ask:

Q *Have you noticed a burning crushing pain in the area?*

A Yes, it sometimes burns when it is sore.

Addressing axillary nerve compression we ask:

Q *Have you had recent trauma to or dislocation of your shoulder?*

A No.

Q *Have you noticed weakness or an abnormal sensation over your deltoid (indicate the site)?*

A No.

Addressing long thoracic nerve palsy we ask:

Q *Have you noticed any weakness working overhead?*

A No real weakness, it's more pain.

Addressing scapular fracture we ask:

Q *Have you had a high-energy injury to the area (fall from a height, football tackle from behind)?*

A No.

Addressing quadrilateral space syndrome we ask:

Q *Is there numbness at the back of the shoulder?*

A No.

Addressing snapping scapula syndrome we ask:

Q *Have you noticed any clicking or cracking from beneath the shoulderblade?*

A No.

This will narrow or differential diagnosis somewhat, and we proceed to examination to narrow it further. By palpating painful structures, and recreating the pain through diagnostic maneuvers, we move toward a diagnosis (step 3).

Differential diagnosis

More likely
> m trapezius myalgia
> rotator cuff pathology:
    – m supraspinatus
    – m infraspinatus
> internal impingement
> SICK scapula syndrome
> neuro-myofascial
> suprascapular nerve palsy

Less likely
> referred pain from cervical spine/thoracic spine
> levator scapulae syndrome

> axillary nerve compression
> long thoracic nerve palsy
> quadrilateral space syndrome
> snapping scapula syndrome
> scapular

Step 3: Palpate and re-create

Palpation of the trapezius muscle, especially middle and lower fibers, is effective, as is measuring the cervical spine range of motion. If areas of tightness are palpable, massage, digital ischaemic pressure, or dry-needling may release these. There is no discernable difference between sides.

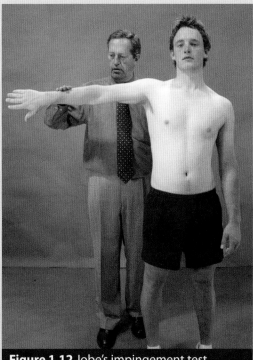

Figure 1.12 Jobe's impingement test

To assess the supraspinatus, the most evidence-based test is Jobe's test: measuring strength at 90° of abduction and neutral rotation first assesses the deltoid. The shoulder is then internally rotated, and angled forward 30°: the thumb should be pointing toward the floor. Muscle testing against resistance is then performed.[72]

Jobe's empty can test was negative.

To assess the infraspinatus, Patte's dropping test is recommended: the examiner supports the patient's elbow in 90° of forward elevation in the plane of the scapula (abducted from the body to 90°); the patient is asked to externally rotate the shoulder against resistance. Pain and/or weakness indicate tendinopathy or a partial tear; a gradual dropping of the shoulder, or inability to maintain elevation, indicates tendon rupture.[73]

Weakness of external rotation was noted and Patte's test recreated symptoms felt during pitching; the dropping sign was not noted, however.

Assessment for internal impingement is best done using the internal impingement test: the patient lies supine, and positions the arm into external rotation; reproduction of the postero-superior pain experienced on throwing indicates a positive test. The examiner may then exert a force on the anterior shoulder, to relocate the humeral head into the glenoid, then symptoms are diminished.[70]

The internal impingement test was negative.

The athlete with SICK scapula syndrome will have a shoulder which appears lower than the unaffected side, a protracted scapula, and a positive scapula retraction test. Here, the patient is positioned supine, and forward flexion in the affected shoulder is limited when compared to the contralateral side. The patient feels pain over the coracoid due to tightness of the pectoralis minor (due to coracoid malposition). The scapula is retracted (repositioned from a protracted to neutral position), and full forward flexion gives resolution of coracoid pain.[64]

Scapular positioning was normal and the retraction test was negative.

Suprascapular nerve palsy may result from a labral injury (SLAP lesion) within the shoulder. The biceps load test or new pain provocation test are recommended; these are described in Case 1. The suprascapular nerve may also be entrapped at the spinoglenoid notch, and this may be palpated. Where denervation has occurred, the physician may note the absence of infraspinatus contraction on resisted external rotation. Normal muscle contraction is seen on observation.

Although the other pathologies are less likely, a complete examination of the cervical spine and thoracic spine is mandatory, assessing for recreation of any symptoms.

Palpation of all of the borders of the scapula, particularly the scapular spine, for tenderness and bruising will help to exclude fracture, but without high-energy trauma this is unlikely. In snapping scapula syndrome, the patient may often voluntarily reproduce the crepitus.

"Regimental badge" numbness and weakness of the deltoid and teres minor are seen in axillary nerve palsy. Bear in mind that teres minor weakness may manifest as weakness of external rotation when compared to the contralateral arm.

Long thoracic nerve palsy will manifest initially as pain in the neck and shoulder, followed by winging of the scapula, demonstrated by having the patient press against the wall, and observing separation of the scapula from the thoracic wall.

Cervical spine range of motion was normal; there are no areas of dysesthesia or muscle wasting.

Differential diagnosis

More likely

> pathology of infraspinatus

> internal impingement

Less likely

> suprascapular nerve palsy

> SICK scapula syndrome

> neuro-myofascial

> pathology of supraspinatus

> m trapezius myalgia

> referred pain from cervical spine/thoracic spine

> levator scapulae syndrome

> axillary nerve compression long thoracic nerve palsy

> quadrilateral space syndrome

> snapping scapula syndrome

> scapular

Or findings above make pathology of the infraspinatus likely; given the athlete's sport, internal impingement may be possible, but testing does not confirm a diagnosis.

We may now proceed to step 4 to confirm our clinical suspicion via imaging. Ultrasonography is effective, but the most evidence-based test is MRI. If, despite clinical findings, internal impingement is still suspected, the use of gadolinium intra-articular contrast will elucidate any articular surface infraspinatus pathology.

References

1. Margo M, Astrid J, Manuel AJ et al. Sports injuries and illnesses in the 2009 FINA World Aquatics Championships. *Br J Sports Med*. May 10.

3. Speer KP. Anatomy and pathomechanics of shoulder instability. *Clin Sports Med*. Oct 1995; 14(4):751–60.

4. Rios CG, Mazzocca AD. Acromioclavicular joint problems in athletes and new methods of management. *Clin Sports Med*. Oct 2008; 27(4):763–88.

5. Fukuda K, Craig EV, An KN, Cofield RH, Chao EY. Biomechanical study of the ligamentous system of the acromioclavicular joint. *J Bone Joint Surg Am*. Mar 1986; 68(3):434–40.

6. Urist MR. Complete dislocation of the acromioclavicular joint. *J Bone Joint Surg Am*. Dec 1963; 45:1750–53.

7. Vangsness CT, Jr., Jorgenson SS, Watson T, Johnson DL. The origin of the long head of the biceps from the scapula and glenoid labrum. An anatomical study of 100 shoulders. *J Bone Joint Surg Br*. Nov 1994; 76(6):951–54.

8. Hsu SH, Miller SL, Curtis AS. Long head of biceps tendon pathology: management alternatives. *Clin Sports Med*. Oct 2008; 27(4):747–62.

9. Darrow CJ, Collins CL, Yard EE, Comstock RD. Epidemiology of severe injuries among United States high school athletes: 2005–2007. *Am J Sports Med*. Sep 2009; 37(9):1798–1805.

9. Glousman R, Jobe F, Tibone J, Moynes D, Antonelli D, Perry J. Dynamic electromyographic analysis of the throwing shoulder with glenohumeral instability. *J Bone Joint Surg Am*. Feb 1988; 70(2):220–26.

10. Ajmani ML. The cutaneous branch of the human suprascapular nerve. *J Anat*. Oct 1994; 185 (Pt 2):439–42.

11. Madsen M, Marx RG, Millett PJ, Rodeo SA, Sperling JW, Warren RF. Surgical anatomy of the triceps brachii tendon: anatomical study and clinical correlation. *Am J Sports Med*. Nov 2006; 34(11):1839–43.

12. Van L, Mulder JD. Function of the supraspinatus muscle and its relation to the supraspinatus syndrome. An experimental study in man. *J Bone Joint Surg Br*. Nov 1963; 45:750–54.

13. Otis JC, Jiang CC, Wickiewicz TL, Peterson MG, Warren RF, Santner TJ. Changes in the moment arms of the rotator cuff and deltoid muscles with abduction and rotation. *J Bone Joint Surg Am*. May 1994; 76(5):667–76.

14. Ogston JB, Ludewig PM. Differences in 3-dimensional shoulder kinematics between persons with multidirectional instability and asymptomatic controls. *Am J Sports Med*. Aug 2007; 35(8):1361–70.

15. Bahu MJ, Trentacosta N, Vorys GC, Covey AS, Ahmad CS. Multidirectional instability: evaluation and treatment options. *Clin Sports Med*. Oct 2008; 27(4):671–89.

16. Neer CS, 2nd, Foster CR. Inferior capsular shift for involuntary inferior and multidirectional instability of the shoulder: a preliminary report. *J Bone Joint Surg Am*. Oct 1980; 62(6):897–908.

17. Procacci P, Zoppi M, Maresca M. Clinical approach to visceral sensation. In: Cervero F, Morrison JFB, eds. *Visceral sensation*. Amsterdam: Elsevier; 1986:21–28.

18. Procacci P, Maresca M. Referred pain from somatic and visceral structures. *Current Pain and Headache Reports*. 1999; 3(2):96–99.

19. Mehta S, Gimbel JA, Soslowsky LJ. Etiologic and pathogenetic factors for rotator cuff tendinopathy. *Clin Sports Med*. Oct 2003; 22(4):791–812.

20. van der Windt DA, Koes BW, de Jong BA, Bouter LM. Shoulder disorders in general practice: incidence, patient characteristics, and management. *Ann Rheum Dis*. Dec 1995; 54(12):959–64.

21. Khan KM, Cook JL, Bonar F, Harcort P, Astrom M. Histopathology of common tendinopathies. Update and implications for clinical management. *Sports Med*. Jun 1999; 27(6):393–408.

22. Curl W. Clinical relevance of sports-induced inflammation. In: Leadbetter W, Buckwalter J, Gordon S, eds. *Sports-induced inflammation*. Park Ridge: American Academy of Orthopaedic Surgeons; 1990:149–54

23. Pfahler M, Branner S, Refior HJ. The role of the bicipital groove in tendopathy of the long biceps tendon. *J Shoulder Elbow Surg*. Sep–Oct 1999; 8(5):419–24.

24. Ahrens PM, Boileau P. The long head of biceps and associated tendinopathy. *J Bone Joint Surg Br*. Aug 2007; 89(8):1001–9.

25. Gill HS, El Rassi G, Bahk MS, Castillo RC, McFarland EG. Physical examination for partial tears of the biceps tendon. *Am J Sports Med*. Aug 2007; 35(8):1334–40.

26. Neer CS. Cuff tears, biceps lesions, and impingement. In: Neer CS, ed. *Shoulder reconstruction*. Philedelphia: WB Saunders; 1990.

27. Warren RF. Lesions of the long head of the biceps tendon. *Instr Corse Lect*. 1985; 34:204–09.

28. Malone TR. Standardized shoulder examination – Clinical and functional approaches. In: Wilk KE, Reinold MM, Andrews JR, eds. *The athlete's shoulder*. 2nd ed. Philadelphia, PA: Churchill Livingstone Elsevier; 2009:45–71.

29. Ogilvie–Harris DJ, Myerthall S. The diabetic frozen shoulder: arthroscopic release. *Arthroscopy*. Feb 1997; 13(1):1–8.

30. Neviaser JS. Adhesive capsulitis and the stiff and painful shoulder. *Orthop Clin North Am*. Apr 1980; 11(2):327–31.

31. Sheridan MA, Hannafin JA. Upper extremity: emphasis on frozen shoulder. *Orthop Clin North Am*. Oct 2006; 37(4):531–39.

32. Kibler WB, Murrell GA. Shoulder pain. In: Brukner P, Khan K, eds. *Clinical sports medicine*. 3rd ed. Sydney: McGraw–Hill Professional; 2006:243–88.

33. Wang RY, Mazzocca AD, Bicos J, Arciero RA. Management of the first-time shoulder dislocation in the athlete. In: Wilk KE, Reinold MM, Andrews JR, eds. *The athlete's shoulder*. Philadelphia, PA: Churchill Livingstone Elsevier; 2009:239–55.

34. Cain EL, Kocaj SM, Wilk KE. Adhesive capsulitis of the shoulder. In: Wilk KE, Reinold MM, Andrews JR, eds. *The athlete's shoulder*. Philadelphia, PA: Churchill Livingstone Elsevier; 2009:293–301.

35. McLaughlin HL, Cavallaro WU. Primary anterior dislocation of the shoulder. *Am J Surg*. Nov 15 1950; 80(6):615–21, passim.

36. Bedi A, Allen AA. Superior labral lesions anterior to posterior-evaluation and arthroscopic management. *Clin Sports Med*. Oct 2008; 27(4):607–30.

37. Barber A, Field LD, Ryu R. Biceps tendon and superior labrum injuries: decision-marking. *J Bone Joint Surg Am*. Aug 2007; 89(8):1844–55.

38. Snyder SJ, Karzel RP, Del Pizzo W, Ferkel RD, Friedman MJ. SLAP lesions of the shoulder. *Arthroscopy*. 1990; 6(4):274–79.

39. Nam EK, Snyder SJ. The diagnosis and treatment of superior labrum, anterior and posterior (SLAP) lesions. *Am J Sports Med*. Sep–Oct 2003; 31(5):798–810.

40. Ellenbecker TS, Bailie DS. Shoulder athroplasty in the athletic shoulder. In: Wilk KE, Reinold MM, Andrews JR, eds. *The athlete's shoulder*. Philadelphia, PA: Churchill Livingstone Elsevier; 2009:315–24.

41. Parsons IMt, Campbell B, Titelman RM, Smith KL, Matsen FA, 3rd. Characterizing the effect of diagnosis on presenting deficits and outcomes after total shoulder arthroplasty. *J Shoulder Elbow Surg*. Nov–Dec 2005; 14(6):575–84.

42. Malanga GA, Nadler SF. Physical examination of the shoulder. *Musculoskeletal physical examination, an evidence based approach*. Philedelphia: Elsevier Mosby; 2006.

43. Mair SD, Viola RW, Gill TJ, Briggs KK, Hawkins RJ. Can the impingement test predict outcome after arthroscopic subacromial decompression? *J Shoulder Elbow Surg*. Mar–Apr 2004; 13(2):150–53.

44. Armstrong A, Teefey SA, Wu T et al. The efficacy of ultrasound in the diagnosis of long head of the biceps tendon pathology. *J Shoulder Elbow Surg*. Jan–Feb 2006; 15(1):7–11.

45. Rokous JR, Feagin JA, Abbott HG. Modified axillary roentgenogram. A useful adjunct in the diagnosis of recurrent instability of the shoulder. *Clin Orthop Relat Res*. Jan–Feb 1972; 82:84–86.

46. Steinbach LS. Magnetic resonance imaging of glenohumeral joint instability. *Semin Musculoskelet Radiol*. Mar 2005; 9(1):44–55.

47. Kim SH, Ha KI, Ahn JH, Choi HJ. Biceps load test II: A clinical test for SLAP lesions of the shoulder. *Arthroscopy*. Feb 2001; 17(2):160–64.

48. Mimori K, Muneta T, Nakagawa T, Shinomiya K. A new pain provocation test for superior labral tears of the shoulder. *Am J Sports Med*. Mar–Apr 1999; 27(2):137–42.

49. Liu SH, Henry MH, Nuccion SL. A prospective evaluation of a new physical examination in predicting glenoid labral tears. *Am J Sports Med.* Nov–Dec 1996; 24(6):721–25.

50. Bencardino JT, Beltran J, Rosenberg ZS, et al. Superior labrum anterior-posterior lesions: diagnosis with MR arthrography of the shoulder. *Radiology.* Jan 2000; 214(1):267–71.

50. Kibler WB. Specificity and sensitivity of the anterior slide test in throwing athletes with superior glenoid labral tears. *Arthroscopy.* Jun 1995; 11(3):296–300.

51. Dodds SD, Wolfe SW. Injuries to the pectoralis major. *Sports Med.* 2002; 32(14):945–52.

52. Connell DA, Potter HG, Sherman MF, Wickiewicz TL. Injuries of the pectoralis major muscle: evaluation with MR imaging. *Radiology.* Mar 1999; 210(3):785–91.

53. McFarland EG, Tanaka MJ, Papp DF. Examination of the shoulder in the overhead and throwing athlete. *Clin Sports Med.* Oct 2008; 27(4):553–78.

54. Baker CW, Busconi BD. Tensile failure of the rotator cuff. In: Wilk KE, Reinold MM, Andrews JR, eds. *The athlete's shoulder.* Philadelphia, PA: Churchill Livingstone Elsevier; 2009:111–14.

55. Jenp YN, Malanga GA, Growney ES, An KN. Activation of the rotator cuff in generating isometric shoulder rotation torque. *Am J Sports Med.* Jul–Aug 1996; 24(4):477–85.

56. Walch G, Boulahia A, Calderone S, Robinson AH. The 'dropping' and 'hornblower's' signs in evaluation of rotator-cuff tears. *J Bone Joint Surg Br.* Jul 1998; 80(4):624–28.

57. Bencardino JT, Rosenberg ZS. Entrapment neuropathies of the shoulder and elbow in the athlete. *Clin Sports Med.* Jul 2006; 25(3):465–87, vi–vii.

58. Jobe FW, Moynes DR, Antonelli DJ. Rotator cuff function during a golf swing. *Am J Sports Med.* Sep–Oct 1986; 14(5):388–92.

59. Ryu RK, McCormick J, Jobe FW, Moynes DR, Antonelli DJ. An electromyographic analysis of shoulder function in tennis players. *Am J Sports Med.* Sep–Oct 1988; 16(5):481–85.

60. Pink M, Jobe FW, Perry J, Kerrigan J, Browne A, Scovazzo ML. The normal shoulder during the butterfly swim stroke. An electromyographic and cinematographic analysis of twelve muscles. *Clin Orthop Relat Res.* Mar 1993; (288):48–59.

61. Piasecki DP, Nicholson GP. Tears of the subscapularis tendon in athletes – diagnosis and repair techniques. *Clin Sports Med.* Oct 2008; 27(4):731–45.

62. Lo IK, Burkhart SS. The etiology and assessment of subscapularis tendon tears: a case for subcoracoid impingement, the roller-wringer effect, and TUFF lesions of the subscapularis. *Arthroscopy.* Dec 2003; 19(10):1142–50.

63. Habermeyer P, Magosch P, Pritsch M, Scheibel MT, Lichtenberg S. Anterosuperior impingement of the shoulder as a result of pulley lesions: a prospective arthroscopic study. *J Shoulder Elbow Surg.* Jan–Feb 2004; 13(1):5–12.

64. Burkhart SS, Morgan CD, Kibler WB. The disabled throwing shoulder: spectrum of pathology Part III: The SICK scapula, scapular dyskinesis, the kinetic chain, and rehabilitation. *Arthroscopy.* 2003; 19(6):641–61.

65. Taylor SA, Drakos MC, O'Brien SJ. Anterior instability of the shoulder. In: Wilk KE, Reinold MM, Andrews JR, eds. *The athlete's shoulder.* Philadelphia, PA: Churchill Livingstone Elsevier; 2009:191–208.

66. Robinson CM, Aderinto J. Recurrent posterior shoulder instability. *J Bone Joint Surg Am.* Apr 2005; 87(4):883–92.

67. Boyce RH, Wang JC. Evaluation of neck pain, radiculopathy, and myelopathy: imaging, conservative treatment, and surgical indications. *Instr Corse Lect.* 2003; 52:489–95.

68. Duralde XA. Neurologic injuries in the athlete's shoulder. *J Athl Train.* Jul 2000; 35(3):316–28.

69. Walch G, Liotard JP, Boileau P, Noel E. [Postero-superior glenoid impingement. Another shoulder impingement]. *Rev Chir Orthop Reparatrice Appar Mot.* 1991; 77(8):571–74.

70. Meister K, Buckley B, Batts J. The posterior impingement sign: diagnosis of rotator cuff and posterior labral tears secondary to internal impingement in overhand athletes. *Am J Orthop* (Belle Mead NJ). Aug 2004; 33(8):412–15.

71. Reinold MM, Wilk KE, Dugas JR, Andrews JR. Internal impingement. In: Wilk KE, Reinold MM, Andrews JR, eds. *The athlete's shoulder.* Philadelphia, PA: Churchill Livingstone Elsevier; 2009:123–141.

72. Jobe FW, Jobe CM. Painful athletic injuries of the shoulder. *Clin Orthop Relat Res.* Mar 1983; (173):117–24.

73. Naredo E, Aguado P, De Miguel E et al. Painful shoulder: comparison of physical examination and ultrasonographic findings. *Ann Rheum Dis.* Feb 2002; 61(2):132–36.

74. Bencardino JT, Garcia AI, Palmer WE. Magnetic resonance imaging of the shoulder: rotator cuff. *Top Magn Reson Imaging.* Feb 2003; 14(1):51–67.

75. Lunn JV, Castellanos–Rosas J, Tavernier T, Barthelemy R, Walch G. A novel lesion of the infraspinatus characterized by musculotendinous disruption, edema, and late fatty infiltration. *J Shoulder Elbow Surg.* Jul–Aug 2008; 17(4):546–53.

76. Lintner D, Noonan TJ, Kibler WB. Injury patterns and biomechanics of the athlete's shoulder. *Clin Sports Med*. Oct 2008; 27(4):527–51.

77. Barth JR, Burkhart SS, De Beer JF. The bear-hug test: a new and sensitive test for diagnosing a subscapularis tear. *Arthroscopy*. Oct 2006; 22(10):1076–84.

78. Deutsch A, Altchek DW, Veltri DM, Potter HG, Warren RF. Traumatic tears of the subscapularis tendon. Clinical diagnosis, magnetic resonance imaging findings, and operative treatment. *Am J Sports Med*. Jan–Feb 1997; 25(1):13–22.

79. Chronopoulos E, Kim TK, Park HB, Ashenbrenner D, McFarland EG. Diagnostic value of physical tests for isolated chronic acromioclavicular lesions. *Am J Sports Med*. Apr–May 2004; 32(3):655–61.

80. Walton J, Mahajan S, Paxinos A et al. Diagnostic values of tests for acromioclavicular joint pain. *J Bone Joint Surg Am*. Apr 2004; 86–A(4):807–12.

81. Zanca P. Shoulder pain: involvement of the acromioclavicular joint. (Analysis of 1,000 cases). *Am J Roentgenol Radium Ther Nucl Med*. Jul 1971; 112(3):493–506.

82. Liu SH, Henry MH, Nuccion S, Shapiro MS, Dorey F. Diagnosis of glenoid labral tears. A comparison between magnetic resonance imaging and clinical examinations. *Am J Sports Med*. Mar–Apr 1996; 24(2):149–54.

83. Provencher MT, Bell SJ, Menzel KA, Mologne TS. Arthroscopic treatment of posterior shoulder instability: results in 33 patients. *Am J Sports Med*. Oct 2005; 33(10):1463–71.

84. Beltran J, Kim DH. MR imaging of shoulder instability injuries in the athlete. *Magn Reson Imaging Clin N Am*. May 2003; 11(2):221–38.

86. Ott JW, Clancy WG, Wilk KE. Soft tissue injuries of the shoulder. In: Wilk KE, Reinold MM, Andrews JR, eds. *The athlete's shoulder*. 2nd ed. Philadelphia, PA: Churchill Livingstone Elsevier; 2009:283–292.

87. Zehetgruber H, Noske H, Lang T, Wurnig C. Suprascapular nerve entrapment. A meta-analysis. *Int Orthop*. 2002; 26(6):339–43.

88. Jee WH, McCauley TR, Katz LD, Matheny JM, Ruwe PA, Daigneault JP. Superior labral anterior posterior (SLAP) lesions of the glenoid labrum: reliability and accuracy of MR arthrography for diagnosis. *Radiology*. Jan 2001; 218(1):127–32.

89. Witvrouw E, Cools A, Lysens R et al. Suprascapular neuropathy in volleyball players. *Br J Sports Med*. Jun 2000; 34(3):174–80.

90. Jung JY, Jee WH, Chun HJ, Ahn MI, Kim YS. Magnetic resonance arthrography including ABER view in diagnosing partial-thickness tears of the rotator cuff: accuracy, and inter- and intra-observer agreements. *Acta Radiol*. Mar; 51(2):194–201.

91. Waling K, Jarvholm B, Sundelin G. Effects of training on female trapezius myalgia: An intervention study with a 3-year follow-up period. *Spine* (Phila Pa 1976). Apr 15 2002; 27(8):789–96.

92. Thompson DA, Flynn TC, Miller PW, Fischer RP. The significance of scapular fractures. *J Trauma*. Oct 1985; 25(10):974–77.

93. Lapner PC, Uhthoff HK, Papp S. Scapula fractures. *Orthop Clin North Am*. Oct 2008; 39(4):459–74, vi.

94. Neviaser JS. Traumatic lesions; injuries in and about the shoulder joint. *Instr Corse Lect*. 1956; 13:187–216.

95. Ettlin T, Schuster C, Stoffel R, Bruderlin A, Kischka U. A distinct pattern of myofascial findings in patients after whiplash injury. *Arch Phys Med Rehabil*. Jul 2008; 89(7):1290–93.

96. Visser CP, Coene LN, Brand R, Tavy DL. The incidence of nerve injury in anterior dislocation of the shoulder and its influence on functional recovery. A prospective clinical and EMG study. *J Bone Joint Surg Br*. Jul 1999; 81(4):679–85.

97. Price MR, Tillett ED, Acland RD, Nettleton GS. Determining the relationship of the axillary nerve to the shoulder joint capsule from an arthroscopic perspective. *J Bone Joint Surg Am*. Oct 2004; 86–A(10):2135–42.

98. Safran MR. Nerve injury about the shoulder in athletes, part 2: long thoracic nerve, spinal accessory nerve, burners/stingers, thoracic outlet syndrome. *Am J Sports Med*. Jun 2004; 32(4):1063–76.

99. Foo CL, Swann M. Isolated paralysis of the serratus anterior. A report of 20 cases. *J Bone Joint Surg Br*. Nov 1983; 65(5):552–56.

100. Redler MR, Ruland LJ, 3rd, McCue FC, 3rd. Quadrilateral space syndrome in a throwing athlete. *Am J Sports Med*. Nov–Dec 1986; 14(6):511–13.

101. Cahill BR, Palmer RE. Quadrilateral space syndrome. *J Hand Surg Am*. Jan 1983; 8(1):65–69.

102. Parsons TA. The snapping scapula and subscapular exostoses. *J Bone Joint Surg Br*. May 1973; 55(2):345–49.

103. Larsson B, Sogaard K, Rosendal L. Work related neck-shoulder pain: a review on magnitude, risk factors, biochemical characteristics, clinical picture and preventive interventions. *Best Pract Res Clin Rheumatol*. Jun 2007; 21(3):447–63.

104. Dreyfuss P, Tibiletti C, Dreyer SJ. Thoracic zygapophyseal joint pain patterns. A study in normal volunteers. *Spine* (Phila Pa 1976). Apr 1 1994; 19(7):807–11.

106. Viikari–Juntura E, Porras M, Laasonen EM. Validity of clinical tests in the diagnosis of root compression in cervical disc disease. *Spine* (Phila Pa 1976). Mar 1989; 14(3):253–57.

107. Boswell MV, Trescot AM, Datta S et al. Interventional techniques: evidence-based practice guidelines in the management of chronic spinal pain. *Pain Physician.* Jan 2007; 10(1):7–111.

108. Hassankhani A, Bencardino JT. Magnetic resonance imaging of sports injuries of the spine. *Top Magn Reson Imaging.* Feb 2003; 14(1):87–102.

109. de Laat EA, Visser CP, Coene LN, Pahlplatz PV, Tavy DL. Nerve lesions in primary shoulder dislocations and humeral neck fractures. A prospective clinical and EMG study. *J Bone Joint Surg Br.* May 1994; 76(3):381–83.

109. Malanga GA, Nadler SF. Physical examination of the cervical spine. *Musculoskeletal physical examination, an evidence-based approach.* Philedlphia, PA: Elsevier Mosby; 2006:33–58.

110. Anderson J, Read J, Lucas P. The shoulder, shoulder-girdle, and thoracic cage. In: Anderson J, Read J, eds. *Atlas of imaging in sports medicine.* 2nd ed. Sydney: McGraw–Hill Australia; 2008:186–284.

111. Milch H. Partial scapulectomy for snapping of the scapula. *J Bone Joint Surg Am.* Jul 1950; 32-A(3):561–66.

112. Sisto DJ, Jobe FW. The operative treatment of scapulothoracic bursitis in professional pitchers. *Am J Sports Med.* May–Jun 1986; 14(3):192–94.

113. Zeman SC, Rosenfeld RT, Lipscomb PR. Tears of the pectoralis major muscle. *Am J Sports Med.* Nov–Dec 1979; 7(6):343–47.

114. Cahir J, Saifuddin A. Calcific tendonitis of pectoralis major: CT and MRI findings. *Skeletal Radiol.* Apr 2005; 34(4):234–38.

115. Bhatia DN, de Beer JF, van Rooyen KS, Lam F, du Toit DF. The "bench-presser's shoulder": an overuse insertional tendinopathy of the pectoralis minor muscle. *Br J Sports Med.* Aug 2007; 41(8):e11.

116. Anderson K. Evaluation and treatment of distal clavicle fractures. *Clin Sports Med.* Apr 2003; 22(2):319–26, vii.

117. Walsh RM, Sadowski GE. Systemic disease mimicking musculoskeletal dysfunction: a case report involving referred shoulder pain. *J Orthop Sports Phys Ther.* Dec 2001; 31(12):696–701.

118. Arendt–Nielsen L, Svensson P. Referred muscle pain: basic and clinical findings. *Clin J Pain.* Mar 2001; 17(1):11–19.

119. Allen GM, Wilson DJ. Ultrasound in sports medicine – a critical evaluation. *Eur J Radiol.* Apr 2007;62(1):79–85.

120. Lazarus MD, Seon C. Fractures of the clavicle. In: Buckholz RW, Heckman JD, Cort–Brown C, Tornetta P, eds. *Rockwood and Green's fractures in adults.* 6th ed. Philadelphia: Lippincott Williams & Wilkins; 2005:1211–55.

121. Sheeran SR, Hallizey MJ, Murphy TP, Faberman RS, Sherman S. Local thrombolytic therapy as part of a multidisciplinary approach to acute axillosubclavian vein thrombosis (Paget–Schroetter syndrome). *J Vasc Interv Radiol.* Mar–Apr 1997; 8(2):253–60.

122. Baker (Jr) CL, Baker (III) CL. Neurovascular compression syndromes of the shoulder. In: Wilk KE, Reinold MM, Andrews JR, eds. *The athlete's shoulder.* Philadelphia, PA: Churchill Livingstone Elsevier; 2009:325–35.

123. Rohrer MJ, Cardullo PA, Pappas AM, Phillips DA, Wheeler HB. Axillary artery compression and thrombosis in throwing athletes. *J Vasc Surg.* Jun 1990; 11(6):761–68, discussion 768–69.

124. Schneider K, Kasparyan NG, Altchek DW, Fantini GA, Weiland AJ. An aneurysm involving the axillary artery and its branch vessels in a major league baseball pitcher. A case report and review of the literature. *Am J Sports Med.* May–Jun 1999; 27(3):370–75.

125. Sotta RP. Vascular problems in the proximal upper extremity. *Clin Sports Med.* Apr 1990; 9(2):379–88.

126. Todd GJ, Benvenisty AI, Hershon S, Bigliani LU. Aneurysms of the mid axillary artery in major league baseball pitchers – a report of two cases. *J Vasc Surg.* Oct 1998; 28(4):702–07.

127. Shaffer BS. Painful conditions of the acromioclavicular joint. *J Am Acad Orthop Surg.* May–Jun 1999; 7(3):176–88.

128. Scavenius M, Iversen BF. Nontraumatic clavicular osteolysis in weight lifters. *Am J Sports Med.* Jul–Aug 1992; 20(4):463–67.

129. O'Brien SJ, Pagnani MJ, Fealy S, McGlynn SR, Wilson JB. The active compression test: a new and effective test for diagnosing labral tears and acromioclavicular joint abnormality. *Am J Sports Med.* Sep–Oct 1998; 26(5):610–13.

130. Walton KA, Buono LM. Horner syndrome. *Curr Opin Ophthalmol.* Dec 2003; 14(6):357–63.

131. Wright CD, Mathisen DJ. Superior sulcus tumors. *Curr Treat Options Oncol.* Feb 2001; 2(1):43–49.

132. Mughal M, Longmuir R. Current pharmacologic testing for Horner syndrome. *Curr Neurol Neurosci Rep.* Sep 2009; 9(5):384–89.

2

The elbow triangle

Introduction

G olf, tennis and baseball are popular upper-limb dominated sports where overhead activity exposes the athlete to injury. These activities are associated with a significant incidence of elbow pathology; while 1–3% of the general population suffer elbow pain, up to 50% of overhead sports athletes have elbow pain.[1] Elbow injuries are significant in terms of morbidity, time lost from sport, and impairment of function.[2] Lateral elbow pain is more common than medial elbow pain.[1] The anatomy of both areas is complicated and crowded; the authors believe that a thorough knowledge of the anatomy of the area is necessary to correctly differentiate a diagnosis from within the many pathologies.

A comprehensive knowledge of the sport or activity involved is of course important, as training load and technique play a role in the pathogenesis of both medial and lateral elbow pain. Both age and level of performance contribute to the development of elbow pain; 30–50% of recreational tennis players may expect to suffer from "tennis elbow" or common extensor origin tendinopathy (the most common cause of lateral elbow pain) in their playing lifetime.[3]

This chapter will guide the clinician through the anatomy of the elbow joint, forming a reference guide for those wishing to improve their knowledge of the anatomy and pathology of the elbow joint, using the familiar triangle relationships to construct a differential diagnosis.

Learning objectives
The landmarks of the elbow
The pain-generating structures of the region
Significant joints, ligaments, and muscle actions and properties
The presenting symptoms of pathology of each of these structures, to allow differentiation between them
Discriminative examinations and maneuvers to alter (reduce/increase) the presenting pain
evidence-based examinations to confirm the clinical diagnosis

The joint

The elbow joint is the union of three bones, the humerus, radius and ulna. It is a synovial, hinged joint which flexes and extends in one plane. The **ulnohumeral joint** is the main weightbearing joint; the articulation is between the trochlea of the distal humerus and the trochlear notch of the proximal ulna. The trochlear surface is smooth and lined with hyaline cartilage. The anatomy of this articulation means that the elbow flexes at a fixed angle; the carrying angle generally ranges between 5–10° in men and 10–25° in women.

The **radiohumeral joint** is the articulation of the radial head and the capitellum on the lateral aspect of the humerus; movement at this joint combines with that of the **proximal radioulnar joint** to allow pronation and supination. This occurs due to rotation of the radial head within the annular ligament. The rotation of the radius at the elbow facilitates pronation and supination of the forearm. Effectively the radius moves around the ulna, bringing the muscles and neurovascular structures with it, and preventing their twisting, which would occur if there were a single forearm bone.[4]

The stability of the elbow joint is ensured primarily by the bony congruency of the joint and the collateral ligaments and, to a lesser extent, the joint capsule and surrounding muscles and their tendons. The elbow joint has a more restricted range of movement than the ankle, a similar hinge joint. Its ligamentous structures are therefore not as prone to injury. The collateral ligaments of the elbow are nonetheless a source of injury, in particular on the medial aspect of the arm. The medial collateral ligament (MCL) is prone to large valgus forces in overhead throwing sports like baseball (MCL provides 54% valgus stability, while osseous articulation provides 33%)[5].

The ligaments

Medial
The **ulnar** or **medial collateral ligament complex** is composed of anterior, posterior, and oblique (transverse) bands. The posterior band passes from the posterior aspect of the medial epicondyle to the medial edge of the olecranon. The anterior band passes from the medial epicondyle to the medial aspect of the coronoid process; this provides the primary constraint to valgus stress. It is injured in athletes who frequently use a throwing motion. The oblique band (transverse band or ligament of Cooper) bridges the attachments of the anterior and posterior bands, between the olecranon and the coronoid process. This ligament is in relation with the triceps brachii and flexor carpi ulnaris, and the ulnar nerve, and gives origin to part of the flexor digitorum superficialis.

Lateral
The **lateral ligament complex** is formed of four ligaments: the lateral ulnar collateral ligament; the radial collateral ligament; the annular ligament of the radial head; and the accessory lateral collateral ligament.

The lateral ulnar collateral ligament

The lateral ulnar collateral ligament (LUCL) runs from the lateral epicondyle across the annular ligament, to attach to the ulna as a broad attachment along the supinator crest.

The radial collateral ligament

The radial collateral ligament (RCL) is a short, narrow, fiberous band attached superiorly to the lateral epicondyle of the humerus, and inferiorly to the annular ligament and the lateral margin of the ulna. It blends with the tendinous origin of the supinator.

The annular ligament

The annular ligament is an incomplete ligamentous cylinder which is responsible for maintaining the position of the proximal radial head; it is attached to the radial notch at its anterior and posterior margins. Proximally, its fibers blend with the elbow joint capsule. Its inner surface is smooth, lined with a synovial membrane around the radial head.

The accessory collateral ligament

The accessory lateral collateral ligament helps to stabilize the annular ligament, but is inconsistently present.[6]

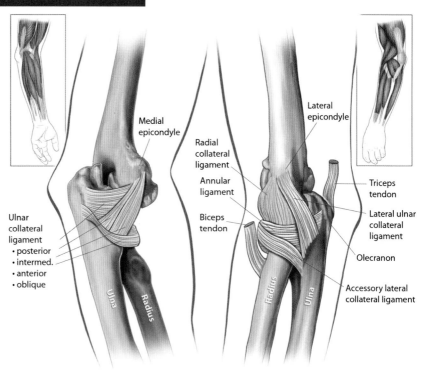

Figure 2.1 Elbow and bony ligaments

Secondary ossification centers

The ossification of the cartilaginous structures to form secondary ossification centers in the developing elbow, occur in a predictable sequence: capitellum; radial head; epicondyle; trochlea; olecranon; lateral epicondyle (CRETOL).

| Table 2.1 Secondary ossification centers ||
Center	Age
Capitellum	1–2 yrs
Radial head	3 yrs
Epicondyle (medial)	5 yrs
Trochlea	7 yrs
Olecranon	9 yrs
Lateral epicondyle	11 yrs

Reproduced from Anderson IF, Read JW, 2008, *Atlas of imaging in sports medicine*, 2nd ed., Sydney, McGraw–Hill, Australia.

These centers of ossification are prone to injury in childhood, resulting in damage to the epiphysis, and subsequent malformation. This stage of childhood development is completed with the appearance of all secondary ossification centers.[7]

These ossification centers are exposed to greater forces in the adolescent athlete, potentially causing avulsion of the epiphyses and avascular necrosis (AVN) of the capitellum. This stage ends when the ossification centers fuse.

In adults, muscular development is complete and fusion of the epiphyses has occurred. This means that musculotendinous and avulsion fractures occur, rather than at ossification sites.

Landmarks of the elbow triangle

The anatomical apex points of the triangle are as follows:

> the lateral epicondyle

> the medial epicondyle

> 3G point (located at the surface markings of the cross-section of the brachioradialis and pronator teres muscles)

Anatomical relations of the borders of the elbow triangle

A line drawn between the lateral epicondyle and the medial epicondyle forms the **superior border** of the triangle. The majority of the structures encountered in the elbow triangle cross the superior border of the triangle. Moving laterally to medially, the structures encountered are:

> common extensor tendon

> extensor carpi radialis longus

> cephalic vein

> brachioradialis muscle

> brachialis muscle; this forms a base on which we encounter:
  - biceps brachii tendon
  - brachial artery
  - bicipital aponeurosis

> median nerve, lies just medial to the medial border of the brachialis

> pronator teres muscle

> medial cubital vein

> common flexor origin, of which the most superficial is the flexor carpi radialis muscle

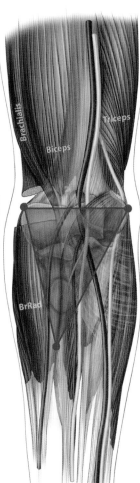

Figure 2.2 The elbow triangle

BrRad	=	Brachioradialis
Biceps	=	Biceps brachii

Lateral epicondyle (Common extensor origin)

Medial epicondyle (Common flexor origin)

The lateral epicondyle of the humerus is a small, tuberculated eminence giving attachment to the radial collateral ligament (originates from the lateral epicondyle and attaches distally to the annular ligament which surrounds the radial head) of the elbow joint, and to the common origin of the supinator and the common extensor origin.

Common extensor tendon

The common extensor tendon arises from the lateral epicondyle of the humerus, and is a tendon shared by a number of extensor muscles in the forearm:

> extensor carpi radialis brevis

> extensor digitorum communis

> extensor digiti minimi

> extensor carpi ulnaris

Acting with the extensor carpi radialis longus, these five muscles control extension and medial and lateral movements of the wrist.

Extensor carpi radialis longus is quite long, starting on the lateral side of the humerus, superior to (but palpable medial to) the common extensor origin. It initially runs along with the brachioradialis, but becomes mostly tendon early on, running between the brachioradialis and extensor carpi radialis. The radial nerve innervates the extensor muscles of the forearm.

The **Cephalic vein** is located in the superficial fascia along the anterolateral surface of the biceps brachii muscle. It crosses the elbow joint and lies on the brachioradialis; it communicates with the basilic vein via the median cubital vein at the elbow.

Brachioradialis arises from the upper two-thirds of the lateral supracondylar ridge of the humerus and the anterior aspect of the lateral intermuscular septum. It inserts distally into the radius, laterally at the base of the styloid process. Supplied by the radial nerve, it acts synergistically with the biceps brachii to flex the elbow when the forearm is in neutral, and acts to stabilize the elbow during rapid flexion or extension. When pronated, the brachioradialis is more active during elbow flexion, since the biceps brachii is in a mechanical disadvantage.

The **brachialis muscle** arises from the anterior surface of the distal half of the humerus, and the adjacent intermuscular septa, more so medially. It inserts distally into the anterior surface of the coracoid process of the ulna. Because it inserts into the ulna, the brachialis flexes the elbow, with the forearm pronated or supinated. Supplied by the radial and musculocutaneous nerves, it is the most powerful elbow flexor, and plays no role in pronation or supination.

The **biceps brachii tendon** is the distal insertion of the **biceps brachii** muscle. It traverses that elbow joint, inserting into the radial tuberosity. Because the ulnar and radial bones can rotate about each other, the biceps can powerfully supinate the forearm. The biceps also connects with the fascia of the medial side of the forearm, via the bicipital aponeurosis. As a forearm flexor, the biceps brachii is most effective when the forearm is supinated. When the forearm is pronated, the brachialis, brachioradialis, and supinator function to flex the forearm, with minimal contribution from the biceps brachii. It is supplied by the musculocutaneous nerve.

The **brachial artery** overlies the triceps proximally and the brachialis distally. The biceps lies lateral to the artery, which becomes more superficial in the antecubital fossa, lying beneath the bicipital aponeurosis with the median nerve. The brachial artery terminates by dividing into the radial and ulnar arteries in the cubital fossa.

The **bicipital aponeurosis** stretches from the medial side of the biceps tendon, and passes obliquely downward and medially across the brachial artery. It is continuous with the antebrachial fascia, covering the origins of the flexor muscles of the forearm. The aponeurosis reinforces the antecubital fossa, and helps to protect the brachial artery and the median nerve running underneath.

Median nerve

The course of the median nerve and of the brachial artery are closely related; proximally, the median nerve is immediately lateral to the brachial artery, and the median nerve crosses over the artery to the medial side, lying anterior to the elbow joint. Here it passes beneath the bicipital aponeurosis, leaving the elbow between the humeral and ulnar heads of the pronator teres (which it supplies). Arising from the lower three cervical and first thoracic roots (C6–8, T1) at the elbow, it supplies the pronator teres, flexor carpi radialis (FCR), palmaris longus and flexor digitorum superficialis (FDS), and the superior radioulnar joint.

Deep to the FDS, it gives off the anterior interosseus branch, which supplies the flexor pollicis longus (FPL) part of the flexor digitorum profundus (FDP) and pronator quadratus. It continues to the wrist deep into the flexors, to supply some of the muscles of the hand (½LOAF – first and second lumbricals, opponens pollicis, abductor pollicis brevis, and flexor pollicis brevis), which will be discussed in Chapter 3.

Pronator teres acts synergistically with the pronator quadratus (at the wrist), the pronator teres serves to pronate the forearm (turning it so the palm faces downward).

The muscle originates from two heads; the humeral head, the larger and more superficial, arises immediately above the medial epicondyle, and from the common flexor tendon. The ulnar head is the thinner, arising from the medial side of the coronoid process of the ulna, and joins the more superior humeral head at a sharp angle.

The median nerve enters the forearm between these two heads. The muscle passes obliquely across the forearm, and ends in a flat tendon, which inserts to the lateral border of the radius, just below the insertion of the supinator. Entrapment of the median nerve between the head of the pronator teres may cause symptoms along the distribution of the median nerve, called pronator teres syndrome, a rare cause of wrist pain.

The medial cubital vein connects the basilic and cephalic veins, and is a common site for venepuncture. It lies in the cubital fossa, superficial to the bicipital aponeurosis.

There exists a fair amount of variation of the median cubital vein. It may adopt an H- or M-pattern in bridging the cephalic and basilic veins.

The **medial epicondyle** forms the palpable tip of the humerus. It is larger and more prominent than the lateral epicondyle, and it is directed in a slightly posterior direction.

It gives attachment to the ulnar collateral ligament of the elbow joint, to the pronator teres, and to the tendon of the common flexor origin:

> pronator teres

> flexor carpi radialis

> palmaris longus

> flexor digitorum superficialis

> flexor carpi ulnaris

The ulnar nerve runs in a groove on the back of the medial epicondyle.

Although not palpable, we will discuss the anatomy of **supinator**, which is a significant muscle in the forearm. As its name suggests, it aids the biceps in supinating a pronated forearm.

It consists of two planes of fibers, between which lies the deep motor branch of the radial nerve. The superficial plane arises from the lateral epicondyle via a tendinous origin (the arcade of Frohse); the deeper portion is a muscular origin arising from the lateral epicondyle, from the radial collateral and annular ligaments, and from the ulna.

Both planes insert into the radius, the superficial fibers into the lateral edge of the radial tuberosity and the oblique line of the radius, and the deeper fibers into the dorsal and lateral surfaces of the body of the radius.

The deep motor branch of the radial nerve mentioned above diminishes considerably, and becomes the **posterior interosseus nerve**, as it passes through the supinator muscle. It supplies all the muscles on the radial side and dorsal surface of the forearm, excepting the anconæus, brachioradialis, and extensor carpi radialis longus. Entrapment of the nerve may occur, resulting in weakness of extension of the wrist, and pain similar to extensor tendinopathy. The anatomical sites where nerve entrapment may occur are more easily recalled as follows; FREAS[8]

> Fibrous bands about the radiocapitellar joint

> Radial recurrent vessels

> Extensor carpi radialis brevis

> Arcade of Frohse

> Supinator

Borders of the triangle

A line drawn from the medial epicondyle, following the pronator teres, to the 3G point, where the pronator teres passes beneath the brachioradialis, forms the **medial border** of the triangle. The pronator teres is easily visualized and palpated when the patient is asked to move from a supine to a pronated position against resistance.

The **lateral border** of the triangle is formed by a line drawn from the lateral epicondyle, following the body of the brachioradialis, to the 3G point, where the brachioradialis passes over the pronator teres. The brachialis is visible and palpable along the lateral border of the forearm when the patient flexes the elbow against resistance.

The extensor aspect of the elbow contains the structures encountered **posterior to the triangle**. Moving posterior from the lateral epicondyle, the capitellum of the humerus is palpable in the depression, lateral to the olecranon of the ulna. The anconæus also fills this space, inserting into the lateral aspect of the olecranon. The upper border of the olecranon is the insertion site of the triceps tendon. The most superior fibers of the ulnar origin of the flexor carpi ulnaris (FCU) are palpable when this muscle contracts (flexion and ulnar deviation of the wrist). The ulnar nerve and the superior ulnar collateral artery pass between the ulnar and humeral (lateral epicondyle) heads of the FCU.

Anconaeus is palpable in the lateral groove between the lateral epicondyle and the olecranon, where it inserts, this small muscle arises from the posterior aspect of the lateral epicondyle of the humerus, and is a weak extensor of the elbow. It is supplied by the radial nerve (C7,8).

The three heads of the **triceps** arise at the infraglenoid tubercle of the scapula (long head), and upper (lateral head) and lower halves (medial heads) of the posterior aspect of the humerus. The insertion of its conjoint tendon into the olecranon of the ulna makes it the primary extensor of the elbow. The medial head also serves to retract the capsule of the elbow joint on extension. It is supplied by the radial nerve (C6–8).

The ulnar nerve arises from the C8 and T1, entering the elbow between the intermuscular septum and the medial head of the triceps. It supplies the elbow joint and FCU, through which it passes, and subsequently runs beneath, with the ulnar artery on its medial side from one-third down the forearm. The ulnar nerve supplies muscles of the hand which will be discussed in Chapter 3.

Nomenclature

Extensor tendinopathy

"Tennis elbow" is the term commonly used to describe the pathology affecting the lateral epicondyle, hence the term "lateral epicondylitis"; studies have shown, however, that the primary pathology is collagen disarray, rather than inflammation of the common extensor origin.[9] Extensor tendinopathy therefore more accurately describes the pathology often localized to the first 1–2 cm of the extensor carpi radialis brevis (ECRB) tendon.[10]

Flexor tendinopathy

This is the medial equivalent of extensor tendinopathy; it is often called "golfer's elbow". Similar pathological processes affect the pronator teres and the flexor tendon.[10]

Pronation

Pronation is rotation of the forearm, and it occurs at the radioulnar joint. In the anatomical position, pronation moves the palm of the hand from an anterior-facing position (supine) to a posterior-facing position (prone). This corresponds to a counter-clockwise twist for the right forearm, and a clockwise twist for the left.

This action is performed by the pronator quadratus and pronator teres muscles. The brachioradialis puts the forearm into a mid-pronated/supinated position from either

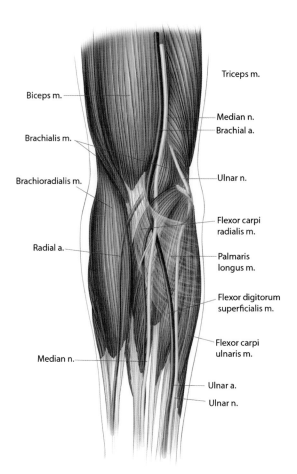

Biceps m.

Brachialis m.

Brachioradialis m.

Radial a.

Median n.

Triceps m.

Median n.
Brachial a.

Ulnar n.

Flexor carpi
radialis m.

Palmaris
longus m.

Flexor digitorum
superficialis m.

Flexor carpi
ulnaris m.

Ulnar a.

Ulnar n.

Figure 2.3 Muscles and nerves at the elbow		
m.	=	muscle
n.	=	nerve
a.	=	artery

full pronation or supination. The examiner should always check this movement with the patient's elbow by their side, to exclude medial rotation of the shoulder, which partly pronates the arm.

Supination

Supination is the opposite motion to pronation. It moves the palm from the prone to supine position. This action is performed by the biceps brachii and the supinator muscle.

Bursitis

Bursitis may occur in the elbow in the olecranon bursa, posteriorly or anteriorly, in either the bicipitoradial bursa, or the interosseus bursa. It may be impossible to differentiate between these structures. For the purpose of this text, when the symptoms are within the triangle, it is termed "cubital bursitis", and when it is lateral, it is termed "radiohumeral bursitis".

Lateral to the triangle

Lateral to the triangle, the bulk of extensor muscles, "the extensor wad", lies above the lateral epicondyle. This bony landmark is the origin of the common extensor tendon, and much of the pathology associated with the lateral aspect of the arm is associated with it. By far the most common pathology is extensor tendinopathy, the subject of much debate.[I]

Common extensor origin (CEO) tendinopathy is a chronic degenerative process occurring due to excessive use of the wrist extensors. Repetitive microtrauma leads to fiberoelastic degeneration, and mucinoid degeneration of the extensor origin, and subsequent failure of the tendon.[II] The athlete will complain of lateral elbow pain, worsened by activity, and pain on palpattion of both the epicondyle and the extensor tendons, particularly the extensor carpi radialis brevis (ECRB).

Muscle	Origin	Insertion	Nerve	Root
Extensor digitorum		Base of 3rd metacarpal		
Extensor carpi radialis brevis		Base of 3rd metacarpal		
Extensor digitorum	Humerus; lateral epicondyle	Extensor expansion of fingers	Posterior interosseus n.	
Extensor digiti minimi		Extensor expansion 4th finger	C7, C8	
Extensor carpi ulnaris		Base of 3rd metacarpal		
Extensor carpi radialis longus	Lateral supracondylar ridge (lower ⅓)	Posterior of base of 2nd metacarpal	Radial n.	C6, C7
Brachioradialis	Lateral supracondylar ridge (upper ⅔)	Radius; styloid process	Radial n.	C5, C6
Brachialis	Humerus, lower half, intermuscular septum	Ulna; coronoid process and tuberosity	Musculo-cutaneous n.	C5, C6
Biceps brachii	Long head – scapula; supraglenoid tubercle; Short head – scapula; coracoid process	Radius; bicipital tuberosity, bicipital aponeurosis, deep fascia, subcutaneous ulna	Musculo-cutaneous n.	C5, C6
Pronator teres	Humerus; medial epicondyle, supracondylar ridge; Ulna; coronoid process	Radius; lateral aspect, mid-shaft	Median n.	C6, C7
Flexor carpi radialis	Medial epicondyle	Base 2nd and 3rd metacarpals	Median n.	C6, C7
Palmaris longus		Flexor retinaculum and palmar aponeurosis	Median n.	C7, C8

Table 2.2 Origins, insertions, and nerve supply to the main movers of the elbow joint

Table 2.2 *(continued)*				
Muscle	**Origin**	**Insertion**	**Nerve**	**Root**
Flexor digitorum superficialis	Humerus; medial epicondyle, ulna; coronoid process, radius; anterior oblique line	Middle phalanges of medial 4 fingers	Median n.	C7, C8, T1
Flexor carpi ulnaris	Humerus; medial epicondyle Ulna; medial olecranon, medial border of ulna	Pisiform, hook of hamate, base of 5th metacarpal	Ulnar n.	C7, C8, T1
Flexor digitorum profundus	Anterior and medial surface of upper ⅔ of ulna	Distal phalanges of medial 4 fingers	Median n. Ulnar n.	C8, T1 and C8, T1
Flexor pollicis longus	Radius, anterior surface of middle ⅓	Distal phalanx of thumb	Anterior interosseus n.	C7, C8
Supinator	Deep head; ulna, supinator crest Superficial head; lateral epicondyle, lateral collateral ligament	Neck and shaft of radius	Posterior interosseus n.	C6, C7
Triceps brachii	Long head; scapula infraglenoid tubercle Lateral head; posterior humerus lower ½ Medial head;	Olecranon of ulna	Radial n.	C6–8
Anconæus	Posterior aspect of lateral epicondyle	Olecranon lateral side	Radial n.	C6–8

Table 2.3 Muscles responsible for the movements of the elbow			
Flexion	**Extension**	**Pronation**	**Supination**
Brachialis	Triceps brachii	Pronator quadratus	Supinator
Biceps brachii	Anconæus	Pronator teres	Biceps brachii
Brachioradialis		Flexor carpi radialis	
		Anconæus	

The clinician will be aware that other pathologies may be present, rather than CEO tendinopathy. A thorough history will differentiate pathology such as osteochondritis or Panner's disease. Subtle presentations, which may mimic localized elbow pain lateral to the triangle, include referred pain. Pain referred from the cervical and thoracic spine (particularly C6/7) must be excluded on thorough examination of the cervical spine and peripheral nervous

Table 2.4 A pathoanatomic approach; lateral to the triangle				
Define and align	**Pathology**	**Listen and localize**	**Palpate and recreate**	**Alleviate and Investigate**
Lateral to the triangle	Extensor tendinopathy	Lateral elbow pain at epicondyle and more distal	Extensor carpi radialis brevis test[23]	Ultrasound, MRI[1]
	Referred pain > cervical (C6/7)/ thoracic spine	Persistent, unpredictable, related to posture, dysesthesia	Neurological examination, neural tension testing	Manipulation of C-spine[24], plain film, MRI
	> myofascial	Trigger points within extensor compartment[25]	Pain recreated by palpation of trigger point	Dry-needling, digital pressure[25]
	> visceral	Poorly localized, C6/7 dermatome pain	Pain unrelated to elbow movement/ muscle contraction	Appropriate medical assessment[26]
	Osteochondritis dessicens	Adolescent patient, history of sport/ activity with excessive lateral compressive forces, movement limited, locking/clicking[11], adolescents 11–16 yrs	Loss of extension, crepitus on forced movement, anterolateral pain	Plain film[7], MRI[27]
	Panner's disease	Children aged < 11 yrs, vague dull aching lateral arm pain, aggravated by activity and eased with rest, limited movement[14]	Lateral tenderness over radiocapitellar joint, 10–20° flexion contracture, crepitus, effusion rare[14]	
	Radial head fracture	Adult, fall on outstretched hand, loss of extension[28]	Pain on pronation supination, loss of extension[10]	Plain film[7]
	Lateral epicondyle fracture	Children 6–10 yrs, varus tensile force on a supinated forearm	Loss of extension, swelling, ecchymosis	Plain film[7], MRI[29]
	Radiohumeral joint pathology	Pain closely related to activity levels, history of trauma	Pain on passive pronation/ supination	Plain film, MRI[30]
	Radial head subluxation (pulled/ nursemaid"s elbow)	Child 2–6 yrs pulled sharply by the arm or hand when the arm is pronated and extended; sharp pain and refusal to move arm[31]	Arm held flexed and pronated Point tenderness but this may be absent[19]	Plain film (to outrule fracture if suspected)[19]

Define and align	Pathology	Listen and localize	Palpate and recreate	Alleviate and investigate
	Radial nerve entrapment > radial tunnel syndrome	Weakness rare, lateral dorsal forearm pain, vague, deep, night pain[8]	Pain on resisted supination with extended elbow[8] Tenderness along radial tunnel[20]	Diagnostic local anesthetic injection[8], nerve conduction studies[32] (negative in 90% of cases of radial tunnel syndrome[33])
	> posterior interosseus nerve syndrome	Lateral forearm pain, progressive weakness of digit extension and wrist adduction[8]	Weakness on resisted digit extension[8], resisted middle finger extension test[34*]	
	Radiohumeral bursitis	Anterolateral elbow pain, tends to worsen with activity	Pain anterolateral aspect of radial head[10, 35]	Ultrasound[10]

Table 2.4 (continued)

* Interpret with caution as may be positive in common extensor origin (CEO) tendinopathy (50% of patients with radial tunnel syndrome may have concomitant CEO tendinopathy[18])

system. Myofascial trigger points in the trapezius, supraspinatous, and infraspinatous may all generate upper-limb and elbow pain. Visceral pain due to cardiac ischaemia may also be appreciated in the left elbow.

Osteochrondral injuries

In the younger age group, osteochondritis dessicens (OCD) and Panner's dizease both may cause degeneration of the articular cartilage of the capitellum, but they tend to affect different age groups and need to be differentiated.

Osteochondritis dessicens is a common cause of lateral elbow pain in children and adolescents, characteristically occurring between the ages of 11–16 yrs. It is commonly seen in throwing athletes, where the pathology is thought to be due to repetitive trauma from valgus stress and lateral trauma, and gymnasts, where the upper limb acting as a weightbearing structure is subjected to shear stress.[12] The etiology is thought to be due to focal injury to the subchondral bone; this causes a loss in structural support for the overlying cartilage, with subsequent fragmentataion and destruction.[13] The natural history of OCD is difficult to predict, but loose body formation, and loss of range of movement are both poor prognosticating factors.[14]

Panner's disease tends to affect younger children, being the most common cause of lateral pain in the age group of 10 years and younger. The etiology is thought to be similar to that of Perthes' disease, and relates to changes in the vascularity of the developing capitellum.[15] Although late complications and joint deformity may occur, the outcome of this condition is usually benign and self-limiting, warranting only conservative management.[14]

Figure 2.4 Lateral to the triangle

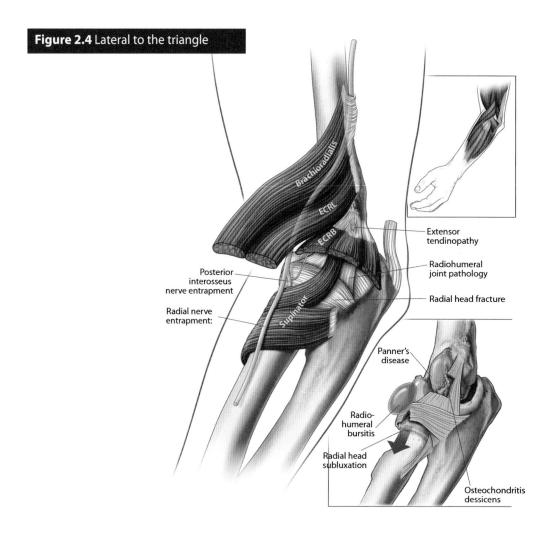

Brachioradialis

ECRL

ECRB

Supinator

Posterior
interosseus
nerve entrapment

Radial nerve
entrapment:

Extensor
tendinopathy

Radiohumeral
joint pathology

Radial head fracture

Panner's
disease

Radio-
humeral
bursitis

Radial head
subluxation

Osteochondritis
dessicens

Radial head fracture commonly occurs from a fall on the outstretched arm, where the load is transferred through the radial head. The radial head behaves as a stabilizing force against valgus stress, complementing the more important MCL.[16] Management depends on the degree of displacement; the physician must always endeavor to avoid excessive joint stiffness, while ensuring that adequate healing has occurred.

Lateral epicondyle fracture is a common pediatric fracture, with an age peak of 6–10 yrs.[16] This is a traction injury which causes injury to the lateral physis.[17] The fracture usually involves the physis and articular surface (Salter-Harris).

Pathology of the radiohumeral joint and entrapment of the radial nerve may both present similarly to extensor tendinopathy, and should be considered when usual treatment measures fail; all three may in fact co-exist.[18]

Radial head subluxation or "pulled elbow" is a common condition with many alternative names, including "temper tantrum elbow", as it usually involves the child (1–6 years) either

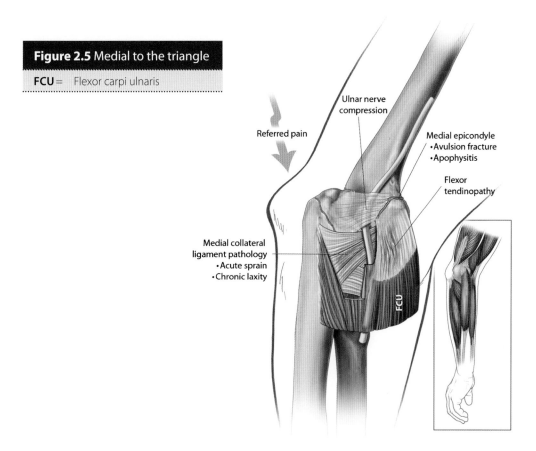

Figure 2.5 Medial to the triangle

FCU =   Flexor carpi ulnaris

Ulnar nerve
compression

Referred pain

Medial epicondyle
•Avulsion fracture
•Apophysitis

Flexor
tendinopathy

Medial collateral
ligament pathology
•Acute sprain
•Chronic laxity

FCU

being pulled from above, or throwing itself to the ground while being held by the hand.[19] The diagnosis is a clinical one, although if a fracture is suspected, an x-ray is useful. Partial subluxation of the radial head from the annular ligament is seen. Relocation is straightforward, either by supination or pronation of the forearm during extension, with subsequent flexion.

Radial nerve entrapment at the elbow most often involves the posterior interosseous nerve. Compressive neuropathy of the posterior interosseous nerve at the radial tunnel, without motor deficit, is the hallmark of radial tunnel syndrome.[20] A vague, deep pain is described on the radial aspect of the elbow and forearm; confusingly, this may co-exist with CEO tendinopathy, the very condition it often masquerades as![21] Posterior intersosseous nerve syndrome is by definition a motor neuropathy; pain and muscle weakness, with loss of extension of all the digits, and decrease of wrist dorsiflexion, can be noted.[21]

Radiohumeral bursitis may be differentiated from CEO tendinopathy on palpation; the point of maximal tenderness is predominantly over the radial head.[10] A careful history is important; as with other forms of bursitis, symptoms often sharply worsen with exercise. Symptoms may result from repetitive inflammatory arthropathies, infection, chemical synovitis, bone proliferation, or synovial chondromatosis.[22]

| Table 2.5 A pathoanatomic approach; medial to the triangle ||||
Define and align	Pathology	Listen and localize	Palpate and recreate	Alleviate and investigate
Medial to the triangle	Flexor tendinopathy	Pain 1–2 cm distal to medial epicondyle[36]	Resisted wrist flexion and pronation[23]	Ultrasound, MRI[1]
	Medial collateral ligament pathology: > acute sprain	Medial swelling, pain. History of repetitive valgus stress	Valgus stress (Jobe"s) test[40], tenderness over the anterior band of ligament[11]	Valgus stress plain film,[43] MRI, magnetic resonance arthrography,[44] arthroscopy[42]
	> chronic laxity	Loss of performance, function decreased ± pain[41]	Moving valgus stress test[42]	
	Ulnar nerve compression	Posteromedial pain, paresthesia (ulnar border of arm, 4th and 5th fingers) prior to weakness, loss of manual dexterity	Tinels test at the elbow,[45] tenderness to palpate nerve posterior to medial epicondyle[38]	Nerve conduction studies[46]
	Medial epicondyle > avulsion fracture	Medial pain, swelling, loss of function[47]	Pain on resisted wrist flexion and pronation	Plain film (comparative views),[49] MRI[49, 50]
	> apophysitis (Little League elbow)	Pediatric 9–12 yrs,[39] overtraining[48]		
	Referred pain > cervical spine/ thoracic spine (C8, T1)	Persistent, unpredictable, related to posture, dysesthesia	Neurological examination, neural tension testing	Manipulation of C-spine,[51] plain film, MRI
	> myofascial	Trigger points within extensor compartment[25]	Pain recreated by palpation of trigger point	Dry-needling, digital pressure[25]
	> visceral	Poorly localized, C8, T1 dermatome, somatic symptoms	Unrelated to elbow movement/muscle contraction	Appropriate medical assessment[26]

*Interpret with caution; symptoms related to ulnar nerve injury are present in over 40% of patients undergoing surgery for MCL insufficiency[52]

Medial to the triangle

Flexor tendinopathy is the best known cause of medial elbow pain commonly termed "golfer's elbow"; flexor tendinopathy is five times less common than its lateral counterpart, but it is the most common cause of medial elbow pain and, confusingly, quite common in professional tennis players![28] Wrist flexion and pronation are painful. Repetitive stress on medial soft tissues in golf and tennis are etiological factors. Occurring in all ages, it is most often seen in the 4th and 5th decades.[36] Research has shown this to be a degenerative, rather than inflammatory, process;[37] the etiology is generally chronic repetitive stress, but a single pre-disposing traumatic event may have occurred. It is common in throwing sports such as baseball. Although common, it is important to differentiate the pathology from the differential diagnoses for elbow pain medial to the triangle.

Medial collateral ligament pathology is the most serious medial elbow pathology for the overhead throwing athlete. The ligament is the primary medial stabilizer of the joint; when this is insufficient, the articular surface of the joint itself acts as a stabilizer. The resultant abnormal stresses lead to injury and degenerative changes, with osteophyte formation which may further produce medial elbow symptoms.[11] Medial insufficiency also increases compressive loads on the lateral joint surface.

MCL injuries may present as the insidious onset of medial elbow pain, or may occur acutely when the athlete feels a "pop" on the medial side of the elbow. The athlete usually complains of pain during the early acceleration phase of throwing, which is usually significant enough to interfere with effective throwing. Throwing at velocities greater than 60% of maximum speed usually causes severe pain.[38] Ulnar nerve entrapment is often associated with chronic MCL injury.

Ulnar nerve compression is second only to carpal tunnel syndrome as the most common entrapment neuropathy of the upper limb.[21] The most common site of entrapment is in the cubital tunnel (formed between the olecranon, the medial epicondyle, and the arcuate ligament/cubital retinaculum). This may occur due to direct trauma, due to the superficial nature of the nerve, or due to flexion of the elbow (the arcuate ligament is most tight at elbow flexion of 90°). Entrapment occurs secondary to lateral ulnar collateral ligament injury in 40% of cases.[38] Overstretching during the early acceleration phase of throwing, or subluxation of the nerve over the medial epicondyle, may occur when ligament damage is present. The clinician should suspect underlying ligament injury when a throwing athlete presents with ulnar nerve symptoms.

Medial epicondyle pathology is common, although fracture at the site is seen less often than at the lateral epicondyle or supra-condylar regions. The epicondyle is the site of origin of the common flexor tendon, and also the MCL. Excessive valgus strain, seen in repetitive throwing, is a common cause of a traction apophysitis of the medial epicondyle termed "Little League elbow". The valgus overload and distraction forces which occur during the cocking and acceleration phases of throwing are causative.[39] Where a true apophysitis occurs, management includes mandatory rest and rehabilitation, limitation of subsequent activity (i.e. the number of pitches per week in baseball), and technique correction. Where the apophysis has widened (3–5 mm), surgical assessment is warranted.

Referred pain
The elbow and forearm may be the site of referred pain from the cervical and thoracic spine (particularly C8 & T1).[53] A thorough examination of the peripheral nervous system of the upper

limbs should be part of any thorough examination of the upper limb. Myofascial trigger points in the trapezius, supraspinatous, and infraspinatous may all generate upper-limb and elbow pain. Visceral pain due to cardiac ischaemia may also be referred to and present as pain in the left elbow.

Posterior to the triangle

Just as the olecranon dominates the area posterior to the triangle on the posterior elbow, so too pathology of both this structure and its appendages are the most common problems encountered.

Posterolateral impingement

Posterolateral impingement is common, not only in the sporting population, but also in the older patient. Repetitive hyperextension valgus stress causes osteophyte formation, secondary to impingement of the olecranon on the olecranon fossa.[10] In the older patient, degenerative osteoarthritis may affect the radiocapitellar joint, with generalized osteophyte formation.

Triceps tendinopathy and the very rare rupture of the triceps tendon are primarily seen in male throwing (repetitive forced extension) athletes in their 4th decade. A traction spur is often present.[1] Avulsion injuries are less common, and differentiated by the acuteness of symptom onset.

Triceps tendon rupture has been more frequently reported in weightlifters, particularly in men in their 4th decade.[1] Local and systemic steroid use has been implicated in collagen derangement; disruption at the musculotendinous junction is described, but avulsion injury is the most common injury seen.[54] Complete rupture has significant implications for the athlete, and in activities of daily living, and warrants surgical intervention.

Acute posterior dislocation of the elbow is rare, but not to be missed, as it may cause neurovascular compromise. Dislocation usually occurs as a result of a fall onto an extended elbow. Dislocations are classified according to the direction of dislocation (posterior the most common, due to the congruency of the olecranon and the olecranon fossa of the humerus). A dislocation is described as "complex" if a fracture occurs; fracture of the radial head is the most common concomitant fracture. Medial epicondyle fracture is seen in younger children, and may involve the ulnar nerve.[16] Neuropraxia is seen in one in five cases. MCL injury is not uncommon and ligamentous laxity may be a consequence, and follow-up is important.

Apparent **posterior subluxation/dislocation** may also exist as a result of chronic instability, where injury to the lateral collateral ligament causes a "chain reaction" from lateral to medial in posterolateral rotatory instability.[51] Rupture of the ulnar part of the lateral collateral ligament, due to dislocation, trauma, or surgery, may lead to chronic posterolateral rotatory instability (PLRI), as described by O'Driscoll.[55] The annular ligament remains intact, so there is no dislocation of the proximal radio-ulnar joint; instead, there is rotation and subluxation of the radiohumeral joint. This manifests as chronic instability; one study described 35% of patients post-simple dislocation suffering chronic instability.[56] The clinician should be vigilant to a subtle diagnosis of exclusion, and a history of recurrent instability episodes.

Olecranon bursitis may arise from persistent low-grade pressure, such as leaning an elbow at a desk, or from acute trauma, such as a blow to the elbow in American football.[57] The bursa may become inflamed or even infected. Although it may respond temporarily to steroid injection, the most effective means of treatment is to remove the inciting event.

The **posterolateral plica** may produce symptoms along the posterolateral aspect of the elbow, where the patient complains of mechanical symptoms such as clicking or popping.[11] Careful examination allows palpation of a capsular thickening in the posterolateral gutter.

Olecranon fracture in the athlete is usually a high-velocity injury. All olecranon fractures involve the articular surface, so a joint effusion and hemorrhage are usually seen. In the older patient, sudden contraction of the triceps and brachialis may cause a low-velocity fracture. In both cases, an ability to extend the elbow against gravity is an important clinical sign; failure to do so signifies discontinuity of the triceps mechanism.[58] Disruption of this mechanism warrants surgical intervention.

Within the triangle

The anterior elbow, or within the elbow triangle, is the least common site of pain in the elbow. The swelling and ecchymosis of a **supracondylar fracture** will often track to this area. This is the

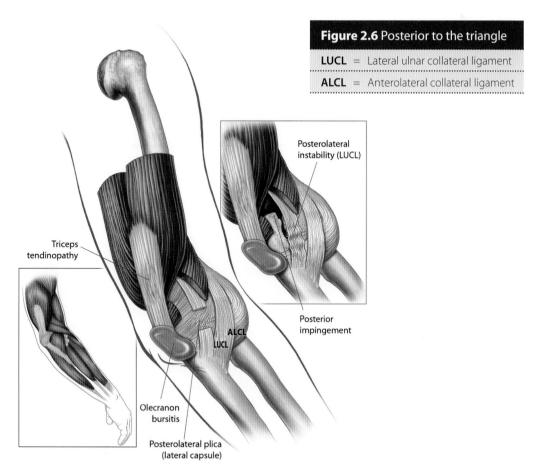

Figure 2.6 Posterior to the triangle

LUCL	=	Lateral ulnar collateral ligament
ALCL	=	Anterolateral collateral ligament

Posterolateral instability (LUCL)

Triceps tendinopathy

Posterior impingement

ALCL

LUCL

Olecranon bursitis

Posterolateral plica (lateral capsule)

Table 2.6 A pathoanatomic approach; posterior to the triangle

Define and align	Pathology	Listen and localize	Palpate and recreate	Alleviate and investigate
Posterior to the triangle	Posterior impingement	Locking, crepitus, loss of extension, Youth – high level throwing sport Older patient – early osteoarthritis[60]	Fixed flexion deformity, pain on forced extension[10]	Plain film axial view, MRI (90% sensitivity with GAD)[60]
	Triceps tendinopathy	Males, 4th decade, throwing athletes[1]	Pain on resisted extension, palpate triceps insertion	Ultrasound,[61] MRI[29]
	Olecranon bursitis	History of repetitive trauma to olecranon, relatively painless[62]	Palpable fluctuant soft tissue swelling over olecranon[62]	Aspiration, ultrasound[1]
	Posterolateral plica	Posterolateral elbow pain, popping, catching[11]	Palpate posterolateral to epicondyle[11]	Local anesthetic injection,[11] MRI[29]
	Olecranon fracture	Direct trauma, high-energy injury	Effused painful joint, inability to extend arm against gravity[58]	Plain film, true lateral
	Posterior dislocation	High impact, fall on outstretched hand, elbow extend, then forced into flexion[8]	Palpate distal pulses! Olecranon more pronounced than normal on flexion	Plain film[63], post-reduction views vital[10]
	Triceps tendon rupture	3rd decade, M: F=3:2,[2] forced contraction against flexing elbow	Weakness of extension, inability to extend against gravity in complete rupture	Plain film for avulsion, ultrasound,[1] MRI[64]
	Posterolateral instability	Prior elbow trauma/surgery. History of popping, giving away on loading the joint[65]	Postero-lateral rotatory instability (PLRI) test[55]	Primarily clinical diagnosis, stress x-ray, MRI[65]

most common fracture around the elbow in children aged 5–10 years, usually occurring due to a hyperextension load on an outstretched arm (body weight fall, landing on the hand with elbow straight).[16] Pain, swelling, and deformity are seen. Careful neurovascular examination is mandatory, paying particular attention to the radial and anterior interosseus nerves (most commonly injured)[65]. Injury to the radial nerve manifests as inability to extend the thumb, proximal phalanges, wrist, or elbow; the hand is held pronated, and the thumb adducted.

The biceps tendon and aponeurosis dominate the space; this is prone to tendinopathy and rupture, although to a much lesser extent than the proximal long head of the biceps tendon. Distal biceps rupture is, however, a more clinically significant injury, and surgical referral

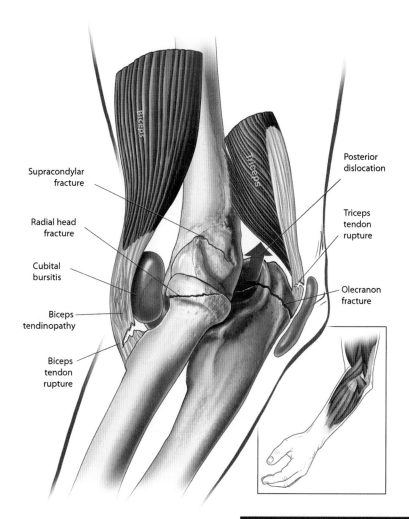

Supracondylar
fracture

Radial head
fracture

Cubital
bursitis

Biceps
tendinopathy

Biceps
tendon
rupture

Posterior
dislocation

Triceps
tendon
rupture

Olecranon
fracture

Figure 2.7 Acute injuries of the elbow

is necessary to ensure future supination and flexion strength. **Tendinopathy of the biceps tendon** has been reported in rock climbers, canoeing, and kayaking,[57] and may be associated with prolonged excessive loading of the tendon. Treatment focuses on technique correction. Although it has been suggested that degenerative changes in the tendon due to impingement at the radial head may be linked to rupture, it is felt that changes in changes in connective tissue related to age, rather than tendinopathic change per se, are the etiological factors in acute rupture.

Cubital bursitis occurs when the bursa between the biceps insertion and the radius becomes enflames and is compressed. The proximity of the median nerve means that pain and swelling in the cubital fossa are sometimes accompanied by symptoms of median nerve irritation.[66]

Define and align	Pathology	Listen and localize	Palpate and recreate	Alleviate and investigate
Table 2.7 A pathoanatomic approach; within the triangle				
Within the triangle	Supracondylar fracture	Diffusely swollen deformed elbow, children 5–10 yrs, fall on hand with elbow hyperextension[16]	Careful neurovascular examination[67]	Plain film
	Biceps tendinopathy	Pain on eccentric loading of tendon, worsened by pronation	Pain at radial tuberosity, pain on resisted supination	Ultrasound[1]
	Cubital bursitis	Painful mass in medial elbow, limitation of movement[66]	Palpate mass/cystic structure, examine for median nerve compression	Plain film,[66] ultrasound, MRI[22]
	Biceps tendon rupture	Contraction against load with elbow flexed to 90°, male, 4th and 5th decade, tearing-type pain[16,67]	Palpable defect in biceps tendon, weakness in supination more than flexion[68]	Ultrasound,[69] MRI[70]

Summary

Injury to the elbow is often caused by direct trauma, such as a fall or contraction against large loads of either the biceps or triceps. Overhead sports generate tremendous valgus force, causing medial ligamentous injury, and posterolateral impingement. The athlete may suffer muscular disruption, osteochondral injury, or instability.

The elbow triangle endeavors to simplify the diagnosis of pathology around the elbow in the active person. A complete, anatomically oriented differential diagnosis facilitates better initial diagnosis and, where a diagnosis is in doubt, allows an easy and complete review of potential pathologies.

In particular, many of these conditions are seen in the growing adolescent athlete and, as such, have significant sequaelae if missed. The clinician must be vigilant about age-group classification and ossification years when assessing the pediatric athlete.

Case histories

Case 1

A 62-year-old woman presents with a six-month history of elbow pain. She is a keen golfer, who recalls initially developing some stiffness over the lateral aspect of her elbow following a number of golf lessons. The sessions had included particular work on her swing. Her pain had been manageable for a number of months, but had worsened following a number of days spent painting her house. It began at the lateral aspect of the elbow but, when severe, may radiate down her arm. She is now not only unable to play golf, but has pain on lifting the kettle at home.

To diagnose the cause of this presentation of elbow pain, proceed to step 1, define and align the elbow triangle.

Step 1: Define and align

Expose the patient properly; a singlet or t-shirt allows an adequate view of the elbow. The patient may be seated or lying at 45°.

Define the triangle: locate the lateral epicondyle, locate the medial epicondyle, locate the 3G point (located at the surface markings of the cross-section of the brachioradialis and pronator teres muscles).

Align the patient's pain on the triangle. Here the pain is quite specific; the patient points to the lateral aspect of the elbow around the lateral epicondyle.

The patient has localized the pain to the area "lateral to the triangle". From this point, we recommend that the reader attempt to exclude the potential pathologies. From Table 2.4, the potential causal structures are:

Differential diagnosis

> extensor tendinopathy
> referred pain:
>   – cervical (C6/7)/thoracic spine
>   – myofascial
>   – visceral
> osteochondritis dessicens
> radial head fracture
> lateral femoral condyle fracture
> radiohumeral joint pathology
> posterior interosseus nerve entrapment
> radial tunnel syndrome
> radiohumeral bursitis

We proceed to differentiate between these structures, step 2.

Step 2: Listen and localize

Addressing extensor tendinopathy we ask:

Q *Is the pain well localized to the lateral epicondyle (demonstrate where you mean)?*

A Yes

Addressing referred pain we ask:

Q *Is the pain of a persistent, unpredictable nature, related to posture?*

A No, I know exactly the things that cause my pain.

Q *Are there painful points in the muscle of your forearms and shoulders?*

A No, my shoulder is fine; when the pain is bad, however, it tends to spread down my arm which is quite sore.

Addressing osteochondritis dessicens we ask:

Q *Do you experience lack of movement, catch, or clicking?*

A Not initially, but I have noticed that I do have pain when I lift heavy things now.

Addressing radiohumeral joint pathology we ask:

Q *Is it painful to pronate your arm? (Demonstrate movement)*

A No.

Addressing radial nerve entrapment we ask:

Q *Have you noticed any abnormal sensation of the skin in the area?*

A No.

Q *Have you noticed any pain or tingling in the hand?*

A No.

Q *Have you noticed any weakness of the muscles of the hand?*

A No.

This will narrow our differential diagnosis somewhat, and we proceed to examination to narrow it further. By palpating painful structures, and recreating the pain through diagnostic maneuvers, we move toward a diagnosis, step 3.

Step 3: Palpate and re-create

The lateral aspect of the elbow is best examined facing the patient, with them seated comfortably. Locate the olecranon; the lateral epicondyle is the next bony prominence palpated when moving laterally. The extensor wad, a large mass of muscle, covers the lateral epicondyle. Flexion of the elbow makes palpation of the epicondyle easier. Moving from proximal to distal (lateral supracondylar ridge to lateral epicondyle), the muscles palpated are the brachioradialis, extensor carpi radialis longus, extensor carpi radialis brevis, and extensor digitorum communis. Pathology of the capitellum may be palpated posterolaterally, deep between the lateral epicondyle and the olecranon.

Assess range of movement; a full, pain-free range of extension, flexion, pronation, and supination makes joint pathology unlikely. A normal neurological examination means that referred pain is unlikely.

The pain is likely either extensor tendinopathy, or radial tunnel syndrome. The most evidence-based examination for extensor tendinopathy is the ECRB test; the patient holds the elbow extended and the forearm pronated, and extends the wrist (making a fist) against resistance. Pain at the ECRB origin is highly suggestive of extensor tendinopathy; the pain is usually worse with an extended elbow, and lessened by flexion of the elbow.[23]

Radial tunnel entrapment is usually most painful 3 cm distal to the lateral epicondyle, and should be obliterated by the injection of local anesthetic into the radial tunnel (between the two layers of the supinator muscle).

We now proceed to step 4 to confirm our clinical suspicion via imaging. Ultrasonography and MRI are both effective in the diagnosis of extensor tendinopathy.

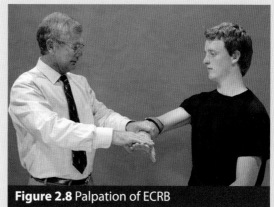

Figure 2.8 Palpation of ECRB

Case 2

A 25-year-old cricket fast bowler presents with medial elbow pain and a loss of form. He is nearing the season's end. Although he has been playing cricket since a very young age, this is his first season in the club's first team, and the numbers of overs he bowls per week has risen significantly.

He has been treated for flexor tendinopathy, with non-steroidal anti-inflammatory medication and two cortisone injections, but has not improved.

This is a presentation of elbow pain; as such proceed to step 1, define and align the elbow triangle.

Step 1: Define and align

Expose the patient properly; a singlet or t-shirt allows an adequate view of the elbow. The patient may be seated or lying at 45°.

Define the triangle: locate the lateral epicondyle, locate the medial epicondyle, locate the 3G point (located at the surface markings of the cross-section of the brachioradialis and pronator teres muscles).

Align the patient's pain on the triangle. Here the pain is vague; the patient points to the medial of the elbow, around the medial epicondyle.

The patient has localized the pain to the area "medial to the triangle". From this point, we recommend that the reader attempt to exclude the potential pathologies. From Table 2.5, the potential causal structures are:

Differential diagnosis

> flexor tendinopathy
> medial collateral ligament pathology:
>   – acute sprain
>   – chronic laxity
> ulnar nerve compression
> medial epicondyle:
>   – avulsion fracture
>   – apophysitis
> referred pain:
>   – cervical spine/thoracic spine (C8, T1)
>   – myofascial
>   – visceral

Step 2: Listen and localize

Regarding flexor tendinopathy we ask:
Q *Is your pain 2 cm inferior to the medial epicondyle?*
A Yes, it is in and around that area.

Regarding acute medial collateral ligament pathology we ask:
Q *Did you notice a sharp pain with bruising and swelling at any time after bowling a ball?*
A No, but it is always much more sore after an over.

Regarding chronic medial collateral ligament pathology we ask:
Q *Have you noticed your bowling speed has suffered recently?*
A Yes.

Regarding ulnar nerve compression we ask:
Q *Do you suffer from tingling or dysesthesia down the outside of your arm?*
A Sometimes, particularly when the pain is bad, and then it goes all the way down to my baby finger.

Regarding the medial epicondyle, the patient is too old to have an apophysitis.

Regarding an avulsion fracture we ask:
Q *Have you been able to bowl lately?*
A Yes, I'm still playing ok, but could do with a little more speed.

Regarding referred pain we ask:

Q *Do you have any neck or back pain?*

A Not particularly, just the usual aches and pains.

Q *Have you had any chest pain or indigestion related to exercise?*

A No.

This narrows our differential diagnosis, and guides our examination; the potential diagnoses are flexor tendinopathy, chronic medial collateral ligament injury, or ulnar neuritis.

Step 3: Palpate and re-create

The medial aspect of the elbow is best examined with the patient comfortably seated with the elbow flexed, and the examiner sitting at the patient's side. The medial epicondyle and the distal belly of the common flexor origin are easily palpable. The ulnar nerve may be palpated in the groove between the medial epicondyle and the olecranon.

Assess range of movement; a full, pain-free range of extension, flexion, pronation, and supination makes joint pathology unlikely.

The most evidence-based test for the flexor tendinopathy is resisted wrist flexion and pronation; the patient extends the elbow, with the forearm supinated and the fist clenched. The examiner resists wrist flexion and forearm supination; in this instance, while this is painful, it is not *the* pain.

Tinel's test at the elbow will reproduce any pathology of the ulnar nerve; the nerve is tapped with a finger in the groove between the medial epicondyle and the olecranon. In this circumstance, symptoms are reproduced in an ulnar nerve distribution. This test is positive.

The integrity of the medial collateral ligament is assessed by Jobe's test; applying a valgus stress to the elbow at 30° of flexion. This reproduces a mild pain.

Functional instability is best assessed by the moving valgus stress test; a valgus stress is applied to the elbow, while the shoulder

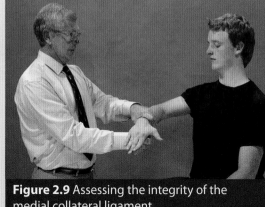

Figure 2.9 Assessing the integrity of the medial collateral ligament

is abducted and externally rotated. The elbow is then taken through a range of flexion and extension. Pain is reproduced within the arc of 80° to 120°. This recreates the patient's pain.

It is likely, given the first three steps, that this athlete has a combination of medial collateral ligament chronic instability, and secondary ulnar neuritis; flexor tendinopathy may, however, be present.

Step 4: Alleviate and investigate

To confirm our clinical suspicion, a valgus stress plain film is sensitive, and MRI will diagnose either tendinopathy, or ligamentous insufficiency. If the ulnar neuritis persists following treatment of underlying medial collateral injury, nerve conduction studies are appropriate.

Case 3

A 15-year-old national standard gymnast presents with a six-month history of posterior elbow pain, and difficulty attaining her normal range of hyperextension at the joint. She has no history of trauma, and has been training largely injury-free for nine years.

A number of enforced rest periods have temporarily eased her symptoms, and she is currently taking regular analgesia prior to competition and practice. She has not had any formal investigation of her problem.

This is a presentation of elbow pain; as such proceed to step 1, define and align the elbow triangle.

Step 1: Define and align

Expose the patient properly; a singlet or t-shirt allows an adequate view of the elbow. The patient may be seated or lying at 45°.

Define the triangle: locate the lateral epicondyle, locate the medial epicondyle, locate the 3G point (located at the surface markings of the cross-section of the brachioradialis and pronator teres muscles).

Align the patient's pain on the triangle. Here the pain is posterior; the patient points to the medial aspect of the olecranon.

The patient has localized the pain to the area "posterior to the triangle". From this point, we recommend that the reader attempt to exclude the potential pathologies. From Table 2.6, the potential causal structures are:

Differential diagnosis
> posterior impingement
> triceps tendinopathy
> olecranon bursitis
> posterolateral plica
> olecranon fracture
> posterior dislocation
> triceps tendon rupture

We proceed to differentiate between these structures, step 2.

Step 2: Listen and localize

Regarding posterior impingement we ask:

Q *Do you have locking, crepitus, or loss of extension?*

A I often hear crackles from the joint, but it has never locked. I cannot hyperextend my elbow beyond 180° as I could in the past.

Regarding triceps tendinopathy we ask:

Q *Do you have pain on resisted extension at the elbow?*

A No.

Olecranon bursitis is not present, as there is no obvious swelling or bursal enlargement at the olecranon.

Regarding posterolateral plica we ask:

Q *Do you have popping or clicking in the posterolateral aspect of the elbow? (demonstrate)*

A No, my pain is on the other side of the olecranon.

Olecranon fracture is extremely unlikely in the absence of acute injury, but a stress fracture may be present. Regarding this we ask:

Q *Do you have pain on extending the elbow?*

A Yes.

Q *Have you noticed swelling in the area, or the joint?*

A No.

Posterior dislocation is not present, given her presentation, but posterolateral rotational instability may be developing. With regard to this we ask:

Q *have you had any previous injury to the ligaments of your elbow?*

A None.

Triceps tendon rupture is very unlikely given this presentation, but we ask:

Q *Can you extend the elbow against gravity? (demonstrate)*

A Yes.

This will narrow our differential diagnosis somewhat, and we proceed to examination to narrow it further. By palpating painful structures, and recreating the pain through diagnostic maneuvers, we move toward a diagnosis, step 3.

Step 3: Palpate and re-create

Although triceps pathology is very unlikely, we must still palpate the insertion to the olecranon, and have the patient extend against resistance/gravity. These are both normal. There is no bursa present. Passive movement of the joint reveals mild crepitus, but no locking or clicking. The contour of the olecranon against the humerus is normal, but there is loss of 5–10° of terminal extension; when this is forced, there is pain.

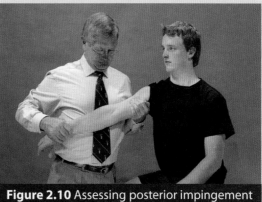

Figure 2.10 Assessing posterior impingement

The pathology is centered on the olecranon; we must differentiate between posterior impingement, and a stress fracture of the olecranon.

Step 4: Alleviate and investigate

A plain film true lateral x-ray of the hip may identify some abnormalities of the body and articular surface of the olecranon. If this is inconclusive, an MRI will differentiate the pathologies.

References

1. Hume PA, Reid D, Edwards T. Epicondylar injury in sport: epidemiology, type, mechanisms, assessment, management and prevention. *Sports Med.* 2006; 36(2):151–70.
2. Sellards R, Kuebrich C. The elbow: diagnosis and treatment of common injuries. *Prim Care.* Mar 2005; 32(1):1–16.
3. Fichez O. Épicondylite: Histoire naturelle et étude critique des différents traitements. *Journal de traumatologie du sport.* 1998; 15(3):163–72.
4. Kapandji A. Biomechanics of pronation and supination of the forearm. *Hand Clinics.* 2001; 17:111–22.
5. Morrey BF, An KN. Articular and ligamentous contributions to the stability of the elbow joint. *Am J Sports Med.* Sep–Oct 1983; 11(5):315–19.
6. Blease S, Stoller DW, Safran MR, Li AE, Fritz RC. The elbow. In: Stoller DW, ed. *Magnetic resonance imaging in orthopaedics and sports medicine.* 3rd ed. Philadelphia: Lippincott, Williams & Wilkins; 2007:1463–1626.
7. Anderson IA, Read JW. The elbow and forearm. *Atlas of imaging in sports medicine.* 2nd ed. Sydney: McGraw–Hill Australia; 2008:127–85.
8. Tsai P, Steinberg DR. Median and radial nerve compression about the elbow. *J Bone Joint Surg Am.* Feb 2008; 90(2):420–28.
9. Khan KM, Cook JL, Bonar F, Harcort P, Astrom M. Histopathology of common tendinopathies. Update and implications for clinical management. *Sports Med.* Jun 1999; 27(6):393–408.
10. Bell S. Elbow and arm pain. In: Brukner P, Khan K, eds. *Clinical sports medicine.* 3rd ed. Sydney: McGraw–Hill Australia; 2007:289–307.
11. Field LD, Savoie FH. Common elbow injuries in sport. *Sports Med.* Sep 1998; 26(3):193–205.
12. Peterson RK, Savoie FH, 3rd, Field LD. Osteochondritis dissecans of the elbow. *Instr Course Lect.* 1999; 48:393–98.
13. Singer KM, Roy SP. Osteochondrosis of the humeral capitellum. *Am J Sports Med.* Sep–Oct 1984; 12(5):351–60.
14. Rudzki JR, Paletta GA, Jr. Juvenile and adolescent elbow injuries in sports. *Clin Sports Med.* Oct 2004; 23(4):581–608, ix.
15. DaSilva MF, Williams JS, Fadale PD, Hulstyn MJ, Ehrlich MG. Pediatric throwing injuries about the elbow. *Am J Orthop* (Belle Mead NJ). Feb 1998; 27(2):90–96.
16. Kandemir U, Fu FH, McMahon PJ. Elbow injuries. *Curr Opin Rheumatol.* Mar 2002; 14(2):160–67.
17. Badelon O, Bensahel H, Mazda K, Vie P. Lateral humeral condylar fractures in children: a report of 47 cases. *J Pediatr Orthop.* Jan–Feb 1988; 8(1):31–34.
18. Kalb K, Gruber P, Landsleitner B. [Compression syndrome of the radial nerve in the area of the supinator groove. Experiences with 110 patients]. *Handchir Mikrochir Plast Chir.* Sep 1999; 31(5):303–10.
19. Broomfield DJ, Maconochie I. The pulled elbow: a review article. *Trauma.* 2004; 6(4):255–59.
20. Barnum M, Mastey RD, Weiss AP, Akelman E. Radial tunnel syndrome. *Hand Clin.* Nov 1996; 12(4):679–89.
21. Bencardino JT, Rosenberg ZS. Entrapment neuropathies of the shoulder and elbow in the athlete. *Clin Sports Med.* Jul 2006; 25(3): vi–vii, 465–87.
22. Liessi G, Cesari S, Spaliviero B, Dell'Antonio C, Avventi P. The US,CT and MR findings of cubital bursitis: a report of five cases. *Skeletal Radiol.* Jul 1996; 25(5):471–75.
23. Budoff JE, Nirschl RP. Tendinopathies about the elbow. In: Garrett WE, Speer KP, Kirkendall DT, eds. *Principles and practice of orthopaedic sports medicine.* Philadelphia: Lippincott Williams & Wilkins; 2000.
25. Simons D, Travell JC, Simons LS. Hand extensor and brachioradialis muscles. *Myofascial pain and dysfunction, the trigger point manual.* Vol 1: Lippincott, Williams & Wilkins; 1992:477–573.
26. Barry M, Jenner JR. ABC of rheumatology. Pain in neck, shoulder, and arm. *BMJ.* Jan 21 1995; 310(6973):183–86.

27. Brunton LM, Anderson MW, Pannunzio ME, Khanna AJ, Chhabra AB. Magnetic resonance imaging of the elbow: update on current techniques and indications. *J Hand Surg* [Am]. Jul–Aug 2006; 31(6):1001–11.
28. Kandemir U, Fu FH, McMahon PJ. Elbow injuries. *Current Opinion in Rheumatology*. 2002; 14(2):7.
29. Thornton R, Riley GM, Steinbach LS. Magnetic resonance imaging of sports injuries of the elbow. *Top Magn Reson Imaging*. Feb 2003; 14(1):69–86.
30. Pike JM, Athwal GS, Faber KJ, King GJ. Radial head fractures – an update. *J Hand Surg Am*. Mar 2009; 34(3): 557–65.
31. Krul M, van der Wouden JC, van Suijlekom-Smit LW, Koes BW. Manipulative interventions for reducing pulled elbow in young children. *Cochrane Database Syst Rev*. 2009(4):CD007759.
32. Feinberg JH, Nadler SF, Krivickas LS. Peripheral nerve injuries in the athlete. *Sports Med*. Dec 1997; 24(6):385–408.
33. Rinker B, Effron CR, Beasley RW. Proximal radial compression neuropathy. *Ann Plast Surg*. Feb 2004; 52(2):174–80; discussion 181–83.
34. Roles NC, Maudsley RH. Radial tunnel syndrome: resistant tennis elbow as a nerve entrapment. *J Bone Joint Surg Br*. Aug 1972; 54(3):499–508.
35. Cyriax JH. The pathology and treatment of tennis elbow. *The Journal of Bone and Joint Surgery* [AM]. Oct 1936; 18:921–40.
36. Ciccotti MC, Schwartz MA, Ciccotti MG. Diagnosis and treatment of medial epicondylitis of the elbow. *Clin Sports Med*. Oct 2004; 23(4):693–705, xi.
37. Leach RE, Miller JK. Lateral and medial epicondylitis of the elbow. *Clin Sports Med*. Apr 1987; 6(2):259–72.
38. Rettig AC. Elbow, forearm and wrist injuries in the athlete. *Sports Med*. Feb 1998; 25(2):115–30.
39. Benjamin HJ, Briner WW, Jr. Little league elbow. *Clin J Sport Med*. Jan 2005; 15(1):37–40.
40. Jobe FW, Stark H, Lombardo SJ. Reconstruction of the ulnar collateral ligament in athletes. *J Bone Joint Surg Am*. Oct 1986; 68(8):1158–63.
41. Richard MJ, Aldridge JM, 3rd, Wiesler ER, Ruch DS. Traumatic valgus instability of the elbow: pathoanatomy and results of direct repair. *J Bone Joint Surg Am*. Nov 2008; 90(11):2416–22.
42. O'Driscoll SW, Morrey BF, Korinek S, An KN. Elbow subluxation and dislocation. A spectrum of instability. *Clin Orthop Relat Res*. Jul 1992; (280):186–97.
43. Ellenbecker TS, Mattalino AJ, Elam EA, Caplinger RA. Medial elbow joint laxity in professional baseball pitchers. A bilateral comparison using stress radiography. *Am J Sports Med*. May–Jun 1998; 26(3):420–24.
44. Munshi M, Pretterklieber ML, Chung CB, et al. Anterior bundle of ulnar collateral ligament: evaluation of anatomic relationships by using MR imaging, MR arthrography, and gross anatomic and histologic analysis. *Radiology*. Jun 2004; 231(3):797–803.
45. Posner MA. Compressive neuropathies of the ulnar nerve at the elbow and wrist. *Instr Course Lect*. 2000; 49:305–17.
46. Frostick SP, Mohammad M, Ritchie DA. Sport injuries of the elbow. *Br J Sports Med*. Oct 1999; 33(5):301–11.
47. Cassas KJ, Cassettari-Wayhs A. Childhood and adolescent sports-related overuse injuries. *Am Fam Physician*. Mar 15 2006; 73(6):1014–22.
48. Hogan KA, Gross RH. Overuse injuries in pediatric athletes. *Orthop Clin North Am*. Jul 2003; 34(3):405–15.
49. Behr CT, Altchek DW. The elbow. *Clin Sports Med*. Oct 1997; 16(4):681–704.
50. Hang DW, Chao CM, Hang YS. A clinical and roentgenographic study of Little League elbow. *Am J Sports Med*. Jan–Feb 2004; 32(1):79–84.
51. Vicenzino B, Collins D, Wright A. The initial effects of a cervical spine manipulative physiotherapy treatment on the pain and dysfunction of lateral epicondylalgia. *Pain*. Nov 1996; 68(1):69–74.
52. Conway JE, Jobe FW, Glousman RE, Pink M. Medial instability of the elbow in throwing athletes. Treatment by repair or reconstruction of the ulnar collateral ligament. *J Bone Joint Surg Am*. Jan 1992; 74(1):67–83.
53. Singer K. Thoracic and chest pain. In: Brukner P, Khan K, eds. *Clinical sports medicine*. 3rd ed. Sydney: McGraw–Hill Australia; 2007:240–51.
54. Stannard JP, Bucknell AL. Rupture of the triceps tendon associated with steroid injections. *Am J Sports Med*. May–Jun 1993; 21(3):482–85.
55. O'Driscoll SW, Bell DF, Morrey BF. Posterolateral rotatory instability of the elbow. *J Bone Joint Surg Am*. Mar 1991; 73(3):440–46.
56. Mehlhoff TL, Noble PC, Bennett JB, Tullos HS. Simple dislocation of the elbow in the adult. Results after closed treatment. *J Bone Joint Surg Am*. Feb 1988; 70(2):244–49.
57. Magra M, Caine D, Maffulli N. A review of epidemiology of paediatric elbow injuries in sports. *Sports Med*. 2007; 37(8):717–35.

58. Cain EL, Jr., Dugas JR, Wolf RS, Andrews JR. Elbow injuries in throwing athletes: a current concepts review. *Am J Sports Med.* Jul–Aug 2003; 31(4):621–35.

59. O'Driscoll SW, Lawton RL, Smith AM. The "moving valgus stress test" for medial collateral ligament tears of the elbow. *Am J Sports Med.* Feb 2005; 33(2):231–39.

60. Eygendaal D, Safran MR. Postero-medial elbow problems in the adult athlete. *Br J Sports Med.* May 2006; 40(5):430–34; discussion 434.

61. Tran N, Chow K. Ultrasonography of the elbow. *Semin Musculoskelet Radiol.* Jun 2007; 11(2):105–16.

62. Cardone DA, Tallia AF. Diagnostic and therapeutic injection of the elbow region. *Am Fam Physician.* Dec 1 2002; 66(11):2097–100.

63. Feldman DR, Schabel SI, Friedman RJ, Young JW. Translational injuries in posterior elbow dislocation. *Skeletal Radiol.* Feb 1997; 26(2):134–36.

64. Kijowski R, Tuite M, Sanford M. Magnetic resonance imaging of the elbow. Part II: Abnormalities of the ligaments, tendons, and nerves. *Skeletal Radiol.* Jan 2005; 34(1):1–18.

65. Singleton SB, Conway JE. PLRI: posterolateral rotatory instability of the elbow. *Clin Sports Med.* Oct 2004; 23(4): ix–x, 629–42.

66. Karanjia ND, Stiles PJ. Cubital bursitis. *J Bone Joint Surg Br.* Nov 1988; 70(5):832–33.

67. Dormans JP, Squillante R, Sharf H. Acute neurovascular complications with supracondylar humerus fractures in children. *J Hand Surg Am.* Jan 1995; 20(1):1–4.

67. Safran MR, Graham SM. Distal biceps tendon ruptures: incidence, demographics, and the effect of smoking. *Clin Orthop Relat Res.* Nov 2002; (404):275–83.

68. Morrey BF, Askew LJ, An KN, Dobyns JH. Rupture of the distal tendon of the biceps brachii. A biomechanical study. *J Bone Joint Surg Am.* Mar 1985; 67(3):418–21.

69. Weiss C, Mittelmeier M, Gruber G. Do we need MR images for diagnosing tendon ruptures of the distal biceps brachii? The value of ultrasonographic imaging. *Ultraschall Med.* Dec 2000; 21(6):284–86.

70. Le Huec JC, Moinard M, Liquois F, Zipoli B, Chauveaux D, Le Rebeller A. Distal rupture of the tendon of biceps brachii. Evaluation by MRI and the results of repair. *J Bone Joint Surg Br.* Sep 1996; 78(5):767–70.

The hand and wrist triangle

Introduction

Chronic wrist pain is reported in up to 79% of young gymnasts under the age of 14 years,[1] and the hand and wrist are exposed in many ball and racquet sports. It is not surprising that they are commonly injured, either traumatically in sports such as hockey, cricket, and skiing,[2] or from overuse in golf or rowing.[3]

Although the wrist anatomy often appears so complex as to be impenetrable to the generalist, it is the decline of anatomy teaching[4] which has meant that, almost certainly to most nonspecialists, the wrist ligaments are a distant memory, if indeed ever found, and understanding of the biomechanics of injury is not easily accessed.

Commonly, clinicians suggest the commonly known wrist injuries, such as triangular fibrocartilage complex (TFCC) injury or scapho-lunate disruption, without fully understanding the wider differential injury, or, indeed, the anatomical basis for this differential. It is prefereable to have a more structured approach to understanding the anatomy, and hence differential diagnosis, as this underpins all diagnoses, and can lead to more targeted investigation and clinical accuracy.

There has been a recent focus on the wrist in the literature regarding the ossification times of the carpal bones becoming popular, for the assessment of skeletal maturity[5, 6] and age-group assessment of players in international soccer, but also for the consideration of maturity and ultimate musculoskeletal attributes in terms of athletic development.

This chapter utilizes the triangle concept again, to delineate the anatomically important structures, while taking the reader through the more complex anatomical structures, and making them relevant to the pathologies encountered. The hand is distal to the triangles, but again is neatly subdivided by the relationship to the triangle and, as such, we feel this is a useful way to combine the approach.

The wrist joint

The wrist consists of the distal radius and ulna of the forearm, eight carpal bones, and the proximal bases of the five metacarpals. The hand then consists of the remainder of the metacarpals and phalanges, and is made up of a series of joints, allowing it a complex movement capacity.

The wrist joint itself allows both marginal movements of radial abduction and ulna abduction, along with dorsiflexion and palmarflexion by the extrinsic hand muscles in the forearm, acting via the flexor and extensor retinaculum as slings.

Proximally, the distal **radioulnar** joint lies between the ulna notch of the radius, and the head of the ulna. The joint is discrete from the radiocarpal joint, separated by the fibrocartilaginous disc between the radius and styloid process of the ulna (Fig. 3.1).

The **radiocarpal** joint is the largest joint of the wrist, an elliptical joint between the radius, ulna, triquetrium, lunate, and scaphoid bones. It is a synovial joint (Fig. 3.1) between five articular surfaces and two mensical ones. Lewis et al.[9] highlight the similarities between the Homo sapiens, wrist and that of the primates, as it retains its complex structure, more than just having an articulation between the radius and ulna.

It is the carpal bones themselves which form the intercarpal joints; they are all synovial plane joints, and the small degree of movement between these contributes to wrist mobility. Together, they form an arch in the transverse plane which is concave palmarly; this flattens with wrist extension, and deepens with wrist flexion.

The **midcarpal** joint separates the first row of carpal bones (triquetrium, lunate, scaphoid, and pisiform) from the distal row (triquetral, trapezium, capitate, and hamate). This joint is controlled by the capitate; as the axis of movement, the carpal bones work as a unit, due to the intercarpal ligaments of each row. The proximal row has been described as an intercalated segment, as no tendinous insertions are located in these carpals, and their motion is dependent on the articulation of surrounding joints.[8] Those of the distal row all have strong intercarpal ligaments connecting them, and movement within the row is little or none, or, indeed, between the capitate in the second row and the second and third metacarpals. The kinematics of this row suggests that they are under the direct control of the forearm muscles.

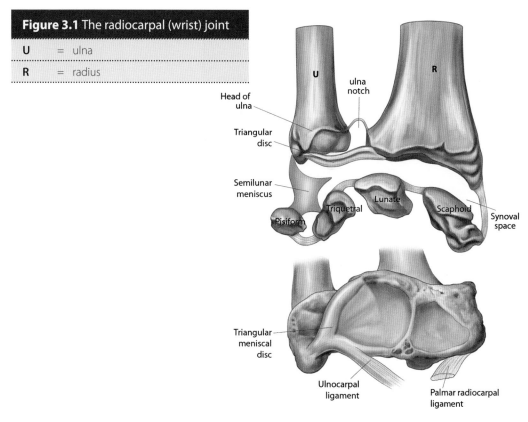

Figure 3.1 The radiocarpal (wrist) joint

U	= ulna
R	= radius

Distally, the second row of carpal bones forms the **carpometacarpal** joints, which articulate with the metacarpals, in turn forming the five phalanges with their **proximal** and **distal interphalangeal** joints.

The triangular fibrocartilaginous complex (TFCC; Fig. 3.2)[9] refers to the structures that suspend the distal radius and carpal bones from the distal ulna. The TFCC is the significant stabilizer of the distal radioulnar joint (DRUJ), and extends ulnarly to insert into the base of the ulna styloid. Distally, it inserts into the lunate via the ulnolunate ligament, and into the triquetrum via the ulnotriquetral ligament, hamate, and base of the fifth metacarpal.

The normal ranges of movement of the wrist joint are 80° of flexion and 70° of extension, with ulna deviation of 30° and radial deviation of 20°. The normal range of motion for the second to fifth digits is 80° of flexion at the distal inter-phalangeal joint (DIPJ), 100° of flexion at the proximal inter-phalangeal joint (PIPJ), and 90° of flexion at the proximal metacarpal phalangeal joint.

Ligaments of the wrist

The carpal ligaments are grouped as extrinsic ligaments, connecting the carpal bones to the distal radius and ulna, and intrinsic ligaments, which have their origins and insertions within the carpal bones.[10]

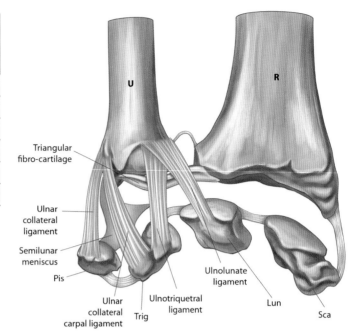

Figure 3.2 The triangular fibrocartilaginous complex (TFCC)

U	=	ulna
R	=	radius
Pis	=	pisiform
Trig	=	Triquetrium
Lun	=	Lunate
Sca	=	Scaphoid

Triangular fibro-cartilage

Ulnar collateral ligament

Semilunar meniscus

Pis

Ulnar collateral carpal ligament

Trig

Ulnotriquetral ligament

Ulnolunate ligament

Lun

Sca

Extrinsic

The **dorsal radiotriquetral** (Fig. 3.4) or dorsal radiocarpal ligament runs from the dorsal distal end of the ulna and Lister's tubercle of the radius, to insert into the proximal and distal tubercle of the triquetrium and the lunate.

The **volar ligaments** (Fig. 3.3) play a substantial part in wrist stability, where the palmar ligaments are more stabilizing.[11, 12] They consist of the radioscaphocapitate (RSC), the long radiolunate (LRL) or radiolunatetriquetral ligament, and the short radiolunate ligament.

The RSC begins proximally at the radial styloid process, and runs inferiorly to insert at the waist of the scaphoid, and proximal to the distal pole. The LRL originates from the volar border of the scaphoid fossa of the distal radius, its proximal attachment overlaid by the RSC ligament. It attaches distally to the radial border of the lunate, and volarly to the scapholunate interosseus ligament, preventing distal transposition of the lunate. The short radiolunate ligament originates from the ulnar and radius at the lunate fossa, and attaches distally to the volar edge of the lunate.

The radioscapholunate ligament (RSL) is located between the long and short radiolunate ligaments; running from the dorsal surfaces of the radius, it attaches at the interfossal ridge between the scaphoid and lunate fossa of the ulnar. This is part of the triangular fibrocartilaginous complex, and reinforces the fibrocartilaginous disc, and maintains the radiocarpal joint integrity.

The **ulnolunate ligament** arises from the proximal radioulnar joint, and attaches on the ulnar border of the lunate. The **ulnocapitate ligament** arises from the fovea of the ulnar head and proximal radioulnar ligament, running to cover the ulnotriquetral and ulnolunate

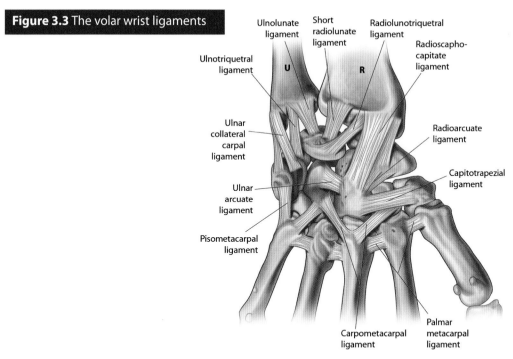

Figure 3.3 The volar wrist ligaments

Ulnolunate ligament

Short radiolunate ligament

Radiolunotriquetral ligament

Radioscapho-capitate ligament

Ulnotriquetral ligament

U

R

Ulnar collateral carpal ligament

Radioarcuate ligament

Ulnar arcuate ligament

Capitotrapezial ligament

Pisometacarpal ligament

Carpometacarpal ligament

Palmar metacarpal ligament

ligaments, and attaches to the capitate on its volar surface. The **ulnar collateral carpal ligament** runs from the ulnar styloid, distally to the palmar component, attaching to the pisiform and the dorsal component, which attaches to the triquetrium. The **radial collateral carpal ligament** originates on the tip of the styloid process of the radius, and inserts into the scaphoid at its waist radially.

Intrinsic ligaments

Interosseous

The **scapholunate interosseus ligament** joins the scaphoid and lunate along the proximal joint line, and has three parts: a volar; proximal; and dorsal part. It combines to provide rotational stability of the scapholunate joint, and hence is clinically important. The dorsal scapholunate part is the strongest and most critical.[13]

The **luntotriqetral interosseous** and **trapeziotrapezoid interossei** run between the respective carpal bones.

Volar (Fig. 3.3)

The deltoid ligament is divided into the radial arcuate ligament, which runs from the capitate to the distal pole of the scaphoid, and the ulnar arcuate ligament, running from the lunate and triquetrium to the neck of the capitate. They play a significant part in limiting the volar flexion of the proximal row of carpal bones.

The **lunotriquetral ligament** is strong and important; it originates from the distal and ulnar side of the lunate, and attaches to the ulnolunate ligament and interosseus ligament.

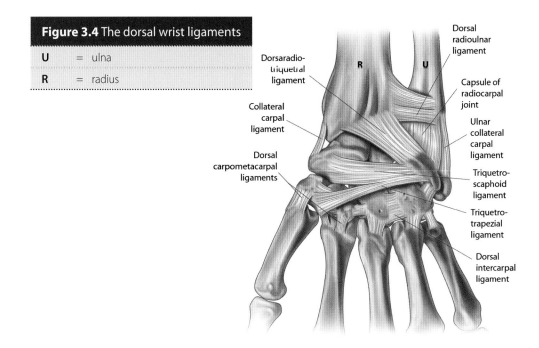

Figure 3.4 The dorsal wrist ligaments

U	= ulna
R	= radius

Dorsal radioulnar ligament

Dorsaradio-triquetral ligament

Collateral carpal ligament

Dorsal carpometacarpal ligaments

Capsule of radiocarpal joint

Ulnar collateral carpal ligament

Triquetro-scaphoid ligament

Triquetro-trapezial ligament

Dorsal intercarpal ligament

The lunotriquetral, trapeziotrapezoid, **scaphotrapezial**, **scaphotrapezoidal**, **scaphocapitate**, and **capitotrapezoid** ligaments all run intercarpally.

The **capitohamate**, **triquetrocapitate**, and **triquetrohamate** complete the volar intrinsics.

The **dorsal intercarpal ligament** originates proximally at the distal and radial aspect of the dorsal tubercle of the triquetrium; the thickest portion of this ligament inserts on the scaphoid, with thinner parts inserting into the trapezium and trapezoid. This ligament gives dorsal stability to the scapholunate in flexion, and prevents segment instability. The **triquetroscaphoid** part of the dorsal intercarpal ligament runs from the scaphoid to the triquetrium, and is joined by the **triquetrotrapezial ligament**, running between the respective carpal bones.

The dorsal **trapeziotrapezoid**, **capitotrapezoid**, and **capitohamate** ligaments run, as their names suggest, along with the **triquetrohamate**.

The carpal bones appear usually at the rate of one per year of age of the developing child, starting with the first one at one year, etc. The order of appearance is: capitate, hamate, triquetral, lunate, trapezium, trapezoid, navicular, scaphoid, and pisiform.

Landmarks of the hand and wrist triangles

The triangle landmarks are the same both in volar and dorsal positions:

> base of third metacarpal

> distal ulnar styloid

> distal radius

This triangle divides the wrist into a number of areas. For the purposes of anatomical function and pathological differentiation, we use:

1. within the triangle (volar)
2. within the triangle (dorsal)
3. radial to the triangle
4. ulnar to the triangle
5. distal to the triangle
6. proximal to the triangle

We describe, as in other chapters, the anatomy one encounters while passing along the borders of the triangles, with respect to both volar and dorsal aspects, and then expand fully within the triangles, utilizing the clockface approach also seen in the greater trochanter, groin and gluteal triangles, to create a more memorable approach to this important area. The relationships to the radial and ulnar aspects, and distally and proximally to the triangles, are again described in more detail in the tables relating to these regions.

The proximal border (volar)

Structures encountered:

> flexor retinaculum

> extensor pollicis brevis

> abductor pollicis brevis

> superficial branch of radial artery

> palmar cutaneous branch of median nerve

> flexor carpi radialis

> palmaris longus

> flexor digitorum superficialis

> ulnar artery

> flexor carpi ulnaris

Moving along the volar surface, from the distal radius to the ulnar, we palpate at the distal radius, the origin of the flexor retinaculum, running from the anterolateral border of the radius, immediately proximal to the radial stylus, running medially to the pisiform and triquetrium. Palpable beneath this is the sheath carrying the tendons of the extensor pollicis brevis and abductor pollicis brevis.

The American Society for Surgery of the Hand has named the tiered, complex arrangement of arcuate fibers A1–A5, and the cruciate fibers C1–C3, which support the structure of the flexor tendons. As the flexor tendons pass down the fingers, they pass through a fibro-ossseus canal constructed by this arrangement, distal to the flexor retinaculum in the wrist. Cruciate ligamentous fibers act as pulleys, and cross the phalanges at the interphalangeal joints, allowing a fixed point of flexion, essential for finger flexion.[14]

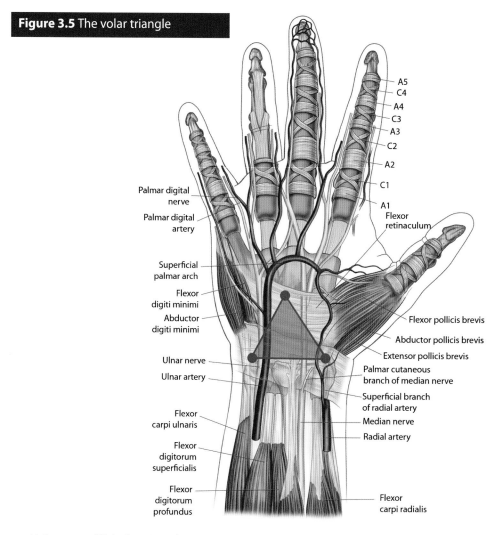

Figure 3.5 The volar triangle

A5
C4
A4
C3
A3
C2
A2
C1
A1
Flexor retinaculum

Palmar digital nerve
Palmar digital artery

Superficial palmar arch
Flexor digiti minimi
Abductor digiti minimi

Ulnar nerve
Ulnar artery

Flexor carpi ulnaris

Flexor digitorum superficialis

Flexor digitorum profundus

Flexor pollicis brevis
Abductor pollicis brevis
Extensor pollicis brevis
Palmar cutaneous branch of median nerve
Superficial branch of radial artery
Median nerve
Radial artery

Flexor carpi radialis

Abductor pollicis brevis (AbPB) originates from the scaphoid tubercle and the base of the trapezium; along with the flexor retinaculum, it runs distally to insert on the base of the proximal phalanx of the thumb. Abducting the thumb against resistance enhances the muscle's palpation, and it is supplied by the median nerve (C8, T1).

Extensor pollicis brevis (EPB) originates from the posterior and distal third of the radius and the interosseus membrane, and runs laterally across the forearm, to insert in the base of the proximal phalanx of the thumb. Supplied by the radial nerve (C7, C8), the muscle makes up the lateral border of the "anatomical snuffbox" with the abductor pollicis longus, the medial border being made up of the extensor pollicis longus. The muscle is most palpable in the forearm, in extension and adduction of the thumb.

The superficial branch of the radial artery is now crossed and a pulse palpable, before crossing the palmar cutaneous branch of the median nerve, before the tendinous sheath of the flexor carpi radialis. **Palmaris longus**, where present, is next, more medially, before the median nerve passes below the retinaculum. The common tendons of the flexor digitorum superficialis are medially located along the posterior border.

Flexor carpi radialis (FCR) originates at the medial epicondyle of the elbow, via the common flexor tendon, and runs distally down the forearm, to pass over the wrist, to insert into the bases of the second and third metacarpals. Acting to flex and radially deviate the wrist, it is supplied by the median nerve (C6, C7) and is palpably best located at the elbow, while flexing and radially deviating the wrist.

Palmaris longus (PL) arises from the common flexor tendon at the medial epicondyle, and descends distally through the forearm, before inserting into the palmar aponeurosis and the flexor retinaculum. It may be absent (in 10–20% of population) and, on occasion, forms fibrous adhesions to the coronoid head, flexor carpi radialis and flexor digitorum superficialis. It lies superficial to the flexor retinaculum, and acts to flex the wrist. It is supplied by the median nerve (C7, C8), and can be palpated best when the thumb and fifth finger are opposed, and the wrist is flexed.

Flexor digitorum superficialis (FDS) arises from two heads, the humero-ulnar head from the medial epicondyle, via the common flexor tendon and the coranoid process of the ulna and medial ulnar collateral ligament, and the radial head, which arises from the oblique line of the radius along its upper anterior border. The muscle belly runs in the forearm, before dividing into four tendinous slips in the mid-forearm. The tendons split into lateral and medial slips, to insert in the base of the middle phalanges of the second to fifth fingers, allowing the central tendon of the flexor digitorum profundus to pass through. The muscle acts to flex the second to fifth fingers, and also weakly flexes the wrist. It is supplied by the median nerve (C7, C8, T1), and is palpated best in the mid-forearm, when flexing the fingers while maintaining DIP (distal interphalangeal joint) extension.

Ulnar artery, the larger terminal branch of the brachial artery, runs down the forearm on the flexor digitorum profundus, and crosses the border of the triangle, just medial to the ulnar nerve. The tendon of the flexor carpi ulnaris is the last muscular structure to encounter before the distal ulnar is palpable.

Flexor digitorum profundus (FDP) originates from the anterior and medial surface of the proximal ulna and the interosseus membrane, running distally down the forearm. It splits into four tendinous slips, which pass under the flexor retinaculum to insert into the base of the distal second to fifth phalanges. The muscle acts to flex the fingers at the DIP (distal interphalangeal), PIP (proximal interphalangeal) and MCP (metacarpophalangeal) joints. The muscle is dually innervated, and the radial bulk of the muscle is supplied by the median nerve and the ulnar bulk by the radial nerve. The bellies are best palpated by palpating the forearm when flexing the fingers at the DIPJ.

Flexor carpi ulnaris (FCU) arises from two heads, the humeral head from the common flexor tendon at the medial epicondyle, and the ulnar head arising from the medial aspect of the olecranon and proximal two-thirds of the lateral ulna.

The muscle inserts into the pisiform, hook of hamate, and base of the fifth metacarpal, acting to flex the wrist and ulnar deviate. It is supplied by the ulnar nerve (C7, C8) and is best palpated while flexing and ulnar ulnarly deviating the wrist.

Deep to the muscle layer from the radius, one is crossing the origins of the radiolunotriquetral ligament, short radiolunate, ulnolunate, then ulnotriquetral ligament, before reaching the ulnar styloid.

The ulnar border (volar)

Structures encountered:

> radioulnar ligament

> meniscal homologue TFCC

> flexor carpi ulnaris

> ulnar artery

> flexor digiti minimi brevis

> opponens digiti minimi

> flexor digitorum superficialis

Moving from the ulnar styloid to the base of the third metacarpal, one crosses the volar radioulnar ligament and the variously named, meniscus homolgue (Fig. 3.4 on page 102) originating from the distal corner of the sigmoid notch of the the ulna, and inserting into the base of the triquetrium and base of the fifth metacarpal, part of the TFCC. Moving distally, we encounter the tendinous part of the flexor carpi ulnaris, as it inserts into the pisiform bone, and hook of the hamate. Running radially is the ulnar artery, but progressing down the line of the triangle, we cross the origins of the flexor digiti minimi brevis, as it originates from the hook of the hamate and the flexor retinaculum. The next palpable structure is the muscle belly of the opponens digiti minimi and then, as one reaches the base of the third metacarpal, the overlying structure is that of the tendon of the flexor digitorum superficialis.

Flexor digiti minimi (FDmi) originates from the flexor retinaculum and the hook of the hamate, on the ulnar border of the triangle. It runs forward to insert in the base of the proximal fifth phalanx on the ulnar margin. It acts to flex the fifth finger, and is supplied by the ulnar nerve (C8, T1). It is palpable over the lateral part of the hypothenar eminence, when the patient is asked to flex the fifth finger.

Opponens digiti minimi (ODM) also originates at the hook of the hamate and the flexor retinaculum, lies deep to the flexor digiti minimi, and inserts into the anterior and medial surface of the fifth metacarpal. Acting to oppose the little finger, it is supplied by the ulnar nerve (C8, T1), and is palpable when the patient opposes the fifth finger to the thumb.

The radial border (volar)

Structures encountered:

> abductor pollicis brevis

> scaphoid

> flexor pollicis brevis

> adductor pollicis

> flexor digitorum superficialis

> flexor pollicis longus

> flexor carpi radialis

> median nerve; palmar branches

Again starting at the radius, one encounters the belly of the abductor pollicis brevis, as it originates from the scaphoid tubercle, and the flexor pollicis brevis and on occasion the oblique head of the adductor pollicis, originating from the second and third metacarpals.

Flexor pollicis brevis (FPB) originates from the trapezium tubercles and the flexor retinaculum, inserting into the base of the proximal phalanx of the thumb. The muscle acts to flex the thumb at the trapezio-metacarpal joint, and is supplied by the median nerve (C8, T1). The muscle is best palpated over the thenar eminence, when flexing the thumb against resistance.

Adductor pollicis (AP) originates from two heads; the oblique head from the capitate and bases of the second and third metatarsals, and the transverse head from the palmar surface of the third metacarpal (Fig. 3.8). The muscle acts to adduct the thumb, and is supplied by the ulnar nerve (C8, T1). It is palpated best in the "web" of the thumb, when adducting the thumb.

Flexor pollicus longus (FPL) originates from the middle third of the radius and interosseus membrane, and passes distally through the wrist, running below the flexor retinaculum, to insert into the base of the distal phalanx of the thumb. Supplied by the median nerve (C7, C8), it flexes the thumb, and can be palpated in the forearm when flexing the interphalangeal joint of the thumb.

And then there is the flexor tendon of the flexor digitorum superficialis, as it passes under the flexor retinaculum. The flexor pollicus longus and flexor carpi radialis lie deep to the FDS. The palmar branches of the median nerve cross this border of the triangle, but are not fixed in their anatomical relationships, and the base of the third metacarpal is at the apex.

Proximal border (dorsal)

Structures encountered:

> extensor pollicis brevis

> extensor carpi radialis

> extensor carpi radialis longus

> extensor carpi radialis brevis

> joint capsule

> posterior interosseus artery

> extensor digitorum

> extensor digiti minimi

> extensor carpi ulnaris

Moving across the proximal base of the triangle from the radius to the ulnar, one commences at the radius, and then encounters the extensor pollicis brevis under the landmark of the triangle. Moving along this border, the next tendinous structure is the extensor carpi radialis longus, then the thicker tendon of the extensor carpi radialis brevis.

Extensor carpi radialis longus (ECRL) arises from the lower supracondylar ridge of the lateral humerus; it runs distally through the forearm, and inserts after passing beneath the extensor retinaculum into the base of the second metacarpal. It extends the wrist with some radial deviation, and is supplied by the radial nerve, critically above the level of the wrist, so if the radial nerve is injured at the elbow, the ECRL will be spared (C5, C6). It is palpable in resisted wrist extension.

Extensor pollicis brevis (EPB) originates from the posterior surface of the distal third of the radius and the interosseus membrane, running dorsally to insert into the base of the proximal phalanx of the thumb. It makes up the lateral border of the "anatomical snuffbox", with the abductor pollicis longus, and is palpable if the patient is asked to extend and abduct the thumb while the forearm is rested in a neutral position. The muscle acts to extend the proximal phalanx, and is supplied by the radial nerve (C7, C8).

Extensor carpi radialis brevis (ECRB) arises from the common extensor origin at the lateral epicondyle of the humerus, and runs distally down the forearm to insert into the base of the third metacarpal. It acts to both extend and radially deviate the wrist, and is supplied by the radial nerve (C7, C8). It is crossed along the line of the triangle by the tendinous slip of the extensor pollicis longus.

Extensor pollicis longus (EPL) arises from the posterior middle third of the ulna and interosseus membrane, and travels distally to insert into the distal phalanx of the thumb. The muscle acts to extend the thumb, and forms the medial border of the anatomical snuffbox in the wrist. It is supplied by the radial nerve (C7, C8), and is most palpable in thumb extension and abduction.

Deep to the tendons lies the capsule of the radiocarpal joint, and this is directly palpable prior to crossing the extensor digitorum tendons in their sheath beneath the extensor retinaculum. This 2 cm-wide fascial thickening attaches to the radial border, proximal to the styloid process, and runs across the dorsal wrist to the pisiform and triquetrium. Interestingly, the retinaculum divides the extensor tendons into six compartments, by fascial attachments containing the following:

1. abductor pollicis longus and extensor pollicis brevis
2. extensor carpi radialis lingus and brevis
3. extensor pollicis longus
4. extensor digitorum and common sheath
5. extensor digiti minimi
6. extensor carpi ulnaris

As we palpate more toward the ulna, we can again find the joint capsule and the posterior interosseus artery, then encounter the tendon of the extensor digiti minimi and the ulnar collateral carpal ligament, deep to the insertion of the extensor carpi ulnaris. The dorsal digital nerves are superficial to the retinaculum, but do not follow a palpable course.

Extensor digitorum originates at the common extensor origin of the lateral humerus, and passes distally obliquely across the forearm, to pass under the retinaculum as four tendinous slips which insert into the phalanges of the second to fifth fingers. The tendons usually possess intertendinous slips, limiting independent phalanx extension, but act to extend both wrist and fingers. The muscle is supplied by the radial nerve (C7, C8), and the tendons are visible in finger extension with a hand placed palmdown on a flat surface, and the muscle belly palpable in wrist extension.

The tendons of the intersossei muscles expand to form a tendinous canal, which holds down the extensor indices tendon to the phalanges as they extend distally; the extensor tendon insertion is via the extensor apparatus, a complex insertion which can be seen in Figure 3.6. It is made up of lateral and medial conjoined tendon slips, and intertendinous connections.

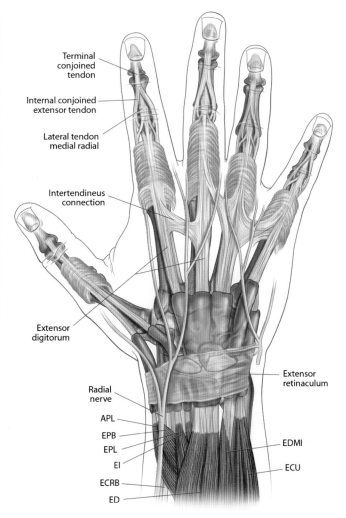

Figure 3.6 The dorsal triangle

APL	=	abductor pollicis longus
EPB	=	extensor pollicis brevis
EPL	=	extensor pollicis longus
EI	=	extensor indicus
ECRB	=	extensor carpi radialis brevis
ED	=	extensor digitorium
EDMI	=	extensor digiti minimi
ECU	=	extensor carpi ulnaris

Terminal conjoined tendon

Internal conjoined extensor tendon

Lateral tendon medial radial

Intertendineus connection

Extensor digitorum

Radial nerve

APL

EPB

EPL

EI

ECRB

ED

Extensor retinaculum

EDMI

ECU

Extensor digiti minimi arises from the common extensor origin at the lateral epicondyle of the humerus, and is a thin, strap-like muscle inserting into the middle phalanx of the fifth finger. It acts to extend the fifth finger, and is supplied by the radial nerve (C6, C7, C8).

Extensor carpi ulnaris arises from two heads, the humeral head via the common extensor tendon, and the ulnar head arising from the posterior surface of the shaft of the ulna. The muscle is small, and runs under the retinaculum of the wrist, to insert into the base of the fifth metacarpal. The action is to ulnarly deviate the wrist in extension, and is innervated by the radial nerve (C6, C7, C8).

The ulnar border (dorsal)

Structures encountered:

> ulnar collateral ligament

> dorsal digital nerve

> extensor carpi ulnaris

> extensor digiti minimi

> dorsal digital vein

Again commencing at the proximal ulnar, and the ulnar collateral ligament at the lateral margin, the dorsal digital nerve from the dorsal branch of the ulnar nerve supplies the skin and ulnar sides of the fifth finger, and ulnar side of the ring finger. It emerges from the ulnar border, and runs an irregular course, following the digital terminal branches to the fingers. The ulnar border traverses the tendon of the extensor carpi ulnaris, moving distally over the dorsal surface of the hamate, as the tendons of the extensor digiti minimi pass over it toward the capitate bone at the apex of the distal transverse row of carpal bones, as it forms the capitate-metacarpal joint and the extensor digitorum tendon overlying it. The dorsal digital veins run superficially just beneath the skin.

Abductor digiti minimi originates from the pisiform and the tendon of the flexor carpi ulnaris. It runs down the volar side of the fifth finger, but inserts in the ulnar border of the proximal phalanx of the fifth finger. Acting to abduct the little finger, it is supplied by the ulnar nerve (C8, T1), and is palpable over the hypothenar eminence when abducting the fifth finger against resistance.

Opponens digiti minimi originates from the flexor retinaculum and hook of the hamate, inserting into the anteromedial surface of the fifth metacarpal shaft. It acts to oppose the fifth finger against the thumb, and is supplied by the ulnar nerve (C8, T1), and is palpable over the hypothenar eminence.

The radial border (dorsal)

Structures encountered:

> extensor pollicis brevis

> extensor pollicis longus

> abductor pollicis longus

> dorsal digital nerves

> extensor indicis

> scaphoid bone

> base of third metacarpal

As we commence at the radius, the extensor pollicis brevis is palpable, and, moving down the radial border, we cross the extensor pollicis longus as it crosses over ulnar to radially. Deep to this is the abductor pollicis longus under the radius, and the dorsal digital nerves arising from the superficial branch of the radial nerve. Directly under the extensor indicis lies the scaphoid bone, and this is palpable directly, moving distally across to the trapezoid en route to the capitate, with the extensor indicis tendon passing over the carpal bones, until reaching the base of the third metacarpal.

Extensor pollicis longus arises from the posterior middle one-third of the ulna and adjoining interosseus membrane, before passing under the extensor retinaculum of the wrist, and inserting into the distal phalanx of the thumb. It acts to extend the thumb, and is supplied by the radial nerve.

Extensor indicis originates from the posterior surface of the distal third of the ulna and interosseus membrane, running transversely to cross the wrist and pass under the extensor retinaculum to the insertion at the base of the middle and distal phalanx of the index finger. The muscle acts to extend the index finger, and is supplied by the radial nerve (C7, C8). It is palpable in resisted extension.

Opponens pollicis arises from the trapezium and flexor retinaculum, to run distally to the anterolateral border of the metacarpal of the thumb. It is supplied by the median nerve, and acts to oppose the thumb.

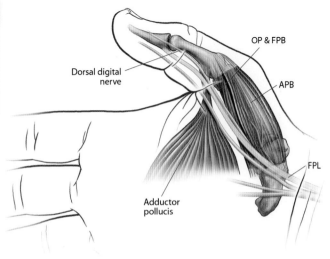

Figure 3.7 The thumb (radial to triangles)

OP	=	opponens pollicis
FPB	=	flexor pollicis brevis
APB	=	abductor pollicis brevis
FPL	=	flexor pollicis longus

OP & FPB

Dorsal digital nerve

APB

Adductor pollucis

FPL

Within the triangles
The volar clockface

Within this triangle, the anatomy of the important structures can be recognized by the use of the "clockface". Starting at the 12 o'clock position, and proximal to the apex of the triangle, lies the capitellum; here the origin of the oblique head of the adductor pollicis is palpable radially. The transverse head is palpable from the radial border of the metacarpal, just distal to the capitate.

At the 1 o'clock position, the trapezoid carpal bone is palpable, and also the tendon of the FCR as it passes just radially to the bone itself. The 3 o'clock position is the trapezium, at the site of the radial insertion of the flexor retinaculum, which covers the clockface. Palpable from the radial border is the origin of the flexor pollicis brevis, deep to the opponens pollicis.

Figure 3.8a The volar clockface		
FDP	=	flexor digitorum profundus
FDS	=	flexor digitorium superficialis
FPL	=	flexor policis longus
FCR	=	flexor carpi radialis
FCU	=	flexor carpi ulnaris
Cap	=	capitate
Tra	=	trapeziod
Trp	=	trapezium
Sc.	=	scaphoid
Lun	=	lunate
P	=	pisiform
H	=	hamate

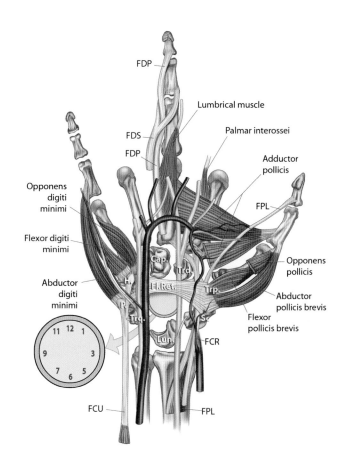

Moving around to the 5 o'clock position, deep to the tendons of the FCR and FPL, is the scaphoid bone, from the radio-distal corner of which arises the abductor pollicis brevis, which is palpable in its muscle belly.

At 6 o'clock is the lunate, lying deep to the common tendons of the flexor digitorum superficialis and profundus, and hence difficult to palpate from the volar aspect.; commonly the bone is best palpated from the dorsal clockface. At 7 o'clock lies the triquetral bone, but between this and the distal ulnar lies the TFCC and the cartilaginous meniscal homologue. At 9 o'clock lies the pisiform bone and at 10 o'clock the hook of the hamate – both sites of attachment of the flexor retinaculum. The pisiform is the origin of the abductor digiti minimi, and the hamate, the origin of the flexor digiti minimi and opponens pollicis, respectively. At 11 o'clock, the FDS/P tendon is palpable as it passes to the fourth metacarpal.

The **lumbricals** originate from the tendons of the flexor digitorum profundus, on the palmar surface of the hand, and insert into the extensor exansion to the radial side of each tendinous slip. They occupy the spaces between the first, second, third, fourth, and fifth, respectively, and they act to flex the metacarpophalangeal joint, and are supplied, the lateral two by the ulnar nerve, and the proximal two by the radial nerve.

The **palmar interossei** originates from the second, fourth, and fifth metacarpals, and insert into the base of the same-digit proximal phalanx. They act to adduct the fingers, and are supplied by the ulnar nerve.

The **dorsal interossei** originate between each metacarpal on the dorsal aspect, and insert into the base of the same-digit proximal phalanges of the second, third, and fourth fingers. They act to cause abduction, and are supplied by the ulnar nerve (C8, T1).

The dorsal clockface

Dorsally, we can utilize the clockface again to identify the insertions of the extensor compartment, and refocus in the carpal bones, particularly in the proximal row. At the 12 o'clock position, we have the capitate bone, and the base of the third metacarpal. Here the insertion of the extensor carpi radialis brevis is palpable, and also the overlying tendons of the extensor digitorum (ED). Moving clockwise, we encounter at 1 o'clock the hamate and here, crossing it, is the tendon slip of the ED. At 2 o'clock, we move to the base of the fifth metacarpal, and the insertion of the extensor carpi ulnaris (ECU); palpable at 3 o'clock is the triquetral carpal bone, under the tendon of the extensor digiti minimi.

At 6 o'clock is the important lunate, commonly seen in dorsal dislocation in wrist flexion, should there be ligamentous disruption. Hence it is important to be able to identify the proximal row, in order to examine the wrist comprehensively.

The scaphoid sits at 8 o'clock, with the scapholunate interosseous ligament at 7 o'clock, and the lunotriquetral at the 5 o'clock position. The scapho-trapezium joint crosses the 9 o'clock position, and the base of the first metacarpal, with the insertion of the abductor pollicis longus. The insertion of the extensor carpi radialis is palpable at the 11 o'clock position, at the base of the first metacarpal.

Figure 3.8b The dorsal clockface

APL	=	abductor pollicis longus
EPB	=	extensor pollicis brevis
ECRL	=	extensor carpi radialis longus
ECRB	=	extensor carpi radialis brevis
EPL	=	extensor pollicis longus
EPB	=	extensor pollicis brevis
ED	=	extensor digitorum
EDM	=	extensor digiti minimi
ECU	=	extensor carpi ulnaris

EI

12 1 2 3 4 5 6 7 8 9

Extensor
pollicis brevis

Abductor
pollicis longus

ECRL

ECRB

EPL

Extensor digitorum

Extensor digiti
minimi

Extensor carpi
ulnaris

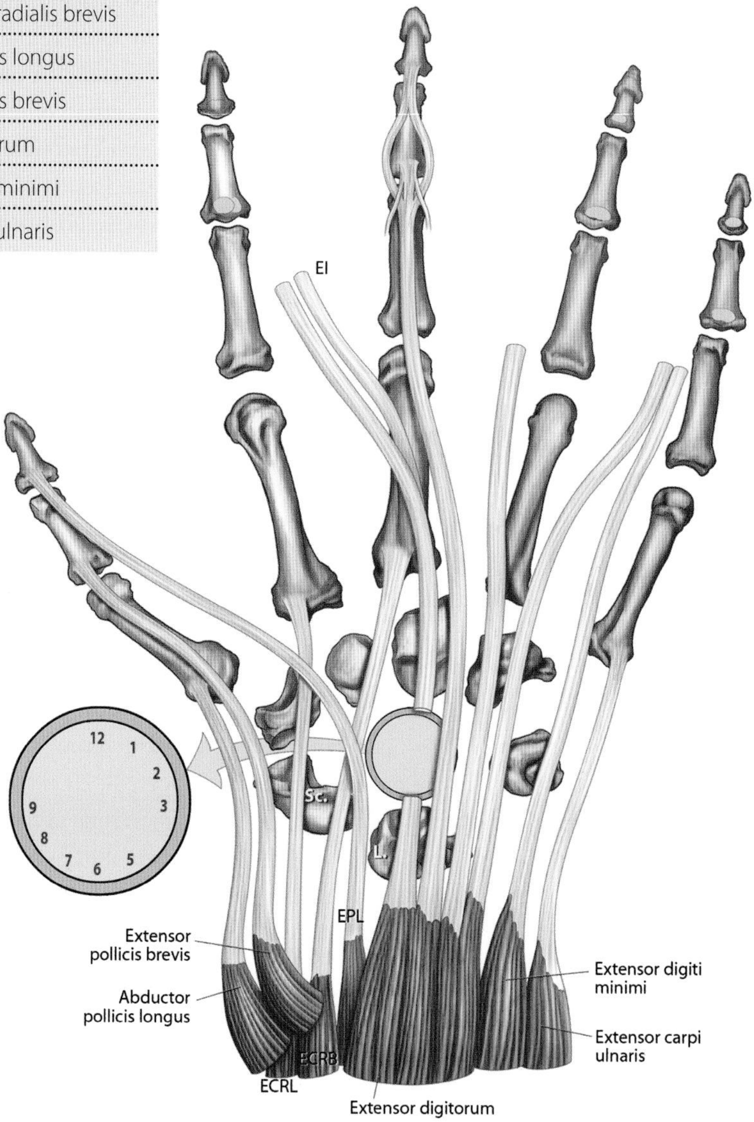

Figure 3.9 Ulnar to the triangle

H	=	hamate
P	=	pisiform
Tra	=	trapeziod
Lun	=	lunate
Sca	=	scaphoid
U	=	ulna
R	=	radius

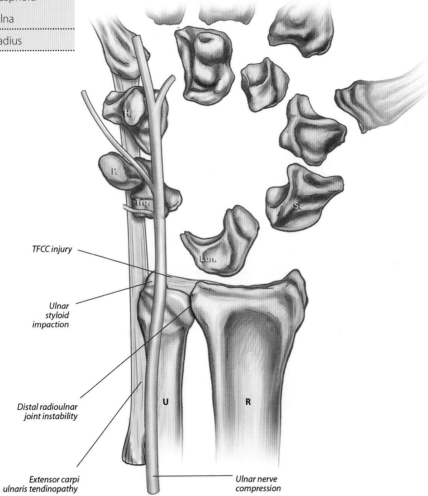

TFCC injury

Ulnar styloid impaction

Distal radioulnar joint instability

Extensor carpi ulnaris tendinopathy

Ulnar nerve compression

U

R

Table 3.1 Muscles of the hand and wrist				
Muscle	**Origin**	**Insertion**	**Nerve**	**Root**
Extensor carpi radialis brevis (ERCB)	Humerus; lateral epicondyle	Base of 3rd metacarpal	Posterior interosseus n. C7, C8	
Extensor digitorum (ED)		Extensor expansion of fingers		
Extensor digiti minimi (EDM)		Extensor expansion of 4th finger		
Extensor carpi ulnaris (ECU)		Base of 3rd metacarpal		
Extensor carpi radialis longus (ECRL)	Lateral supracondylar ridge (lower ⅓)	Posterior of base of 2nd metacarpal	Radial n.	C6, C7
Extensor pollicis brevis (EPB)	Posterior distal ⅓ of radius and interosseous membrane	Base of proximal phalanx of thumb	Radial n.	C7, C8
Extensor pollicis longus (EPL)	Posterior middle ⅓ of ulna and interosseous membrane	Distal phalanx of thumb	Radial n.	C7, C8
Extensor indicis (EI)	Posterior ⅓ of distal ulna and interosseous membrane	Base of 2nd, middle and distal phalanges	Radial n.	C7, C8
Flexor digiti minimi (FDM)	Hook of hamate and flexor retinaculum	Base of proximal phlanx of 5th finger	Ulnar n.	C8, T1
Flexor carpi radialis (FCR)	Medial epicondyle	Base of 2nd and 3rd metacarpals	Median n.	C6, C7
Palmaris longus (PL)		Flexor retinaculum and palmar aponeurosis	Median n.	C7, C8
Flexor digitorum superficialis (FDS)	Humerus; medial epicondyle, ulna; coronoid process, radius; anterior oblique line	Middle phalanges of medial 4 fingers	Median n.	C7, C8, T1
Flexor carpi ulnaris (FCU)	Humerus; medial epicondyle Ulna; medial olecranon, medial border of ulna	Pisiform, hook of hamate, base of 5th metacarpal	Ulnar n.	C7, C8, T1
Flexor digitorum profundus (FDP)	Anterior and medial surface of upper ⅔ of ulna	Distal phalanges of medial 4 fingers	Median n. Ulnar n.	C8, T1 and C8, T1

Table 3.1 *(continued)*				
Muscle	**Origin**	**Insertion**	**Nerve**	**Root**
Flexor pollicus longus (FPL)	Radius, anterior surface of middle third	Distal phalanx of thumb	Anterior interosseus n.	C7, C8
Flexor pollicis brevis (FPB)	Trapezium and flexor retinaculum	Base of lateral proximal phalanx of thumb	Median n.	C8, T1
Opponens digiti minimi (ODM)	Hook of hamate and flexor retinaculum	Anteromedial shaft of distal 5th metacarpal	Ulnar n.	C8, T1
Abductor pollicis longus (AbPL)	Posterior surfaces of ulna, radius and interosseous membrane	Base of 1st metacarpal	Radial n.	C7, C8
Abductor pollicis brevis (AbPB)	Scaphoid and trapezium tubercles	Base of 1st proximal phalanx	Median n.	C8, T1
Abductor digiti minimi (ADM)	Pisiform and flexor carpi ulnaris tendon sheath	Base of proximal phalanx of 5th finger	Ulnar n.	C8, T1
Opponens pollicis (OP)	Trapezium and flexor retinaculum	Anterolateral 1st metacarpal shaft	Median n.	C8, T1
Adductor pollicis (AP)	Oblique head: capitate and base of 2nd/3rd metacarpals Transverse : palmar surface of 3rd metacarpal	Base of proximal 5th phalanx	Ulnar n.	C8, T1
Lumbricals	Tendon of flexor digitorum profundus (radial)	Extensor expansion of proximal phalanges of 2nd, 3rd, 4th, 5th fingers	Median nerve (2nd and 3rd; ulnar nerve (4th and 5th)	C8, T1
Palmar interossei	Ulnar border of 2nd, radial border of 4th and 5th metacarpals	Base of proximal phalanx of same digit	Ulnar n.	C8, T1
Dorsal interossei	Metacarpal shafts between all metacarpals	Base of proximal phalanx of same finger	Ulnar n.	C8, T1
Pronator quadratus (PQ)	Anterior distal ulnar	Anterior distal radius	Median n.	C7, C8

Wrist				Finger		Thumb	
Flexion	**Extension**	**Radial deviation**	**Ulnar deviation**	**Flexion**	**Extension**	**Flexion**	**Extension**
Flexor carpi radialis	Extensor carpi ulnaris	Extensor carpi radialis longus	Flexor carpi ulnaris	Flexor digitorum profundus	Extensor digitorum	Flexor pollicis longus	Extensor pollicis longus
Flexor carpi ulnaris	Extensor digitorum	Extensor carpi radialis brevis	Extensor carpi radialis	Flexor digitorum superficialis		Flexor pollicis brevis	Extensor pollicis brevis
Palmaris longus	Extensor carpi radalis longus	Flexor carpi ulnaris		Lumbricals			
	Extensor carpi radialis brevis						

Table 3.2 Prime movers of the hand and wrist

Ulnar to the triangle

The triangular fibrocartilage complex (TFCC) causes much angst in diagnosis. It is the major stabilizing structure of the distal radioulnar joint, and ulnar carpus, and, alongside being the glide and rotational surface, it also cushions the compressive force. In understanding the anatomy of the region (Fig. 3.3), one can see that the mechanism of injury of this structure usually requires the axial compression seen in falling or fixing on an outstretched wrist, and also the second rotational force, but a ulnar traction can also cause injury, alongside repetitive pronation, ulnar deviation, and compressive grip, such as in gymnastics, golf, and racquet sports.[15]

The blood supply to the meniscus homologue is good[16] and, as such, a surgical repair is often successful.[17]

Palmer[9] classified TFCC into Types 1 and 2, which have been modified by Anderson in the excellent *Atlas of imaging in sports medicine* to:

> Type 1A – traumatic central tear

> Type 1b – traumatic peripheral tear

> Type 2 – degenerative "central" tear

Ulnar impaction syndrome, otherwise known as ulnar-styloid triquetral impaction, is commonly missed.[18] It presents as pain, distal to the tip of the ulna, increased by direct palpation, but not extending onto the dorsal ulnocarpal joint, unlike TFCC injury. The etiology of this condition relates in part to a congenitally long ulnar styloid, or exostosis after repetitive injury, with the normal length of the styloid being 3–6 mm[19], and up to 18 mm being reported in symptomatic patients at radiological examination. It is thought that there is a degree of impingement syndrome, concomitantly with synovium from the capsule, and ulnar collateral ligament trapping in the ulnar space.

The TFCC is the major component of the distal radioulnar joint (DRUJ) stability, aided by the dorsal and ventral radioulnar ligaments, along with the interosseus membrane and pronator quadratus, and also the joint capsule.[20] Injury can occur with both a hyperpronation

Table 3.3 Ulnar to the triangle				
Define and align	Pathology	Listen and localize	Palpate and recreate	Alleviate and investigate
Ulnar to triangle	TFCC tear	Ulnar sided wrist pain, following supination injury[23]	Audible click on forearm rotation[24]. Point tenderness between FCU and ECU distal to ulnar head. +ve ulnar impaction test	MRI arthrogram [25] up to 80% sensitivity, arthroscopy 100% sensitivity[15]
	Ulnar impaction syndrome	Chronic History, not acute. Grinding sound in certain movements and occasional "snap"	Impaction test[26] and palpation deep and volar to ECU tendon, increase in pain when dorsiflexing and supinated	Intra articular LA, plain film shows ulnar variance, subchondral loss in lunate, triquetrium and ulna. MRI[27]
	Distal radioulnar joint (DRUJ) instability	Wrist pain, localized to fovea following injury. Chronicity gives decreased grip strength	Piano key sign, tenderness of fovea ECU when wrist in ulnar deviation and supinated[28] 95% specificity. Pain on compression of DRUJ.	Pronation and supination views plain film
	Ulnar nerve compression	Wide range of symptoms, can be overuse injury or following trauma	Entrapment at Guyon's canal and +ve Tinel's test. Atrophy of hypothenar eminence,[29] burning pain on border of 5th finger	Examination, nerve conduction studies. May need to examine thoracic outlet and elbow with imaging
	ECU tendinopathy	Gradual onset, repeated microtrauma, increase in activity	Pain with forced isometric supination[30]	Peri-tendinous fluid on ultrasound
	ECU subluxation	Occurs acutely "bolt-like" sharp ulnar wrist pain	Pain on passive supination, pain on palpation of ECU groove, local swelling,[31] snapping sensation on palpation of 6th space	Ultrasound dynamic assessment, then MRI T2 FAT and T1 STIR

or supination injury, but also in conjunction with foream fractures such as Galeazzi's or Colles' fractures.

For dorsal radioulnar ligament (dRUL) instability to occur, the interosseus membrane must be torn initially, then the dRUL ligament which, in pronation, demonstrates subluxation on radiological plain film. The situation is reversed in supination, with the volar radioulnar ligamant (V URL) being damaged,[21] and demonstrating subluxation.

Ulnar nerve entrapment at the wrist is focused on Guyon's canal, named after the French urologist in 1861; this divides the course of the ulnar nerve at the wrist into three zones. Zone 1 is proximal to the bifurcation of the ulnar nerve at the wrist, and compression of the nerve here causes sensory and motor loss; it is commonly caused by a fracture of the hook of hamate or a ganglion, causing direct compression. In Zone 2 runs the motor branch, and compression can lead to wasting of the intrinsic and ulnar supplied muscles of the hand. Zone 3 involves the sensory branch, and therefore reduces sensation to the hypothenar eminence, and the fifth and part of the fourth fingers, commonly caused by a ganglion or ulnar artery aneurysm.

Clinicians need to exclude more proximal causes, such as thoracic outlet syndrome, and cubital tunnel syndrome at the elbow, but the nerve is amenable to surgical decompression. These conditions are covered in Chapters 1 and 2, respectively.

Ulnar wrist pain is common, particularly in tennis players, who use the extensor carpi ulnaris (ECU) to develop the spin and control of the ball in a double-handed backhand, and also in spin bowlers in cricket.

As the ECU tendon passes into an osteofibrous sheath, via a groove in the distal ulna, to insert into the fifth metacarpal, it is stabilized in the groove, by fascial attachments formed by the sixth fascia compartment, as described earlier. During pronation, the ECU tendon is in contact with the inner surface of the ulnar head, away from the extensor digiti minimi, creating a space, and, during supination, the tendon moves closer to the EDM, closing this space. The angle of pull is close to 30° and, if the osteofibrous sheath ruptures, the tendon will pull directly, and hence be free to flip over the groove. It can be seen that tendinopathy can result from overuse injury from either learning a new technique, or the recurrence of poor technique.

The 30-item Disabilities Arm Shoulder and Hand (DASH) questionnaire was introduced[22] in order to quantify the degree of impairment of the patient and also to aid diagnosis. The validity of this questionnaire has been tested, and it is reliable across a range of upper-limb and hand conditions in a primary-care setting, and can be a valuable tool for monitoring recovery and rehabilitation.

Within the triangle (dorsal)

Ten to thirty per cent of all wrist injuries result in carpal instability, the most common of which is scapholunate injury.[32] The scaphoid bone acts as a stabilizer between the two carpal rows, acting as a bridge; in the normal wrist, it maintains a flexed position, and is compressed between the trapezium and radial styloid in radial deviation. This is counterbalanced by the extension of the triquetrium on the ulnar aspect.[33]

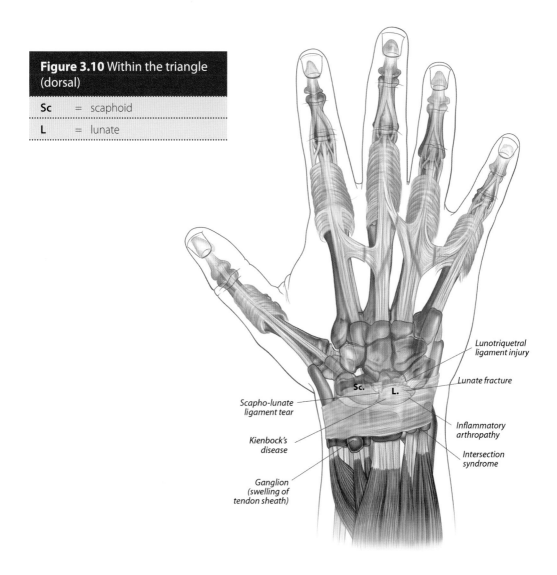

Figure 3.10 Within the triangle (dorsal)

Sc	= scaphoid
L	= lunate

Lunotriquetral ligament injury

Lunate fracture

Scapho-lunate ligament tear

Sc.

L.

Inflammatory arthropathy

Kienbock's disease

Intersection syndrome

Ganglion (swelling of tendon sheath)

The lunate is attached to the scaphoid by the scapholunate interosseus ligament, and similarly to the triquetral via the lunotriquetral interosseous ligament, and these maintain the lunate in its position. Tears of these ligaments allow the dorsal displacement, and subsequent development in the proximal row of carpal bones, or dorsal intercalated segment, of instability.[34]

The Mayfield classification of injury[35] details progressive injury severity:

I. scapholunate interosseus injury
II. dorsal subluxation of capitate
III. luntotriquetral interosseus ligament tear (perilunate dissociation)
IV. dissociation of lunate from its fossa

Scapholunate dissociation is caused by a tear to the scapholunate interosseus ligament, by impact load on an extended, supinated, and ulnarly deviated wrist.[35] Commonly presenting late, due to the supposed trivial injury, patients complain of weakness when loading the wrist, and often swelling, occasionally misdiagnosed as a ganglion, and also on occasion a snap or click with movement[35, 36].

Imaging is best at arthroscopy, where a classification of the injury can be made dependent on physical findings. The four stages of injury have been defined by Watson et al.[37] relating to the degrees of disruption:

1. predynamic instability
2. dynamic instability
3. static instability
4. scapholunate collapse

Luntotriquetral ligament injury is rarely found in isolation. Lunate dislocation occurs as a result of Stage IV, and, as it is a significant traumatic injury, is commonly associated with a distal radius fracture, with significant morbidity, and accelerated post-traumatic arthritis, most commonly dislocating dorsally.

Kienbock's disease is the osteonecrosis of the lunate, typified by lunatomalacia;[38] it was named after Kienböck in 1910. It is characterized by the collapse of the lunate. The condition's etiology is not understood, but it is most frequently seen in the dominant wrists of men aged 20–40. It is possibly related to collective trauma disorders, as repetitive strain certainly plays a part.

Radiological staging:

Stage 1. Normal x-rays; MRI may identify early osteochondral change
Stage 2. Lunate sclerosis
Stage 3. Infarcted bone collapses and breaks up, causing carpal disruption
Stage 4. Osteoarthritis

Lunate fractures are rare, and usually the result of high impact trauma.[39–41]

Ganglion cysts of the wrist are common, with a 3:1 female:male predominance. They occur as an outpouching of the synovium surrounding tendon sheaths, possibly due to collagen disruption. In the wrist, they can present with varied symptoms, due to the small space they occupy, and the potential compression of other structures. They are more common dorsally,[42] where compression of the ulnar nerve can occur in Guyon's canal (described earlier), but also contribute on the volar surface to median nerve compression.

Dorsal ganglions are commonly associated with the scapholunate interosseus ligament and, as such, cause confusion with scapholunate ligament disarticulation.[43] Ultrasound imaging is very helpful in making the diagnosis.

Intersection syndrome is a tenosynovitis of the radial wrist extensors. It is common in weightlifters and rowers.[44] It involves the extensor carpi radialis longus, and extensor carpi radialis brevis. It can also involve the extensor polis brevis, and abductor pollicis longus, but

Table 3.4 Within the triangle (dorsal)				
Define and align	**Pathology**	**Listen and localize**	**Palpate and recreate**	**Alleviate and investigate**
Within triangle, dorsal to triangle	Intercarpal ligament dissociation I. Scapho-lunate ligament dissociation II. Luntotriquetral instability	Poorly differentiated wrist pain, often with insidious onset, decreased grip strength and pain on some resisted movement; pain can be localized to radial side	Swelling, localized pain, Watson's scaphoid shift test[51] Kleinman shear test to distinguish from TFCC tear[55] or Reagan shuck test.[56] Pain exacerbated by dorsiflexion	Supinated AP and lateral view of wrist and Terry-Thomas sign[52] to measure scapholunate gapping > 3mm. Plain stress views in a power grip, false +ve rate high in MR arthrograms,[53] arthroscopy is gold standard[54]
	Kienbock's disease	Manual occupation aged 20–40, male 2:1, dorsal wrist pain, weak grip and dominant hand affected	Swelling over lunate, passive dorsiflexion of middle finger reproduces pain	Plain film staging. Ulnar variance associated[57], wrist arthoscopy
	Lunate fracture	Tenderness on volar wrist over lunate, painful wrist flexion	Ballottement of lunate is painful in Reagan shuck test	Bone scan is 100% sensitive but not specific, MRI arthrogram can be diagnostic
	Ganglion	Varied presentation but complaint chiefly of swelling over wrist	Pain, paresthia and fluctuant (although not always) swelling	Ultrasound[43, 58]
	Intersection syndrome	Pain in wrist extension, repetitive wrist use occupationally or rowing/ weightlifting[44, 59]	Crepitus and pain on resisted extension[45]	Ultrasound examination shows peri-tendinous fluid
	Carpometacarpal dislocation	Localized swelling over carpometacarpal joint	Examine ulnar nerve to exclude deep motor branch of ulnar nerve	Oblique plain x-ray, 30⁰ pronated from AP[60]
	Inflammatory arthropathy	Swollen joint, often symmetrical and polyarthropathy	Tender painful swelling with reduced function, consider reactive arthritis	Aspiration to exclude gout, except if septic contraindications[61]

these present more radially to the triangle. The presentation is one of pain and swelling in the forearm, and pain on resisted extension.[45] It occurs due to the crossing of the extensor pollicus tendon over the ECRL and ECRB, presenting as a lump, and mimicking a ganglion.

Although at first glance one would expect carpometacarpal dislocation to be difficult to misdiagnose, it is actually so,[46] as it is uncommon except for that of the thumb. Oblique plain films can help to identify these, but conservative management, if delayed in their relocation, is complicated by the unstable nature of the joint, and the pull of the extensor and flexor tendons.

Rheumatoid arthritis is the most prevalent inflammatory arthropathy, affecting up to 3% of the US population[47] over 60 years old, and is characterized by inflammatory synovitis. This inflammatory synovitis commonly affects the wrist, metacarpal phalangeal joints, and proximal interphalangeal joints, presenting with swelling, painful movement, and stiffness. This differs from osteoarthritis, which is degenerative, in that radiological x-ray changes show a lack of erosive changes in rheumatoid, unlike osteoarthritis. There is a wide differential, and this includes polymyalgia rheumatica (PMR), gout and pseudogout, and osteoarthritis. PMR typically excludes the upper limb and, as such, wrist presentation is unusual. Gout and pseudogout have very similar presentations, but resolve spontaneously, and it is the persistence of the synovitis for over six weeks seen in rheumatoid arthritis which is pathonomonic.[48] Osteoarthritis more characteristically affects the more proximal joints of the hip and knee, and is characterized by joint space narrowing, subchondral bone cysts, osteopenia, and osteophyte formation. It is degenerative, rather than inflammatory, and, although it does occur in the wrist, is more a sequalae of prior acute injury.

There is an importance to the early detection of rheumatoid arthritis, due to the effectiveness of interventional drug therapies, and, as such, MRI has been shown to be sensitive in early detection.[49]

Inflammatory monoarthritis should always make one consider a reactive arthritis; its incidence has increased, with the concomitant increased prevalence of chlamydia. This should certainly be screened for in the young symptomatic athlete.[50]

Within the triangle (volar)

Carpal tunnel syndrome (CTS) is the most common peripheral neuropathy, responsible for over 90% of all neuropathies.[62] It has a peak incidence between 55 and 60 years of age, and a female to male ratio of 2:1,[63, 64] and is a form in its chronic state of repetitive strain disorder. It is seen occupationally in manual repetitive work, but is also made worse by vibration, poor posture, and external pressure by awkward movements.

The pathophysiology is not well understood, but is thought to involve mechanical compression, vascular insufficiency, and vibration.

Early presenting symptoms are related to the sensory part of median nerve, such as burning pain and numbness in medial nerve distribution; occasionally all five fingers can be involved if the ulnar nerve is also affected. Nocturnal paresthesia is 51–95% sensitive, but only 27–68% specific.[65]

Many signs are reported, with varying degrees of sensitivity and specificity, and a combination is undoubtedly better. Tinel's sign is not precise in CTS, with a sensitivity of 23–67%,[66] while Phalen's test aims to reproduce symptoms within one minute of complete wrist flexion, and

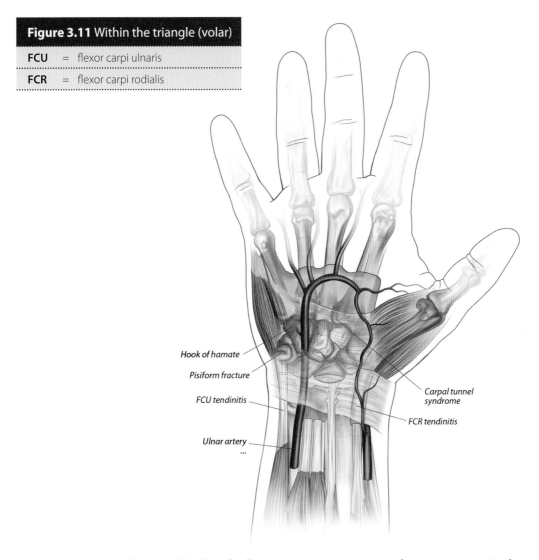

Figure. 3.11 Within the triangle (volar)

| FCU | = | flexor carpi ulnaris |
| FCR | = | flexor carpi rodialis |

Hook of hamate

Pisiform fracture

FCU tendinitis

Ulnar artery
...

Carpal tunnel
syndrome

FCR tendinitis

is more sensitive in chronic CTS, but the literature reports sensitivity between 10–90%. The Katz hand diagram is a self-reported map, where patients draw the symptom location, and this shows 80% sensitivity and 90% specificity, and is probably underutilized.[67]

Nerve conduction studies are the gold standard in diagnosis, but a recent study by Keles[68] suggests that ultrasound examination of the median nerve is promising, as the cross-sectional area was increased in those with positive nerve conduction studies.

The literature represents fractures of the hook of the hamate as less than 2% of all carpal fractures[69], but this may be an underprevalence, as they are frequently missed. The mechanism of injury is commonly due to either a direct blow, or the repetitive load of a bat. In golfers, this can occur in the non-dominant hand if the club hits the ground, or in tennis players in the dominant hand when losing control of the grip. Non-union is common if not immobilized, resulting in persistent pain, and may lead to the need for surgical repair.[70]

Table 3.5 Within the triangle (volar)				
Define and align	**Pathology**	**Listen and localize**	**Palpate and recreate**	**Alleviate and investigate**
Volar to triangle	Carpal tunnel syndrome	Burning pain in thumb index and middle finger	Tinel's, Phalen's, Katz hand diagram, Thener atrophy, late, diminished sensation in median nerve distribution	Nerve conduction studies 96% sensitivity[74, 71] ultrasound[68]
	Hook of hamate fracture/stress fracture	Sudden onset pain after a missed shot or grounding of bat, or persistent pain when gripping bat or racquet handle	Point tenderness over hook of hamate on volar surface at 10 o'clock on volar clockface	Plain film (carpal tunnel view[72] or lateral view with radial deviation) CT may be required if in doubt
	FCR tendinitis/ tendinopathy	Associated with repetitive trauma, pain on gripping	Point tenderness of FCR at wrist flexure, flexion and radial deviation exacerbates pain against resistance. Occasional median nerve pain	Ultrasound, can be calcific deposits[73]
	FCU tendinitis/ tendinopathy	Pain on resisted flexion, pain on hitting tennis ball	Crepitus and pain at insertion of tendon into pisiform, flexion and ulnar deviation	Ultrasound examination shows fluid in tendon sheath
	Traumatic ulnar artery thrombosis	Repetitive trauma by pneumatic compression equipment or acute martial arts injury	Hypothenar swelling, 5th finger pain or paresthesia and poor perfusion occasionally	Ultrasound imaging[74] and MR angiography to confirm[75]
	Pisiform fracture/ Stress fracture	Pain on grip, pain on resisted wrist flexion at the pisiform/hamate flexor retinaculum attachment, CT—computerised tomography, MR—magnetic resonance	Tenderness on palpation, at 9 o'clock on volar clockface	Plain film, carpal tunnel view or oblique view

Flexor carpi ulnaris (FCU) tendinopathy occurs commonly in tennis players, with repetitive forced wrist flexion. It occurs due to the pulley effect of the flexor retinaculum, and pain is felt along the FCU, or at its insertion into the pisiform bone. Ultrasound examination of the tendon may show degenerative changes, although this is less common than fluid in the synovial sheath[59] similar to that found in the flexor carpi radialis. It is interesting that much has been written recently of tendon degeneration, and these two conditions are classically described as tendinitis, i.e. fluid and swelling. Little new in the current evidence suggests otherwise, other than some suggesting shockwave lithotriosy to treat any calcific deposits,[76] and case reports of isolated sclerosing therapy,[77] but this would belie the tendonitis diagnosis, and lean toward tendinopathy, if successful.

Vascular problems in the hypothenar eminence are not common. Traumatic psuedo-aneurysms are rare but important, and related to trauma. The mechanism is usually the tearing of the intimal lining of the radial or ulnar artery, either by repetitive or acute trauma.[75] Presenting as a soft-tissue swelling suggestive of tumor, with concomitant irritation of the ulnar nerve, they can be confused with ulnar nerve entrapment. Patients are at risk of digital ischemia, joint degeneration, and nerve compression.

The pisiform bone is a sesamoid bone within the tendon of the FCU, and articulates with the triquetrium, lying near the deep ulnar nerve and artery. Fractures are rare, but can be painful, due to direct trauma in sports where there is gripping of a club, or after a fall on an outstretched hand.

Radial to the triangle

Scaphoid fractures are the most common of all carpal bone fractures, but are commonly undiagnosed.[78] Delay in treatment can lead to avascular necrosis, due to the distal to proximal blood supply of the bone, pseudoarthrosis, and then wrist instability.

The scaphoid receives its blood supply from the radial artery and branches of the interosseus artery, but the proximal third of the bone receives retrograde flow. The common site of fractures is across the waist of the bone, hence leaving the proximal third without its blood supply.

The scaphoid is injured usually in a fall on an outstretched hand, with an extended and radially deviated wrist. This transmits force through the third metacarpal to the capitate, resulting in compression of the scaphoid against the radius.[79]

Classically, there is tenderness in the anatomical snuffbox, over the scaphoid between the EPB and EPL, but this is not specific. Powell et al.[80] report 100% sensitivity and 66% specificity with pronation of the affected wrist and ulnar deviation, and swelling, discoloration, and axial compression of the index and middle fingers are all thought to contribute to a diagnosis.

De Quervain's disease is a stenosing tenosynovitis of the first extensor compartment of the wrist. It involves the tendons of the abductor pollicis longus and extensor pollicis brevis.[81] Pathologically, effusion is more consistent than hypervascularity, and a hypoechoic retinaculum has been observed.[82] Finkelstein's test of thumb flexion and ulnar deviation reproduces symptoms, whereas a diagnostic injection of local anesthesia into the tendon sheath under ultrasound guidance is effective in its confirmation, should it resolve the symptoms.[83]

Gymnasts at a pre-adolescent age put enormous strain through the distal radial epiphysis, and 79% complain of chronic wrist pain.[1, 84] Whereas acutely the epiphysis can be fractured by a fall on an outstretched wrist between the ages of 6 and 10, they can be more commonly stress reaction overuse injuries in gymnasts. It is the shear force of the hyperextension and supination

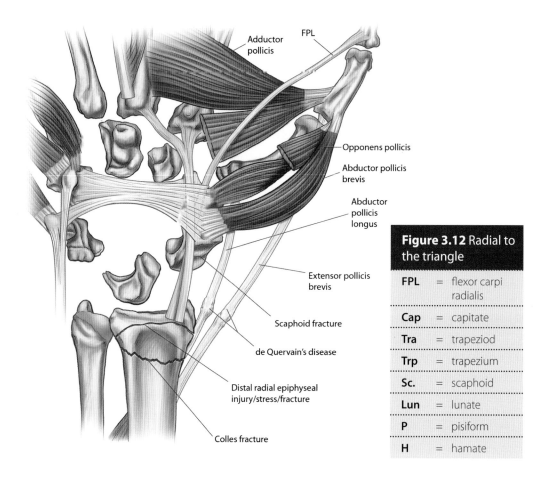

Adductor
pollicis

FPL

Opponens pollicis

Abductor pollicis
brevis

Abductor
pollicis
longus

Extensor pollicis
brevis

Scaphoid fracture

de Quervain's disease

Distal radial epiphyseal
injury/stress/fracture

Colles fracture

Figure 3.12 Radial to
the triangle

FPL	=	flexor carpi radialis
Cap	=	capitate
Tra	=	trapeziod
Trp	=	trapezium
Sc.	=	scaphoid
Lun	=	lunate
P	=	pisiform
H	=	hamate

which displaces the radial epiphysis dorsally. Fractures are classified radiographically, and most are Type I and II Salter-Harris. The distal radial epiphysis provides 75% of remodeling so, in the acute injury, excellent remodeling is possible. There can be associated greenstick fractures of the metaphysis of the ulna, and it should be carefully examined. Chronically, the gymnast can present withe premature closure of the epiphysis, due to loading, and resultant ulnar variance.[85]

In the adult, a fall on an outstretched wrist can result in a distal radius fracture; these can be associated with significant force, and concomitant injury to ligaments at the distal radioulnar joint should be carefully examined. They are the most common fracture in the elderly, with osteopenic bones, presenting with a 4:1 female:male ratio in the postmenopausal group. Presentation is the predictable deformity and pain, confirmed with plain film x-ray.[86] It is termed a "Colles fracture" when there is dorsal displacement, after Abraham Colles, an Irish surgeon, 1773–1843.

Table 3.6 Radial to the triangle				
Define and align	**Pathology**	**Listen and localize**	**Palpate and recreate**	**Alleviate and investigate**
Radial to triangle	Scaphoid fracture	Fall on outstretched hand with non-specific pain, reduced grip strength	Tenderness in anatomical snuffbox, Powell's test[80]	Plain film, scaphoid views, bone scan has 0% false negative if > 48 hrs post injury [87]
	De Quervain's disease	Local tenderness and swelling with painful grip	Finkelstein's test reproduces symptoms	Local anesthetic and cortisone injection[83] USS guidance
	Distal radial epiphyseal injury/ stress fracture	Fall on outstretched hand, unwillingness to move wrist, painful, age <10–12[84]	Tenderness over distal radius, compression painful	Lateral plain film for dorsal displacement. Look for pronator fat pad sign
	Distal radius fracture, Colles'	Pain and obvious deformity are the common presenting symptoms	Tenderness over deformity, confirm distal neurovascular integrity prior to manipulation	PA, lateral and oblique plain film. Radial height and angle < 9 mm[86], > 10–25° respectively diagnostic of comminuted fracture

Distal to the triangle

Distal to the triangles refers mainly to the hand; injury to the metacarpal bones is most common in young adults and adolescents, and accounts for 30% of all hand fractures as a result of direct or indirect trauma. It is usually as a result of axial and torsional loading.

Edward Bennett coined the term "Bennett fracture" in 1882, referring to the base of the first metacarpal fracture. The thumb is critical for pinch, and opposition fractures at this carpo-metacarpal joint are commonly surgically repaired. The strong traction of the abductor pollicis longus leads to unstable fractures; and greater than 1 mm of incongruity after conservative management should lead to repair.[88]

Damage to the ulnar collateral ligament of the thumb (Fig. 3.2) is often referred to as "gamekeeper's" or "skier's" thumb.[89] Acutely, it can tear the ligament, which is amenable to direct surgical repair if caught early, otherwise a ligament reconstruction is required.[23] Injury can significantly hamper sporting ability in ball handling, and therefore is not to be ignored.

Frequently seen in the sporting environment is proximal interphalangeal joint dislocation. A hinge joint with the capsular ligament, reinforced by accessory collateral ligaments, the volar plate is a membranous and fibrocartilaginous reinforment of the capsule. The volar plate is always damaged in distal dislocation, but collateral ligaments are likely to be damaged in Type II and III. These can be classified[89] as below:

Figure 3.13 Distal to the triangle

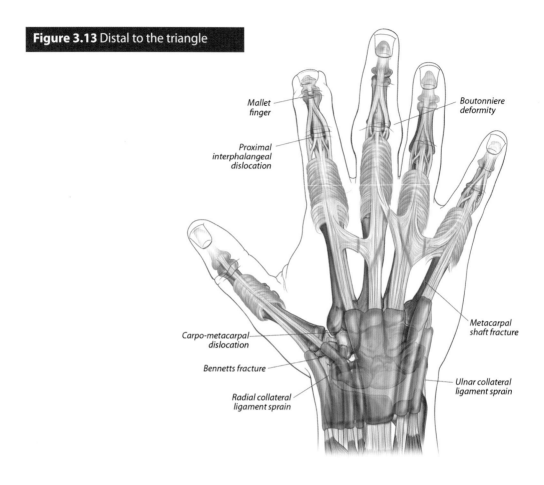

Mallet finger

Boutonniere deformity

Proximal interphalangeal dislocation

Metacarpal shaft fracture

Carpo-metacarpal dislocation

Bennetts fracture

Ulnar collateral ligament sprain

Radial collateral ligament sprain

> Type I – Hyperextension injury: volar plate damage, ligament damaged but joint surface intact

> Type II – Dorsal dislocation: major ligament damage

> Type III – Fracture dislocation: proximal dislocation with small avulsion; less than 40% of base is stable >40%, then unstable and requires surgery[90]

"Mallet finger" occurs as a result of rupture or avulsion of the extensor insertion at the distal inter-phalangeal joint. Commonly this is due to trauma forcing flexion against contracting extension, for example, when miscatching a ball.

Boutonniere deformity occurs in damage to the central slip of the extensor tendons, allowing it to slip either side of the proximal phalanx, pulling the middle phalanx into flexion, and the DIPJ into extension.

Flexor digitorum profundus avulsion, known as "Jersey finger", commonly affects the fourth finger when grabbing a jersey or shorts. The distal phalanx is hyperextended, while flexing the finger.

Define and align	Pathology	Listen and localize	Palpate and recreate	Alleviate and investigate
Distal to triangle	Carpometacarpal joint fracture/ dislocation	Usually stable due to ligament of distal row of carpal. Metacarpal joints	Swelling and rotational deformity when compared to non-injured hand	Plain film
	Metacarpal shaft fracture / dislocation	Most commonly 5th metacarpal fractured from striking object with closed fist, dorsal dislocation most common	Deformity, shortening and loss of dorsal knuckle control	Plain film
	Bennett's fracture	History of catching thumb and immediate pain	Swelling at base of thumb with instability and pain	Plain film
	Ulnar collateral ligament tear	Pain at base of thumb, history of hyperextension injury.[91] Weakness at pinching grip/key holding	Swelling at base of thumb, difficulty with grip, pain on stressing the ligament and gapping	Ultrasound imaging if in doubt
	PIPJ dislocation	Obvious click and pop and deformity	Deformity with dorsal disruption of joint line[90]	Plain film
	Radial collateral ligament sprain	Weakness in pinch grip	Radial deviation > 20° more than the contralateral side indicates rupture	
	Mallet finger	Stubbing finger with ball or bat. Sudden pain, audible pop	Tenderness over dorsal distal phalanx and DIPJ, inability to actively extend joint	Plain film to exclude >1/3 avulsion fracture or epiphyseal plate in prepubescent children
	Boutonniere deformity	Acute flexion when forced extension normally in ball sports	Finger flexion deformity and pain on extension and hyperextension of distal IPJ	None required, but may exclude plain film. Phalangeal fracture
	Flexor digitorum profundus rupture	Audible pop and hyperextension of finger tip when grabbing shirt	Affected finger extended , inability to flex the DIPJ	Plain film to exclude avulsion injury

Table 3.7 Distal to the triangle

Summary

It can be seen that, by differentiating the common pathological complaints of the wrist and hand into their anatomical origins, the differential diagnosis becomes significantly more manageable. The relationships to the triangles of the wrist and the volar clockfaces aid the clinician in focusing on the pain-generating structures, and exclude through systematic evaluation those normal and not contributory muscles and ligaments.

These cases are designed to lead the reader through the process of the triangle approach and the tables. The real-life clinical situation is not always as clear; in particular, the difference in definitions between acute and chronic presentations may help to narrow the diagnosis further, but the principles are the same.

The localization of the pain always helps with narrowing the diagnosis to the underlying anatomy, and, in the hand, most of the anatomy is directly palpable, assisting in this process. Some of the less common diagnoses have been excluded, so as not to overcomplicate the chapter, but the tables lead the reader to the most evidence-based discriminatory tests, where available in the current literature.

Case histories

Case 1

A 41-year-old full-time mum presents with a six-week history of right-wrist pain. She has been playing netball for the first time in a number of years, for her daughter's team. She was determined to keep up and, despite feeling they were passing the ball very hard, she is quite proud she didn't give up. She has been developing a pain and stiffness in her thumb, which is stopping her driving as she cannot grip the wheel.

Step 1: Define and align

Expose the patient properly; in order to examine the wrist properly, the elbow should also be exposed.

Define the triangle: locate the distal radius and ulna, and the base of the third metacarpal.

Align the patient's pain on the triangles. Here the pain is located to the radial side of the triangle.

The patient has localized the pain to the area "radial to the triangle". From this point, we recommend that the reader attempt to exclude the potential pathologies. From Table 3.6, the potential causal structures are:

Differential diagnosis

> scaphoid fracture
> De Quervain's disease
> distal radial epiphyseal injury
> distal radius fracture, Colles

We proceed to differentiate between these structures, step 2.

Step 2: Listen and localize

Addressing the question of scaphoid fracture we ask:

Q *Have you fallen on your wrist at all?*
A No, not that I remember.
Q *Have you injured your wrist in the past?*
A No, not at all, this is the first thing that has gone wrong.

Addressing the potential for De Quervain's disease we ask:

Q *Does it hurt when you grip?*
A Yes, that is when it is worse, or I notice it when doing up buttons and putting on clothes too.
Q *Does it hurt to move your thumb?*
A Yes, it hurts and feels as if there is sandpaper in my wrist.

Addressing the issue of distal epiphyseal fracture/distal fracture we ask:

Q *No falls or sudden pain in your wrist before the netball?*
A No, I've always been fit and well.

This narrows our differential diagnosis somewhat, and we proceed to examination to narrow it further.

Differential diagnosis

More likely
> De Quervain's disease

Less likely
> scaphoid fracture
> distal radial epiphyseal injury
> distal radius fracture, Colles'

By palpating painful structures, and recreating the pain through diagnostic maneuvers, we move toward a diagnosis, step 3.

Step 3: Palpate and re-create

We palpate the joint line of the CMPJ, and we find no tenderness, although flexing the PIPJ and DIPJ causes pain to be reproduced at the radial part of the thumb over the extensor pollicis brevis and abductor pollicis longus tendons, and tenderness at the posterior part of the line; this is worse in extension but we cannot palpate any clicking or movement.

In Finkelstein's test, the thumb is flexed into the palm of the hand, and the wrist is deviated ulnarly, to reproduce the stretch of the tendons, and re-create the symptoms.

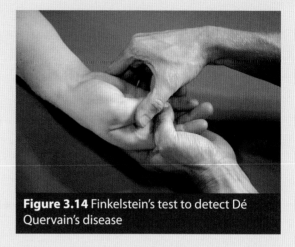

Figure 3.14 Finkelstein's test to detect Dé Quervain's disease

We may now proceed to step 4 to confirm our clinical suspicion, via an ultrasound-guided injection of local anesthetic, which relieves the pain associated with De Quervain's disease. A cortisone injection will also help to settle this down, but it is an overuse injury, and our advice is to graduate the return to sport to avoid such overuse injuries.

Case 2

A 23-year-old world-champion downhill mountain-bike racer complains of left-wrist pain. It started gradually, and he used to notice it at the end of a race but not during it; now it feels as if the damping of his front bike forks are not doing their job, as he feels a sharp pain in the wrist when descending and on big hills. He tells you that he struggles to grip the bars by the end of a race.

Step 1: Define and align

Expose the patient properly; in order to examine the wrist properly, the elbow should also be exposed.

Define the triangle: locate the distal radius and ulna, and the base of the third metacarpal.

Align the patient's pain on the triangles. Here the pain is located to the ulnar side of the triangle.

The patient has localized the pain to the area "ulnar to the triangle". From this point we recommend that the reader attempt to exclude the potential pathologies. From Table 3.3, the potential causal structures are:

Differential diagnosis
> TFCC tear
> ulnar impaction syndrome
> distal radioulnar joint instability
> ulnar nerve compression

> ECU tendinopathy
>
> ECU subluxation

We proceed to differentiate between these structures, step 2.

Step 2: Listen and localize
Addressing the question of TFCC injury we ask:
Q *Have you fallen on your wrist at all?*

A (Laughs) Yes, about 15 times a week, but it has never done this before. It does seem to swell now after racing, and is a bit stiff.

Q *Have you injured your wrist in the past?*

A No, I've never broken it before, but have dislocated my right elbow, had a broken clavicle on the left twice, and a humerus on right. My legs as well.

Q *Have you noticed a click or clunk?*

A Yes, when I move my hand to the side, it sometimes clunks and the pain gets better.

Q *Can you grip things the same with both hands?*

A No, I can't get the bike off the ute with my left hand by itself, as my grip feels a bit weaker.

Addressing the potential for ulnar impaction syndrome we ask:
Q *Has the range of movement of your wrist changed?*

A No, not really, I've always been tight in wrist extension, but that seems to be just related to how much time I spend gripping the bars.

Q *Does it hurt to move your fingers?*

A No, not at all.

Addressing the issue of ulnar nerve compression we ask:
Q *Any burning pain or numbness in your hand or fingers at all?*

A No, no tingling or numbness, some pain under the bones of the wrist, but I can't put my finger on it.

Addressing the issue of the extensor carpi ulnaris tendon we ask:
Q *Is there a snapping or flicking sensation in your wrist, or was there a sudden sharp pain?*

A No, just the occasional click.

Q *Have you been riding more recently?*

A Yes, this last year I've been riding double the amount of previous years, but it's paid off!

Q *Did you get wrist pain before this year?*

A Yes, I think it's been there for over a year, on and off. Only now is it stopping me riding.

This will narrow our differential diagnosis somewhat, and we proceed to examination to narrow it further.

Differential diagnosis

More likely
> TFCC tear
> ulnar impaction syndrome
> distal radioulnar joint instability

Less likely
> ulnar nerve compression
> ECU tendinopathy
> ECU subluxation

By palpating painful structures, and recreating the pain through diagnostic maneuvers, we move toward a diagnosis, step 3.

Step 3: Palpate and re-create

We palpate the ulnar border of the triangle, and find some point tenderness at the ulna between the flexor carpi ulnaris tendon and extensor carpi ulnaris tendon, We progress to perform a piano-key test, which is normal, and also a Tinel's test, which does not reproduce the pain he gets, but does cause some irritation. An ulnar impaction test reproduces the pain, and he confirms that this is his pain.

We may now proceed to step 4 to confirm our clinical suspicion via an MR arthrogram. It is possible that a plain

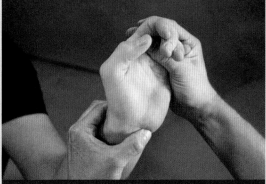

Figure 3.15 Triangular fibrocartilage complex integrity

film prior to this would confirm an elongated ulnar styloid, but, given that he has previously been asymptomatic despite riding for long periods, it is more likely that this is a TFCC tear, sustained either in a fall or due to the repetitive microtrauma of controlling the bike handlebars in descents. It is likely that this will require a surgical approach, in order to manage his pain. It is common to get some ulnar nerve irritation from a TFCC injury and, as such, not unusual to have a mixture of symptoms.

Case 3

A 30-year-old woman presents with pain in her dorsal wrist. She describes a fall from her mountain bike when her dogs ran in front of her front wheel, while out exercising them in the country, approximately two years ago, which she puts this down to. She grazed her elbows, arm, and hip, and was more concerned with the dogs at the time, but now has noticed a pain in her wrist when doing pushups at her "boot camp" class, and finds her tennis grip has weakened.

Step 1: Define and align

Expose the patient properly; in order to examine the wrist properly, the elbow should also be exposed.

Define the triangle: locate the distal radius and ulna, and the base of the third metacarpal.

Align the patient's pain on the triangles. Here the pain is located within the dorsal triangle.

The patient has localized the pain to the area "within the dorsal triangle". From this point we recommend that the reader attempt to exclude the potential pathologies. From Table 3.4, the potential causal structures are:

Differential diagnosis
> scapholunate ligament dissociation
> luntotriquetral instability
> Kienbock's disease
> lunate fracture
> ganglion
> intersection syndrome
> carpometacarpal dislocation/fracture
> inflammatory arthropathy

We proceed to differentiate between these structures, step 2.

Step 2: Listen and localize

Addressing the question of scapholunate ligament injury we ask:

Q *Do you remember the mechanism of the fall at all?*

A No, not really, but I think I put my hand out to break the fall.

Q *Have you injured your wrist in the past?*

A No, prior to this fall I had been relatively injury-free.

Q *Have you noticed any swelling on the back of your wrist?*

A Yes, when the pain is at its worst, there is a swelling at the back of the wrist, which stops me moving it through a full range.

Addressing the potential for lunotriquetral injury we ask:

Q *Have you noticed any clicks or clunks in the wrist?*

A Not really, just a swelling when it flares up.

Kienbock's disease is not appropriate; so addressing the issue of possible lunate fracture we ask:

Q *Has the range of movement of your wrist changed?*

A Yes, on occasions I cannot extend my wrist as normal.

Addressing the possibility of ganglion we ask:

Q *Is the swelling soft or hard at the back of your wrist?*

A It seems hard, it is not there all the time though.

Q *Do you have any burning pain or loss of sensation in your hand?*

A No, it feels normal.

Addressing the possibility of intersection syndrome we ask:

Q *Do you have a sensation of rubbing or creaking at the back of your wrist?*

A No, just a sharp pain when I get into position to do a pushup.

Q *Is your grip affected?*

A Yes, my grip strength is weaker, and my tennis grip is suffering.

Addressing the possibility of carpo-metacarpal fracture is unlikely, given the time until presentation, so we move on to inflammatory arthropathy; we ask:

Q *Are any other joints affected by swelling?*

A No, just the wrist; I do get some back pain at times, but I think this is an old injury.

Q *Is the joint painful and stiff in the morning when you wake up?*

A No, I only really notice it when training, or occasionally shopping.

Q *Do you have any eye irritation, eczematous skin changes, or other symptoms?*

A No, nothing like that.

This will narrow our differential diagnosis somewhat, and we proceed to examination to narrow it further.

Differential diagnosis

More likely

> scapholunate ligament dissociation

> lunotriquetral instability

Less likely

> Kienbock's disease

> lunate fracture

> ganglion

> intersection syndrome

> carpometacarpal dislocation/fracture

> inflammatory arthropathy

By palpating painful structures, and recreating the pain through diagnostic maneuvers, we move toward a diagnosis, step 3.

Step 3: Palpate and re-create

We palpate the joint line of the proximal border of the triangle, and find no distal radioulnar joint instability, with a normal piano-key test, and no tenderness at the ulnar collateral ligament.

On examining the joint range of movement, we see a bony excursion in the dorsal triangle on wrist flexion, and a reduction in extension by 15°. Moving on to special tests, we perform Watson's and Kleinman's shear tests.

When perfoming Watson's test, we recreate the pain, but do not feel the scaphoid move relative to the lunate.

Kleinman's test, with the examiner's contralateral thumb over the dorsal lunate with the wrist in neutral, and the ipsilateral thumb exerting a load through the pisotriqueral joint, re-creates the pain. Reagan's shuck test is also positive, with the examiner's hand ballotting the pisotriquetral bone in one hand, and the lunate in the other, also stressing the lunotriquetral ligament; this reproduces the pain.

Palpation of the lunate itself feels unstable, and is partially ballotable under examinating, but directly is not painful.

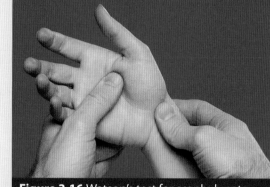

Figure 3.16 Watson's test for scaphulunate instability.

Looking at intersection syndrome, there is no pain on resisted flexion with the wrist in a cocked or extended position, and no synovitis or signs of inflammatory arthropathy.

We may now proceed to step 4 to confirm our clinical suspicion via an MR arthrogram, to identify the extent of injury to the scapholunate and luotriquetral ligaments. One can see that, although the examination can narrow the diagnosis, it is unable to differentiate the extent of the injury clinically.

Case 4

A 16-year-old male golfer presents with wrist pain. He tells you that he has been selected for his country in an international tournament, and that he needs to be fit for next month, but he can't grip the club, and he gets pain on hitting any balls from the mat in the practice nets. It is his non-dominant (left) hand which is affected. He has been playing golf since he was six years old, has not changed clubs recently, and has always hit the same ball, and cannot remember anything else that is relevant.

Step 1: Define and align

Expose the patient properly; in order to examine the wrist properly, the elbow should also be exposed.

Define the triangle: locate the distal radius and ulna, and the base of the third metacarpal.

Align the patient's pain on the triangles. Here the pain is located within the volar triangle.

The patient has localized the pain to the area "within the volar triangle". From this point we recommend that the reader attempt to exclude the potential pathologies. From Table 3.5, the potential causal structures are:

Differential diagnosis

> carpal tunnel syndrome
> hook of hamate fracture
> flexor carpi radialis tendinopathy
> flexor carpi ulnaris tendinopathy
> traumatic ulnar artery thrombosis
> pisiform fracture

We proceed to differentiate between these structures, step 2.

Step 2: Listen and localize

Addressing the question of carpal tunnel syndrome we ask:

Q *Do you get any burning sensations, or pins and needles and numbness, in the thumb or first or second fingers?*
A No, but I do get some numbness to the outside of my hand near the little finger.
Q *Have you injured your wrist in the past?*
A No, I have not missed any practice sessions ever because of injury.
Q *Have you noticed any swelling in your wrist?*
A No, it doesn't feel stiff or swollen, I just get this sharp pain in my grip.

Addressing the potential for hook of hamate injury we ask:

Q *Have you been hitting off a different mat, or do you remember a bad swing where you hit the ground?*
A Not really, I've been hitting maybe 500 more balls a week in the last few months, but can't remember any stub shot.
Q *Can you grip anything in your left hand?*
A Yes, I can clench my fist okay and pick up a bag, but nothing that is hard like a club.

Addressing the possibility of tendinopathy we ask:

Q *Is there pain when you move your wrist?*
A No, not really, it is mainly an impact and grip thing. If I move my wrist outward (he demonstrates ulnar deviation) it can occasionally twinge.
Q *Do you have a sensation of rubbing or creaking at the front or back of your wrist?*
A No, just a sharp pain.
Q *Are any other joints affected by swelling?*
A No.

Addressing the possibility of traumatic ulnar artery thrombosis we ask:

Q *Do you have any pain in the little fingers or do they feel cold?*

A No, the pain is in the wrist. I do get some tingling in the fifth finger, but only after hitting balls, if the wrist pain is already there.

Q *How long has it been painful, and has it become worse?*

A It has been a couple of weeks now that I have struggled, not really worse, but not any better.

This will narrow our differential diagnosis somewhat, and we proceed to examination to narrow it further.

Differential diagnosis

More likely

> hook of hamate injury

> pisiform fracture

Less likely

> carpal tunnel syndrome

> flexor carpi radialis tendinopathy

> flexor carpi ulnaris tendinopathy

> traumatic ulnar artery thrombosis

By palpating painful structures, and recreating the pain through diagnostic maneuvers, we move toward a diagnosis, step 3.

Step 3: Palpate and re-create

As you can see, it is the discrimating questions here which can narrow the diagnosis. It is not certain that the hook of the hamate is injured here, as there is the suggestion of involvement of the ulnar border of the triangle, and we may need to run through the differential diagnosis there, should the examination not prove fruitful. But the history is always extremely important.

The hamate is one of the first carpal bones to appear in the developing child, but does not ossify fully until around the age of 15[92] and, as such, appearances radiologically should be carefully examined, to check for disruption of secondary ossification in the pediatric athlete. Many countries such as Australia and the UK attempt to limit the number of balls hit or bowled in many sports, in order to limit the risk of overuse injuries, but this is difficult to enforce.

On examining the joint range of movement, we see normal flexion and extension, but ulnar deviation is reduced. The volar triangle here is useful, as we can work around the clockface to palpate all the relevant structures. The hamate is at the 10 o'clock position, and is tender to palpation, but it is also tender along the muscle belly of the opponens pollicis. Resisted flexion of the opponens is also painful.

Tinel's test is negative, as is Phalen's test, not causing pain at one minute. There is no swelling palpable, or crepitus beneath the flexor retinaculum on resisted wrist flexion, and hence tendinopathy is unlikely.

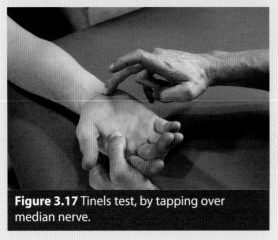

Palpation of the pisiform bone is painful, but resisted flexion of the wrist does not aggravate the symptoms.

We may now proceed to step 4 to confirm our clinical suspicion via a plain film. This is not very discriminatory in stress response, and an MRI may be of more use here in this pediatric athlete. Hook of the hamate fracture is rare, and less likely at the age of ossification, but a stress reaction due to the increase in balls and developing strength is much more likely. Plain film should be taken with carpal tunnel views to exclude a fracture of the body.

Figure 3.17 Tinels test, by tapping over median nerve.

Case 5

A 27-year-old skier complains of persistent pain in her left thumb, following a fall last season. It was swollen and sore after the injury, but seemed to settle down. She works as a schoolteacher, and plays a lot of tennis, and it does not affect her backhand, but she has started some tennis coaching, and finds the thumb is not increasingly sore.

Step 1: Define and align

Expose the patient properly; in order to examine the wrist properly, the elbow should also be exposed.

Define the triangle: locate the distal radius and ulna, and the base of the third metacarpal.

Align the patient's pain on the triangles. Here the pain is located within the dorsal triangle.

The patient has localized the pain to the area "within the dorsal triangle". From this point we recommend that the reader attempt to exclude the potential pathologies. From Table 3.4, the potential causal structures are:

Differential diagnosis
> carpometacarpal joint fracture/dislocation
> metacarpal shaft fracture
> Bennett's fracture
> ulnar collateral ligament of thumb
> radial collateral ligament of thumb

> proximal interphalangeal joint dislocation

> mallet finger

> boutonniere deformity

> flexor digitorum profundus avulsion rupture

We proceed to differentiate between these structures, step 2.

Step 2: Listen and localize

Addressing the question of carpometacarpal fracture or dislocation injury we ask:

Q *Do you remember the mechanism of the fall at all?*

A Yes, I fell and caught my thumb in the dry slope grid. It sort of was pulled backward and outward.

Q *Was it dislocated?*

A No, I could move it, but I didn't go to the emergency room, just didn't use it for a while.

Q *Have you noticed any swelling on the back of your wrist?*

A Yes, when the pain is at its worst, there is a swelling at the back of the wrist, which stops me moving it through a full range.

Addressing the potential for metacarpal shaft fracture we ask:

Q *Was your fist open or closed?*

A It was pulled open, and I lost my ski pole.

Q *You didn't land on the ground with your fist closed?*

A No, I fell and put out the flat of my hand to break the fall.

Addressing the issue of possible Bennett's fracture we ask:

Q *Has the range of movement of your thumb changed?*

A Yes, I think I have not as much flexion of my thumb, and it feels unstable.

Addressing the possibility of the collateral ligaments of the thumb we ask:

Q *Is the swelling soft or hard at the back of your wrist?*

A It seems hard, it is not there all the time though.

Q *Do you have any weakness in your pinch grip?*

A Yes, opening my front door with a key is sometimes difficult.

Addressing the possibility of mallet finger, boutonniere deformity, and flexor digitorium profundus injury are not relevant here, as we are dealing with the thumb.

This will narrow our differential diagnosis somewhat, and we proceed to examination to narrow it further.

Differential diagnosis

More likely

> Bennett's fracture

> ulnar collateral ligament of thumb

> radial collateral ligament of thumb

Less likely

> carpometacarpal joint fracture/dislocation

> metacarpal shaft fracture

> proximal interphalangeal joint dislocation

> mallet finger

> boutonniere deformity

> flexor digitorum profundus avulsion rupture

By palpating painful structures, and recreating the pain through diagnostic maneuvers, we move toward a diagnosis, step 3.

Step 3: Palpate and re-create

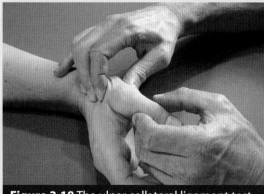

Figure 3.18 The ulnar collateral ligament test with 10 degrees of flexion at MCPJ

We examine the range of movement of the thumb, and find a normal range of movement, but on extension, we find a re-creation of pain under the proximal joint line, and proceed to stress-test the ulnar collateral ligamant of the first metacarpophalangeal joint. The thumb is not rotated, compared to the contralateral side, and, as such, an old fracture of the metacarpal is unlikely, and there is no current swelling.

We may now proceed to step 4 to exclude an old avulsion fracture of a concomitant metacarpal fracture, but there is no radiation. It is likely that this will require a surgical opinion on delayed repair, as the ulnar collateral ligament appears clinically to be ruptured. One can see that, although the examination can narrow the diagnosis, it is unable to differentiate the extent of the injury clinically.

References

1. DiFiori JP, Puffer JC, Aish B, Dorey F. Wrist pain, distal radial physeal injury, and ulnar variance in young gymnasts: does a relationship exist? Am J Sports Med. 2002 Nov–Dec; 30(6):879–85.
2. Rettig AC. Athletic injuries of the wrist and hand. Part I: traumatic injuries of the wrist. Am J Sports Med. 2003 Nov–Dec; 31(6):1038–48.
3. Rettig AC. Athletic injuries of the wrist and hand: part II: overuse injuries of the wrist and traumatic injuries to the hand. Am J Sports Med. 2004 Jan–Feb; 32(1):262–73.
4. Franklyn-Miller A, Falvey E, McCrory P. Problem-based learning in sports medicine: the way forward or a backward step? Br J Sports Med. 2007 October 1, 2007; 41(10):623–24.
5. Hagg U, Taranger J. Skeletal stages of the hand and wrist as indicators of the pubertal growth spurt. Acta Odontol Scand. 1980; 38(3):187–200.
6. Dvorak J, George J, Junge A, Hodler J. Application of MRI of the wrist for age determination in international U-17 soccer competitions. Br J Sports Med. 2007 Aug; 41(8):497–500.
7. Lewis OJ, Hamshere RJ, Bucknill TM. The anatomy of the wrist joint. J Anat. 1970 May; 106(Pt 3):539–52.
8. Kuo CE, Wolfe SW. Scapholunate instability: current concepts in diagnosis and management. J Hand Surg Am. 2008 Jul–Aug; 33(6):998–1013.
9. Palmer AK, Werner FW. The triangular fibrocartilage complex of the wrist – anatomy and function. J Hand Surg Am. 1981 Mar; 6(2):153–62.
10. Taleisnik J. The ligaments of the wrist. J Hand Surg Am. 1976 Sep; 1(2):110–18.
11. Kijima Y, Viegas SF. Wrist anatomy and biomechanics. J Hand Surg Am. 2009 Oct; 34(8):1555–63.
12. Kawamura K, Chung KC. Management of wrist injuries. Plast Reconstr Surg. 2007 Oct; 120(5):73e–89e.
13. Berger RA, Imeada T, Berglund L, An KN. Constraint and material properties of the subregions of the scapholunate interosseous ligament. J Hand Surg Am. 1999 Sep; 24(5):953–62.
14. Hauger O, Chung CB, Lektrakul N, Botte MJ, Trudell D, Boutin RD, et al. Pulley system in the fingers: normal anatomy and simulated lesions in cadavers at MR imaging, CT, and US with and without contrast material distention of the tendon sheath. Radiology. 2000 Oct; 217(1):201–12.
15. Dailey SW, Palmer AK. The role of arthroscopy in the evaluation and treatment of triangular fibrocartilage complex injuries in athletes. Hand Clin. 2000 Aug; 16(3):461–76.
16. Bednar MS, Arnoczky SP, Weiland AJ. The microvasculature of the triangular fibrocartilage complex: its clinical significance. J Hand Surg Am. 1991 Nov; 16(6):1101–05.
17. Anderson ML, Larson AN, Moran SL, Cooney WP, Amrami KK, Berger RA. Clinical comparison of arthroscopic versus open repair of triangular fibrocartilage complex tears. J Hand Surg Am. 2008 May–Jun; 33(5):675–82.
18. Giachino AA, McIntyre AI, Guy KJ, Conway AF. Ulnar styloid triquetral impaction. Hand Surg. 2007; 12(2):123–34.
19. Tomaino MM, Gainer M, Towers JD. Carpal impaction with the ulnar styloid process: treatment with partial styloid resection. J Hand Surg Br. 2001 Jun; 26(3):252–55.
20. Johnston K, Durand D, Hildebrand KA. Chronic volar distal radioulnar joint instability: joint capsular plication to restore function. Can J Surg. 2009 Apr; 52(2):112–18.
21. Kihara H, Short WH, Werner FW, Fortino MD, Palmer AK. The stabilizing mechanism of the distal radioulnar joint during pronation and supination. J Hand Surg Am. 1995 Nov; 20(6):930–36.
22. Beaton DE, Katz JN, Fossel AH, Wright JG, Tarasuk V, Bombardier C. Measuring the whole or the parts? Validity, reliability, and responsiveness of the Disabilities of the Arm, Shoulder and Hand outcome measure in different regions of the upper extremity. J Hand Ther. 2001 Apr–Jun; 14(2):128–46.
23. Morgan WJ, Slowman LS. Acute hand and wrist injuries in athletes: evaluation and management. J Am Acad Orthop Surg. 2001 Nov–Dec; 9(6):389–400.
24. Patel D, Dean C, Baker RJ. The hand in sports: an update on the clinical anatomy and physical examination. Prim Care. 2005 Mar; 32(1):71–89.
25. Golimbu CN, Firooznia H, Melone CP, Jr., Rafii M, Weinreb J, Leber C. Tears of the triangular fibrocartilage of the wrist: MR imaging. Radiology. 1989 Dec; 173(3):731–33.
26. Topper SM, Wood MB, Ruby LK. Ulnar styloid impaction syndrome. J Hand Surg Am. 1997 Jul; 22(4):699–704.
27. Escobedo EM, Bergman AG, Hunter JC. MR imaging of ulnar impaction. Skeletal Radiol. 1995 Feb; 24(2):85–90.
28. Tay SC, Tomita K, Berger RA. The "ulnar fovea sign" for defining ulnar wrist pain: an analysis of sensitivity and specificity. J Hand Surg Am. 2007 Apr; 32(4):438–44.

29. Chan JC, Tiong WH, Hennessy MJ, Kelly JL. A Guyon's canal ganglion presenting as occupational overuse syndrome: A case report. J Brachial Plex Peripher Nerve Inj. 2008; 3:4.

30. Allende C, Le Viet D. Extensor carpi ulnaris problems at the wrist – classification, surgical treatment and results. J Hand Surg Br. 2005 Jun; 30(3):265–72.

31. Montalvan B, Parier J, Brasseur JL, Le Viet D, Drape JL. Extensor carpi ulnaris injuries in tennis players: a study of 28 cases. Br J Sports Med. 2006 May; 40(5):424–29; discussion 9.

32. Jones WA. Beware the sprained wrist. The incidence and diagnosis of scapholunate instability. J Bone Joint Surg Br. 1988 Mar; 70(2):293–97.

33. Weber ER. Concepts governing the rotational shift of the intercalated segment of the carpus. Orthop Clin North Am. 1984 Apr; 15(2):193–207.

34. Manuel J, Moran SL. The diagnosis and treatment of scapholunate instability. Hand Clin. Feb; 26(1):129–44.

35. Mayfield JK. Mechanism of carpal injuries. Clin Orthop Relat Res. 1980 Jun; (149):45–54.

36. Jackson WT, Protas JM. Snapping scapholunate subluxation. J Hand Surg Am. 1981 Nov; 6(6):590–94.

37. Watson HK, Weinzweig J, Zeppieri J. The natural progression of scaphoid instability. Hand Clin. 1997 Feb; 13(1):39–49.

38. Schuind F, Eslami S, Ledoux P. Kienbock's disease. J Bone Joint Surg Br. 2008 Feb; 90(2):133–39.

39. Hofmeister EP, Faruqui S. Two unusual cases of coronal lunate fracture. Orthopedics. 2009 Apr; 32(4).

40. Geissler WB. Carpal fractures in athletes. Clin Sports Med. 2001 Jan; 20(1):167–88.

41. Brolin I. Post-traumatic lesions of the lunate bone. Acta Orthop Scand. 1964; 34:167–82.

42. Chloros GD, Wiesler ER, Poehling GG. Current concepts in wrist arthroscopy. Arthroscopy. 2008 Mar; 24(3):343–54.

43. Thornburg LE. Ganglions of the hand and wrist. J Am Acad Orthop Surg. 1999 Jul–Aug; 7(4):231–38.

44. McNally E, Wilson D, Seiler S. Rowing injuries. Semin Musculoskelet Radiol. 2005 Dec; 9(4):379–96.

45. Browne J, Helms CA. Intersection syndrome of the forearm. Arthritis Rheum. 2006 Jun; 54(6):2038.

46. Henderson JJ, Arafa MA. Carpometacarpal dislocation. An easily missed diagnosis. J Bone Joint Surg Br. 1987 Mar; 69(2):212–14.

47. Rasch EK, Hirsch R, Paulose–Ram R, Hochberg MC. Prevalence of rheumatoid arthritis in persons 60 years of age and older in the United States: effect of different methods of case classification. Arthritis Rheum. 2003 Apr; 48(4):917–26.

48. Arnett FC. Revised criteria for the classification of rheumatoid arthritis. Bull Rheum Dis. 1989; 38(5):1–6.

49. Dalbeth N, Smith T, Gray S, Doyle A, Antill P, Lobo M, et al. Cellular characterisation of magnetic resonance imaging bone oedema in rheumatoid arthritis; implications for pathogenesis of erosive disease. Ann Rheum Dis. 2009 Feb; 68(2):279–82.

50. Carter JD, Hudson AP. The evolving story of chlamydia-induced reactive arthritis. Curr Opin Rheumatol. May 4.

51. Watson HK, Ashmead Dt, Makhlouf MV. Examination of the scaphoid. J Hand Surg Am. 1988 Sep; 13(5):657–60.

52. Frankel VH. The Terry-Thomas sign. Clin Orthop Relat Res. 1977 Nov–Dec; (129):321–22.

53. Herbert TJ, Faithfull RG, McCann DJ, Ireland J. Bilateral arthrography of the wrist. J Hand Surg Br. 1990 May; 15(2):233–35.

54. Bain GI, Munt J, Turner PC. New advances in wrist arthroscopy. Arthroscopy. 2008 Mar; 24(3):355–67.

55. Kleinman WB, Carroll Ct. Scapho-trapezio-trapezoid arthrodesis for treatment of chronic static and dynamic scapho-lunate instability: a 10-year perspective on pitfalls and complications. J Hand Surg Am. 1990 May; 15(3):408–14.

56. Reagan DS, Linscheid RL, Dobyns JH. Lunotriquetral sprains. J Hand Surg Am. 1984 Jul; 9(4):502–14.

57. Chung KC, Spilson MS, Kim MH. Is negative ulnar variance a risk factor for Kienbock's disease? A meta-analysis. Ann Plast Surg. 2001 Nov; 47(5):494–99.

58. Plate AM, Lee SJ, Steiner G, Posner MA. Tumorlike lesions and benign tumors of the hand and wrist. J Am Acad Orthop Surg. 2003 Mar–Apr; 11(2):129–41.

59. Wood MB, Dobyns JH. Sports-related extra-articular wrist syndromes. Clin Orthop Relat Res. 1986 Jan; (202): 93–102.

60. Bora FW, Jr, Didizian NH. The treatment of injuries to the carpometacarpal joint of the little finger. J Bone Joint Surg Am. 1974 Oct; 56(7):1459–63.

61. Punzi L, Cimmino MA, Frizziero L, Gerloni V, Grassi W, Modena V, et al. [Italian Society of Rheumatology (SIR) recommendations for performing arthrocentesis]. Reumatismo. 2007 Jul–Sep; 59(3):227–34.

62. Omer GE, Jr. Median nerve compression at the wrist. Hand Clin. 1992 May; 8(2):317–24.

63. Stevens JC, Sun S, Beard CM, O'Fallon WM, Kurland LT. Carpal tunnel syndrome in Rochester, Minnesota, 1961 to 1980. Neurology. 1988 Jan; 38(1):134–38.

64. Bland JD, Rudolfer SM. Clinical surveillance of carpal tunnel syndrome in two areas of the United Kingdom, 1991–2001. J Neurol Neurosurg Psychiatry. 2003 Dec; 74(12):1674–79.
65. Szabo RM, Slater RR, Jr, Farver TB, Stanton DB, Sharman WK. The value of diagnostic testing in carpal tunnel syndrome. J Hand Surg Am. 1999 Jul; 24(4):704–14.
66. Aroori S, Spence RA. Carpal tunnel syndrome. Ulster Med J. 2008 Jan; 77(1):6–17.
67. Katz JN, Stirrat CR, Larson MG, Fossel AH, Eaton HM, Liang MH. A self-administered hand symptom diagram for the diagnosis and epidemiologic study of carpal tunnel syndrome. J Rheumatol. 1990 Nov, 17(11):1495–98.
68. Keles I, Karagulle Kendi AT, Aydin G, Zog SG, Orkun S. Diagnostic precision of ultrasonography in patients with carpal tunnel syndrome. Am J Phys Med Rehabil. 2005 Jun; 84(6):443–50.
69. Hirano K, Inoue G. Classification and treatment of hamate fractures. Hand Surg. 2005; 10(2–3):151–57.
70. Foucher G, Schuind F, Merle M, Brunelli F. Fractures of the hook of the hamate. J Hand Surg Br. 1985 Jun; 10(2):205–10.
71. Jablecki CK, Andary MT, So YT, Wilkins DE, Williams FH. Literature review of the usefulness of nerve conduction studies and electromyography for the evaluation of patients with carpal tunnel syndrome. AAEM Quality Assurance Committee. Muscle Nerve. 1993 Dec; 16(12):1392–414.
72. Whalen JL, Bishop AT, Linscheid RL. Nonoperative treatment of acute hamate hook fractures. J Hand Surg Am. 1992 May; 17(3):507–11.
73. Ryan WG. Calcific tendinitis of flexor carpi ulnaris: an easy misdiagnosis. Arch Emerg Med. 1993 Dec; 10(4):321–23.
74. Taute BM, Behrmann C, Cappeller WA, Podhaisky H. [Ultrasound image of the hypothenar hammer syndrome]. Ultraschall Med. 1998 Oct; 19(5):220–24.
75. Gimenez DC, Gilabert OV, Ruiz JG, Muns CY, Alter JB, Cubells MD. Ultrasound and magnetic resonance angiography features of post-traumatic ulnar artery pseudoaneurysm: a case report and review of the literature. Skeletal Radiol. 2009 Sep; 38(9):929–32.
76. Wick MC, Weiss RJ, Arora R, Gabl M, Gruber J, Jaschke W, et al. Enthesiopathy of the flexor carpi ulnaris at the pisiform: Findings of high-frequency sonography. Eur J Radiol. Jan 8.
77. Knobloch K, Spies M, Busch KH, Vogt PM. Sclerosing therapy and eccentric training in flexor carpi radialis tendinopathy in a tennis player. Br J Sports Med. 2007 Dec; 41(12):920–21.
78. Munk B, Frokjaer J, Larsen CF, Johannsen HG, Rasmussen LL, Edal A, et al. Diagnosis of scaphoid fractures. A prospective multicenter study of 1,052 patients with 160 fractures. Acta Orthop Scand. 1995 Aug; 66(4):359–60.
79. Kozin SH. Incidence, mechanism, and natural history of scaphoid fractures. Hand Clin. 2001 Nov; 17(4):515–24.
80. Powell JM, Lloyd GJ, Rintoul RF. New clinical test for fracture of the scaphoid. Can J Surg. 1988 Jul; 31(4):237–38.
81. Ilyas AM, Ast M, Schaffer AA, Thoder J. De Quervain tenosynovitis of the wrist. J Am Acad Orthop Surg. 2007 Dec; 15(12):757–64.
82. Volpe A, Pavoni M, Marchetta A, Caramaschi P, Biasi D, Zorzi C, et al. Ultrasound differentiation of two types of De Quervain's disease: the role of retinaculum. Ann Rheum Dis. May; 69(5):938–39.
83. Jeyapalan K, Choudhary S. Ultrasound-guided injection of triamcinolone and bupivacaine in the management of De Quervain's disease. Skeletal Radiol. 2009 Nov; 38(11):1099–103.
84. DiFiori JP, Puffer JC, Aish B, Dorey F. Wrist pain in young gymnasts: frequency and effects upon training over 1 year. Clin J Sport Med. 2002 Nov; 12(6):348–53.
85. Tolat AR, Sanderson PL, De Smet L, Stanley JK. The gymnast's wrist: acquired positive ulnar variance following chronic epiphyseal injury. J Hand Surg Br. 1992 Dec; 17(6):678–81.
86. Hanel DP, Jones MD, Trumble TE. Wrist fractures. Orthop Clin North Am. 2002 Jan; 33(1):35–57, vii.
87. Ganel A, Engel J, Oster Z, Farine I. Bone scanning in the assessment of fractures of the scaphoid. J Hand Surg Am. 1979 Nov, 4(6):540–43.
88. Nagaoka M, Nagao S, Matsuzaki H. Trapeziometacarpal joint instability after Bennett's fracture-dislocation. J Orthop Sci. 2005 Jul; 10(4):374–77.
89. Chinchalkar SJ, Gan BS. Management of proximal interphalangeal joint fractures and dislocations. J Hand Ther. 2003 Apr–Jun; 16(2):117–28.
90. Palmer RE. Joint injuries of the hand in athletes. Clin Sports Med. 1998 Jul; 17(3):513–31.
91. Lee SJ, Montgomery K. Athletic hand injuries. Orthop Clin North Am. 2002 Jul; 33(3):547–54.
92. Andress MR, Peckar VG. Fracture of the hook of the hamate. Br J Radiol. 1970 Feb; 43(506):141–43.

The groin triangle

Introduction

C hronic groin pain is a common presentation in sports medicine practise. Studies in professional sports have found groin injury to be the fourth most common injury affecting soccer players[1] and the third most common injury in Australian rules football.[2] It also has a high prevalence in ice hockey,[3] and rugby,[4,5] and is increasingly diagnosed in American football.[6-8]

To focus purely on the incidence of groin strain provides an incomplete picture, however, as the morbidity attached to chronic groin pain means that it comes behind only fractures, and joint reconstruction, in terms of lost time from sport due to injury.[4,5]

Sports with a high incidence of groin injury often involve kicking and twisting movements while running. These actions place strain on fascial and musculoskeletal structures which are fixed to a number of bony anatomical points in close proximity. The resultant tissue damage, and/or entrapment of anatomical structures, may cause pain.

This chapter discusses the anatomy of the painful groin. The triangle approach allows the clinician to discriminate more easily between pathological conditions, and target their investigation and subsequent management to specific diagnoses.

The joint

The pubic symphysis is a linear (continuous) joint that allows a little movement (amphiarthrodial). It is a non-synovial joint, the pubic ends of which are lined with hyaline cartilage, and separated by a fibrocartilage disc. The union of the superior and inferior pubic ramus forms the pubic bone. The anterior, posterior, superior, and inferior ligaments provide the stability of the joint. The superior ligament receives fibers from the rectus abdominis, external oblique, gracilis, and adductor longus. The pubic symphysis allows small movements in superior and inferior directions, but it may also be compressed or distracted (separated). The main function of the joint is similar to that of the sacroiliac joint: as a shock absorber during walking and running. Relaxation of the ligaments during pregnancy, due to high levels of the hormone relaxin, facilitates expansion of the symphysis width to (in some cases) 9 mm, increasing flexibility, which is helpful during childbirth.

Nerves and blood vessels

As we encounter nerves and blood vessels passing through the triangle they are discussed, but an overview is provided here.

The blood supply (Fig. 4.1)

The **aorta bifurcates** to the left of the midline at the level of the fourth lumbar vertebra. The common iliac artery passes inferolaterally to bifurcate just anterior to the sacroiliac joint, into the internal and external iliac arteries.

The **internal iliac artery** supplies the structures of the pelvis and gluteal area, as well as the reproductive organs, and is the origin of the obturator artery that supplies the muscles of the medial compartment of the thigh.

The **external iliac artery** passes downwards and obliquely along the medial aspect of the psoas major to the mid-point of the inguinal ligament (midway between the ASIS and the pubic symphysis). Here it enters the thigh, and becomes the femoral artery.

The **femoral artery** enters the femoral canal, invested in a sheath of fascia, and gives off the arteria profunda femoris branch. It passes inferomedially above the iliopsoas, pectineus, adductor longus, and adductor magnus, where it enters the adductor canal, and becomes the popliteal artery.

The **arteria profunda femoris** (deep femoral artery) is the largest branch of the femoral artery, supplying most of the muscles of the thigh (extensor and flexor). It arises from the lateral aspect of the femoral artery, about 3–4 cm below the inguinal ligament, medial to the greater trochanter triangle. The artery gives off three or four perforating arteries. These supply the muscles in the flexor and medial compartments of the thigh. Branches include the **lateral circumflex femoral artery**, and the medial circumflex femoral artery, which supply a part of the trochanteric anastomosis and the cruciate anastomosis of the hip.

The nerves (Fig. 4.1)

The **femoral nerve** arises from the second, third, and fourth lumbar nerves. In the pelvis, it descends on the psoas, to pass beneath the inguinal ligament, where it divides into posterior and anterior divisions. The anterior division supplies much of the skin of the thigh, via the intermediate cutaneous nerve and the medial cutaneous nerve; it supplies muscular branches

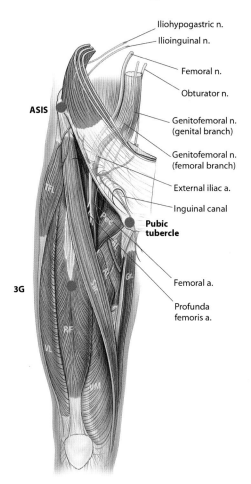

Figure 4.1 Anatomy of the groin		
TFL	=	tensor fasciae latae
Pec	=	pectineus
AL	=	adductor longus
Sar	=	sartorius
Gr	=	gracilis
RF	=	rectus femoris
VL	=	vastus lateralis
VM	=	vastus medialis
ASIS	=	anterior superior iliac spine
3G	=	the 3G point

Iliohypogastric n.
Ilioinguinal n.
Femoral n.
Obturator n.
ASIS
Genitofemoral n. (genital branch)
Genitofemoral n. (femoral branch)
External iliac a.
Inguinal canal
Pubic tubercle
3G
Femoral a.
Profunda femoris a.

to the pectineus and sartorius. The posterior division supplies muscular branches to all of the muscles of the anterior compartment of the thigh (the vasti and the rectus femoris), and articular branches to the knee joint. Its main cutaneous branch is the saphenous nerve, which supplies much of the medial leg below the knee.

The **obturator nerve** arises from the anterior rami of the second, third, and fourth lumbar nerves running along the body of the psoas, exiting the pelvis through the obturator foramen. The nerve divides in the obturator canal into anterior and posterior divisions. The anterior branch innervates the adductor longus, brevis, gracilis, and, occasionally, the pectineus. It supplies sensory innervation to the skin, and the fascia of the inner distal thirds of the medial thigh. The posterior branch supplies the adductor magnus.[9]

Landmarks of the groin triangle

The anatomical apex points of the triangle are as follows:

> anterior superior iliac spine (ASIS)

> pubic tubercle

> 3G point

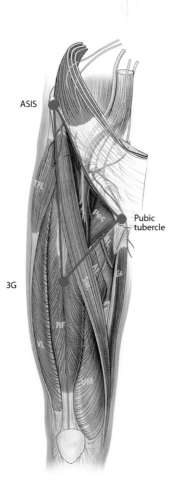

Figure 4.2 The groin triangle		
TFL	=	tensor fasciae latae
Pec	=	pectineus
AL	=	adductor longus
Sar	=	sartorius
Gr	=	gracilis
RF	=	rectus femoris
VL	=	vastus lateralis
VM	=	vastus medialis
ASIS	=	anterior superior iliac spine
3G	=	the 3G point

The **anterior superior iliac spine (ASIS)** is the salient physical landmark when the lower limb is viewed in the lateral decubitus position. From this position, it marks the most anterior projection of the structures responsible for abduction, extension, and lateral rotation of the hip, namely, the gluteals, and tensor fasciae latae. It is the origin of the sartorius and inguinal ligaments. The iliac crest and the ASIS together act as anchor points for the thoracolumbar fascia and its continuation – the fascia lata of the thigh. Just inferior to the ASIS lies the anterior inferior iliac spine (AIIS), the origin of the rectus femoris muscle. Inferior and medial to the ASIS, the lateral femoral cutaneous nerve may be compressed as it passes beneath the inguinal ligament.

The **pubic tubercle** is an anterior projection from the body of the pubis which is the attachment of the inguinal ligament. It is an important structure in the clarification of groin pathology, as it marks the insertion of the rectus abdominis superiorly, and the adductor longus inferiorly, and it forms part of the floor of the superficial inguinal ring.

The **3G point** in the anterior coronal plane is the mid-point between the ASIS and the superior pole of the patella.

Anatomical relations of the borders of the groin triangle

Superior border of the groin triangle

The line between the pubic tubercle and the ASIS forms the superior border of the triangle. This corresponds to the anatomical position of the inguinal ligament – a thickening of the aponeurosis of the external oblique muscle. Superior to this line, and working from the pubic tubercle medially to the ASIS laterally, the following structures will be encountered:

> rectus abdominis and rectus abdominis sheath insertions

> internal oblique, external oblique, and transversus abdominis insertions and aponeuroses

> ilioinguinal, iliohypogastric, and genital branch of the genitofemoral nerve

> superficial inguinal ring and conjoint tendon

> inguinal canal

> pectineus

> femoral vein

> femoral artery

> femoral nerve

> deep inguinal ring

> conjoint tendon of the iliopsoas as it passes under the lateral third of the inguinal ligament

> visceral contents of the abdomen and pelvis

> sartorius

Fascia, canals and aponeuroses

The insertion of the rectus abdominis and its sheath are intimately related to the aponeuroses of the oblique and transversus abdominis. Where these structures converge in the lower abdomen, they "revolve" around the potential space that is the inguinal canal. The inguinal canal is approximately 4 cm in length – a cylindrical potential space which transmits the spermatic cord and the ilioinguinal nerve in males, and the round ligament of the uterus and the ilioinguinal nerve in females.

The inguinal canal commences at the internal inguinal ring, located between the mid-inguinal point (situated midway between the anterior superior iliac spine and the pubic symphysis), and the mid-point of the inguinal ligament.[10] The transversalis fascia blends with the conjoint tendon (a confluence of the internal oblique and the transversalis fasciae) to form the posterior wall of the inguinal canal. The superficial inguinal ring, an opening in the external oblique aponeurosis (the anterior wall of the canal), is situated a centimeter above and lateral to the pubic tubercle. The inguinal ligament, a thickening of the external oblique aponeurosis, forms the floor of the inguinal canal. There is direct continuity with the fascia lata of the thigh.

The **rectus abdominis** are paired muscles, contained within the rectus sheath, which run from the xiphisternum to the pubis, separated by the linea alba (literally "white line" – a joining of the aponeuroses of the recti). The recti are indented by tendinous inscriptions which create the "six pack". This may, however, vary to be an "eight pack" or even be asymmetrical. Supplied by the seventh to twelfth anterior thoracic rami (thoraco-abdominal nerves), the recti are important flexors of the lumbar spine for motions such as an abdominal "crunch".

The **external oblique muscle** arises from the lower eight ribs (fifth to twelfth). The digitations, or slips, arise from the ribs and the costal cartilages, and may be divided into two groups.

The upper five slips interdigitate with the slips of the serratus anterior; they decrease in size from superior to inferior, and run inferiorly and anteriorly. They form an aponeurosis at the mid-clavicular line, passing above the rectus sheath to join the contralateral aponeurosis at the linea alba. The slips from the lower three ribs interdigitate with the latissimus dorsi origins. They diminish in size from superior to inferior. Fibers run directly inferior, inserting into the anterior half of the outer lip of the iliac crest. Nerve supply to the external oblique is via the seventh to twelfth anterior thoracic rami (thoraco-abdominal nerves). Contraction of the external oblique raises intra-abdominal pressure, and may also rotate the trunk to the opposite side.

The **internal oblique muscle** lies directly beneath the external oblique. Fibers arise from the thoracolumbar fascia, the anterior two-thirds of the iliac crest (the upper part of the hip bone) and the lateral half of the inguinal ligament, running superiorly and medially to insert into the length of the linea alba and the inferior borders of the lower three ribs (tenth, eleventh, and twelfth). The internal oblique, for the most part, is supplied by the seventh to twelfth anterior thoracic rami (thoraco-abdominal nerves) but the most inferior section, the conjoint tendon, is supplied by the iliohypogastric and ilioinguinal nerves. It aids respiration by drawing the ribs downward. It is also a "same-side" rotator, acting in conjunction with the contralateral external oblique to pull the trunk toward the ilium, from which it arises.

Transversus abdominis is the deepest of the three abdominal wall muscles. It arises from the lateral aspect of the abdomen, from the lateral third of the inguinal ligament, the ilium, the thoracolumbar fascia, and from the inner surfaces of the cartilages of the lower six ribs, interdigitating with the diaphragm. The transversus aponeurosis (a broad, flattened tendon) inserts along the entire midline at the linea alba. From the xiphisternum to the level of the umbilicus, it passes behind the rectus abdominis. Below this level, it passes in front of the rectus. At its most inferior point, it blends with the internal oblique aponeurosis to form the conjoint tendon. The conjoint tendon is innervated as described above by the iliohypogastric and ilioinguinal nerves. The remainder of the muscle is supplied by the eighth to twelfth anterior thoracic rami (thoraco-abdominal nerves). The function of the transversus is to raise intra-abdominal pressure, and to aid in thoracic[11], abdominal, and pelvic stability (core stability).

Neural structures

The anatomy of the ilioinguinal nerve, the iliohypogastric nerve, and the genital branch of the genitofemoral nerves is extremely variable. Between them, they supply the skin of the lower abdomen, the medial thigh, and the scrotum.[12]

The **pectineus** is the most anterior of the adductors, and also functions as a hip flexor. It arises from the pectineal line on the superior pubic ramus, as far medially as the pubic tubercle. Fibers also derive from the muscle's aponeurosis. A quadrangular, flat muscle, the pectineus, inserts between the lesser trochanter and the linea aspera at the pectineal line of the femur. The femoral nerve supplies the pectineus.

The conjoint tendon of the iliopsoas is discussed in depth in Chapter 5, but we include it here, as it must always be examined in the investigation and management of groin pain. Holmich et al. showed that iliopsoas pathology was present as either a primary or a secondary cause of groin pain in 55% of one series of groin-pain cases reviewed.[11]

The sartorius is a thin, ribbon-like muscle which passes from the ASIS obliquely across the front of the thigh, to join the tendons of the gracilis and the semitendinosus. It inserts into the medial aspect of the tibia at the pes anserinus. Supplied by the femoral nerve, the sartorius assists in the flexion, abduction, and lateral rotation of the hip, and the flexion of the knee.

Medial border of the groin triangle

The inferior line from the pubic tubercle to the 3G point forms the medial border of the triangle. Although neither the medial nor the lateral border of the triangle comprises a muscular line, in both instances they work to separate the clinically important groups of structures that lie on either side of them. Medial to the border lie the adductor muscles, which are encountered in the following order when moving from superficial to deep:

> adductor longus

> gracilis

> adductor brevis

> adductor magnus

> inferior pubic ramus

> long saphenous vein

> obturator nerve

The adductor longus and the gracilis are the most superficial, and the other adductor muscles (the brevis and the magnus) arise more posterolaterally along the inferior pubic ramus. The ramus forms a direct continuum between the pubic body and the ischial tuberosity.

The **adductor longus** arises from the 6–7 o'clock position on the pubic tubercle (see the pubic clock diagram, Fig. 4.4). It arises via a tendinous and muscular origin[13]. At the pubis, there is a tendon: muscle ratio of 2:1, the muscular component increasing distally. The muscle passes inferolaterally in a fan shape, to insert into the medial aspect of the linea aspera. It is supplied by the anterior branch of the obturator nerve, and is a powerful adductor of the femur, as well as a medial rotator. It also aids in the flexion of an extended hip, and it is particularly active in the motion of kicking a ball.

Gracilis arises inferior to the adductor longus on the pubis, and extends along the proximal inferior pubic ramus; it runs along the medial aspect of the thigh, to insert into the medial body of the tibia, below the knee at the pes anserinus. The anterior branch of the obturator nerve supplies the gracilis – a weak adductor of the femur functioning primarily as an extensor of a flexed knee.

Adductor brevis arises from the body of the pubis and the inferior pubic ramus. It inserts in a line to the femur, between the lesser trochanter and the upper half of the linea aspera. Nerve supply is from the obturator nerve (most often the anterior branch) – an adductor of the femur, particularly in the neutral plane.

Adductor magnus is the most posterior and lateral of the adductors, the magnus arises from a curved origin, extending from the lateral inferior pubic ramus to the ischium and the ischial tuberosity. It inserts into the femur inferomedially to the gluteus maximus insertion, and as a linear aponeurosis to the linea aspera, deep to the other adductors. A number of interruptions in the insertion allow the passage of vessels from medial to posterior compartments. The most inferior of these is the adductor hiatus, through which the femoral vessels pass; the most inferior insertion of the aponeurosis is at the posterior aspect of the lateral femoral condyle. The most anterior component of the muscle behaves as an adductor (particularly with the hip extended) and is supplied by the posterior branch of the obturator nerve; the most posterior and lateral part of the muscle serves to extend the femur (in a similar way to a hamstring) and is supplied by the sciatic nerve.

Inferior pubic ramus

The inferior pubic ramus is thin and flattened. It passes laterally and downward from the medial end of the superior ramus and the pubic tubercle; it becomes narrower as it descends, and joins with the inferior ramus of the ischium below the obturator foramen (the space between the pubic rami and the ischium).

Lateral border of triangle

The line from the ASIS superiorly to the 3G point forms the lateral border of the triangle. This runs along the lateral border of the sartorius for the most proximal half, and along the rectus femoris more inferiorly. The structures of import encountered, from superior to inferior, are:

> anterior superior iliac spine (ASIS)

> sartorius

> tensor fasciae latae (TFL) and iliotibial band (ITB)

> rectus femoris

Deep to these structures are:

> femoro-acetabular joint

> trochanteric bursae

Much of the femoro-acetabular joint lies, in fact, within the triangle. Pathology within the joint may be felt medial to the triangle, within the triangle, and lateral to the triangle in the knee and the lower leg. To simplify our approach to the diagnosis of pathologies around the joint, it is considered in this section. The gluteal bursae underlie the gluteus maximus and gluteus medius tendons, proximal to their insertions. The iliotibial band (ITB) or tract is a lateral thickening of the fasciae latae in the thigh. Proximally, it splits into superficial and deep layers, enclosing the tensor fasciae latae, and anchoring this muscle to the iliac crest. The individual anatomy of these structures is described in Chapter 6.

Within the triangle

Within the triangle, the following structures are encountered:

> conjoint tendon of the iliopsoas muscle

> rectus femoris muscle

> femoral canal

The **iliopsoas** is a conjoint muscle of the psoas major, the psoas minor, and the iliacus.

The psoas minor arises as a series of slips, each of which arise from the adjacent margins of the vertebral bodies, and the intervening discs, from the lower border of T12 and L1.

The psoas major arises from the transverse processes of L1–L5, the vertebral bodies of T12–L5, and the intervertebral discs below the bodies of T12–L4.

The iliacus arises from the upper two-thirds of the concavity of the iliac fossa, and the inner lip of the iliac crest, as well as the ventral sacroiliac and iliolumbar ligaments, and the upper surface of the lateral part of the sacrum.

These muscles converge, and pass inferomedially beneath the inguinal ligament, where they join to pass over the hip joint, and into the lesser trochanter of the femur. The passage of this conjoined tendon over the hip joint is facilitated by the iliopsoas bursa, which is, in some cases, in direct communication with the hip joint. The iliopsoas is the primary hip flexor; the psoas minor and major are both supplied by the anterior rami of the lumbar plexus L1, 2, 3; and the iliacus by the femoral nerves L2, 3.

The **rectus femoris** forms part of the quadriceps femoris, arising by two tendons: (a) the anterior head from the anterior inferior iliac spine; and (b) the reflected head from a groove above the brim of the acetabulum. Both heads unite, to form an aponeurosis which is prolonged downward on the anterior surface of the muscle, and, from this, the muscular fibers arise. The muscle ends in a broad and thick aponeurosis, which occupies the lower two-thirds of its posterior surface, and, gradually becoming narrowed into a flattened tendon, is inserted into the base of the patella. The rectus femoris is an extensor of the knee as part of the quadriceps, but, because of its origin above the hip joint, it is also a weak hip flexor. Both of these functions are affected by joint position. Thus, when the knee is extended, the rectus femoris is a weak hip flexor, and when the hip is flexed, it is a weak knee extensor.

Femoral canal

As the femoral vessels pass from the abdomen, they bring with them an investment of fascia that fuses with the adventitia of the vessels 3 cm distal to the inguinal ligament. Within the sheath, a space exists medial to the femoral vein (the nerve is the most medial; remember VAN: Vein, Artery, Nerve). This space is termed the "femoral canal", and is the site of a potential hernia. It is bordered as follows: anterior is the inguinal ligament; posterior is the pectineal ligament; medial is the lacunar ligament; and lateral is the femoral vein.

The origins, insertions, and nerve supplies of the muscle groups encountered in the groin are presented in Table 4.1.

Limitation of movement is often the earliest manifestation of injury. When injury is associated with limitation of a particular movement, it is possible to ascertain which muscles or muscle groups may be limited. The muscles responsible for movement at the hip and the knee are shown in Table 4.2.

Nerve entrapment

The classic distribution of the cutaneous innervation of the area incorporated in the triangle and its potential neuropathies is shown in Figure 4.3. These, however, must serve as a guide only, as, in vivo, considerable variation occurs.[12, 14–17] The clinician will appreciate that, in addition to paresthesia, a compressed nerve can give rise to pain. The additional possibility of referred or radicular pain from T12, L1, L2, and L3 must also be considered.

Pubic tubercle

Because of the numerous anatomical structures that converge at this point, we propose a marking of the structure in a similar fashion to a clockface (Fig. 4.4). This schematic representation of the anatomy of the area serves as a guide to what may be palpable, following invagination of the scrotum. The examining clinician can therefore "walk their finger" around the tubercle, assigning each part of the clockface to the relevant attachment, as highlighted in Figure 4.4. The authors recognize that variability of structures exists in this area. We have based our diagrams on cadaveric studies[18] to represent what the clinician will most often palpate. The adductor longus enthesis is the most commonly affected structure, in an area which is often made even more impenetrable to the clinician by the myriad of differently named pathologies. Enthesopathy of the rectus abdominis insertion at the pubic tubercle may present as pain

Table 4.1 Origins, insertions, and nerve supplies of muscle groups around the groin					
Muscle	**Origin**	**Insertion**	**Nerve**	**Root**
Hip flexors				
Iliacus	Iliac fossa inner surface	Femur – lesser trochanter	Femoral nerve	L2, L3
Psoas major and minor	L1–L5 – transverse processes, T12–L5 – intervertebral discs	Femur – lesser trochanter	Lumbar plexus	L1, L2, L3
Rectus femoris	Anterior head – anterior inferior iliac spine Posterior head – supra acetabular groove	Tibia – tibial tuberosity	Femoral nerve	L2, L3, L4
Sartorius	Ilium – anterior superior iliac spine	Tibia – proximal anteromedial tibia	Femoral nerve	L2, L3
Abdominals				
Rectus abdominis	Pubis – pubic crest and symphysis	Ribs: 5, 6, 7 costal cartilages, medial inferior costal margin Sternum: xiphisternum posterior aspect	Anterior primary rami (T7–12)	T7, T8, T9, T10, T11, T12
External oblique abdominis	Ribs – lower 8 ribs anterior angles	Ilium – iliac crest anterior ½ outer aspect Inguinal ligament Pubis – tubercle and crest Anterior rectus sheath – aponeurosis and linea alba Sternum – xiphisternum	Anterior primary rami (T7–12)	T7, T8, T9, T10, T11, T12
Internal oblique abdominis	Lumbar fascia Ilium–anterior ⅔ of iliac crest Inguinal ligament – lateral ⅔	Ribs – costal margin Rectus sheath – anterior and posterior Pubis – pubic crest and pectineal line (via conjoint tendon)	Anterior primary rami (T7–12) Ilioinguinal nerve (conjoint tendon)	T7, T8, T9, T10, T11, T12 L1

Table 4.1 (continued)				
Muscle	**Origin**	**Insertion**	**Nerve**	**Root**
Transversus abdominis	Ribs – costal margin Lumbar fascia Ilium–anterior ⅔ of iliac crest Inguinal ligament–lateral ½	Rectus sheath – anterior and posterior Pubis–pubic crest and pectineal line (via conjoint tendon)	Anterior primary rami (T7–12) Ilioinguinal nerve (conjoint tendon)	T7, T8, T9, T10, T11, T12 L1
Pyrimidalis	Pubis – crest anterior to rectus abdominis	Linea alba	Subcostal nerve	T12
Adductors				
Pectineus	Pubis – superior pubic ramus – pectineal line	Femur – pectineal line	Femoral nerve and/or obturator nerve	L2, L3 and/or L2, L3, L4
Adductor longus	Pubis – pubic tubercle (6–7 o'clock)	Femur – linea aspera middle ⅓	Obturator nerve	L2, L3, L4
Adductor brevis	Pubis – body and inferior pubic ramus	Femur – linea aspera proximal ⅓	Obturator nerve	L2, L3, L4
Adductor magnus	Anterior head – inferior pubic ramus and ischial ramus Posterior head – ischial tuberosity	Anterior head – linea aspera inferior third Posterior head – adductor tubercle of femur	Anterior–obturator nerve Posterior–sciatic nerve	L2, L3, L4 And L4, L5
Gracilis	Pubis–body and inferior pubic ramus	Tibia–anteromedial (pes anserinus)	Obturator nerve	L2, L3, L4

Table 4.2 Prime movers of the hip and the knee					
Movement					
Hip Flexion	**Hip Lateral rotation**	**Hip Medial rotation**	**Hip Adduction**	**Hip Abduction**	**Knee Extension**
Psoas major	Psoas major	Tensor fascia latae	Adductor magnus	Tensor fascia latae	Rectus femoris
Psoas minor	Psoas minor		Adductor longus		Vastus lateralis
Iliacus	Iliacus		Adductor brevis		Vastus intermedius
Tensor fascia latae			Sartorius		Vastus medialis
Gracilis			Gracilis		

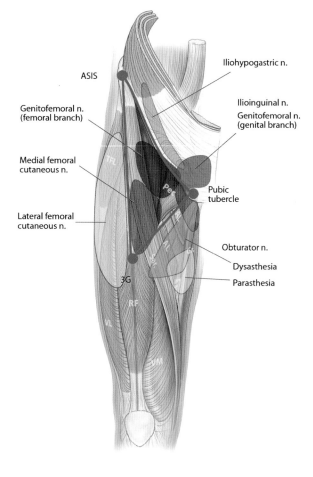

Figure 4.3 Neuropathy of the proximal lower limb

TFL	=	tensor fasciae latae
Pec	=	pectineus
AL	=	adductor longus
Sar	=	sartorius
Gr	=	gracilis
VL	=	vastus lateralis
VM	=	vastus medialis
RF	=	rectus femoris
ASIS	=	anterior superior iliac spine
3G	=	the 3G point

which is very similar to adductor longus enthesopathy – not only due to the proximity of their bony attachment, but also due to their sharing a common aponeurosis.[19]

Nomenclature
Osteitis pubis

We have employed the term "pubic bone stress injury" for what is often in the literature called "osteitis pubis". Osteitis pubis is defined as a non-infectious inflammation of the pubic symphysis, causing varying degrees of lower abdominal and pelvic pain. Osteitis pubis was first described in patients who had undergone suprapubic surgery, and remains a well-known complication of invasive procedures about the pelvis. We feel that "pubic bone stress injury" better reflects the clinical picture in the athlete of excessive stress across the pubic symphysis in the absence of any evidence of an inflammatory process.

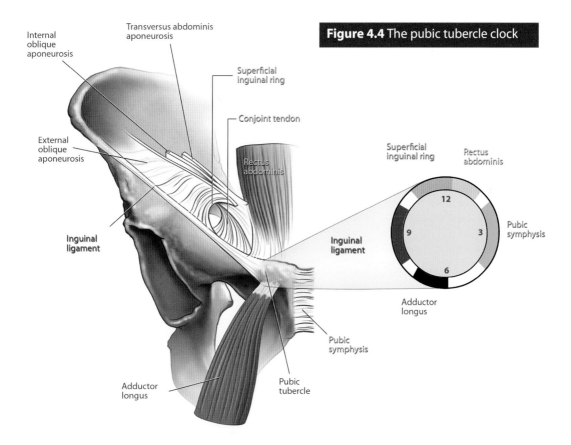

Internal oblique aponeurosis

Transversus abdominis aponeurosis

Superficial inguinal ring

Figure 4.4 The pubic tubercle clock

Conjoint tendon

External oblique aponeurosis

Rectus abdominis

Superficial inguinal ring

Rectus abdominis

Inguinal ligament

Inguinal ligament

Pubic symphysis

12

9

3

6

Adductor longus

Pubic symphysis

Adductor longus

Pubic tubercle

Sportsman's hernia

The topic of incipient hernia is included as disorders of the posterior and anterior inguinal walls. These are diagnoses of exclusion and, outside of the most experienced hands, are probably inseparable. These may represent different ends of a spectrum of pathology in the area owing to differing sporting activity.[3, 20–23]

Medial to the triangle

The hip adductors primarily occupy the space medial to the triangle. Much of the literature to date has focused on the **adductor longus**. Although several factors, including the superficial location of the muscle, its relatively small origin, and poor proximal vascular supply, have been suggested to contribute to the frequent involvement of the adductor longus in groin injuries, the exact cause of adductor strain has yet to be determined.[13, 27] The adductor longus and the gracilis tendons are the most commonly affected, and lie in an almost continuous site of origin along the body of the pubis.[39]

The other **adductor muscles (the brevis and the magnus)** arise more posterolaterally, and are rarely implicated in chronic groin pain.[40, 41] The adductors play an important role – acting with the lower abdominal muscles to stabilize the pelvis. They adduct the femur, and counteract the rotation of the pelvis, particularly during the double support phase, when the anterior limb is flexed and the posterior limb is extended at the hip. They work synergistically with the iliopsoas at the beginning of the swing phase of walking, and with the hamstrings at the end of the swing phase (when the hamstrings contract eccentrically) to prevent further hip flexion.[13]

Table 4.3 Patho-anatomical approach; pubic tubercle region				
Define and align	Pathology	Listen and localize	Palpate and recreate	Alleviate and investigate
Pubic tubercle	Adductor tendon enthesopathy	Insidious onset, warms up with exercise	Guarding on passive abduction,[24] weakness[25] Pubic clock; 6–8	MRI[26]
	Rectus abdominis enthesopathy	Well localized to insertion, acute or insidious onset	Pain from resisted sit-up.[25] Pubic clock; 12	MRI[26]
	Pubic bone stress injury	Non-specific diminished athletic performance, loss of propulsive power	Bone tenderness predominates[27, 28] Diagnosis of exclusion	Plain film.[28] MRI[29]
	Degenerative pubic symphysis	Central pain, associated with stress through symphysis – stair climbing	Tender over symphysis. Pubic clock; 3	Plain film, stress view[30] MRI[29]
	Incipient hernia; conjoint tendon tear	Insidious onset, diminished performance, warms up	Pain on resisted "torsion" of trunk "ipsilateral direction".[31] Pubic clock; 11	Ultrasound[32] MRI[33] Confirmation by direct vision at arthroscopy[22, 34, 35]
	Incipient hernia; external oblique aponeurosis tear	Acute onset, related to sport specific movement e.g. "slap shot"[21]	Pain on resisted "torsion" of trunk "contralateral direction"[31] Tenderness and dilation of superficial inguinal ring on invagination of scrotum[20] Pubic clock; 12–1	
	Nerve entrapment; Ilioinguinal nerve; Genitofemoral nerve (genital branch)	Altered skin sensation Post inguinal surgery?[36]	Superficial pain ± hyper/dysesthesia to skin over pubis[37] Absence of muscular component[15]	Relief of pain by ultrasound-guided local anesthetic infiltration[38] Nerve conduction studies[12]

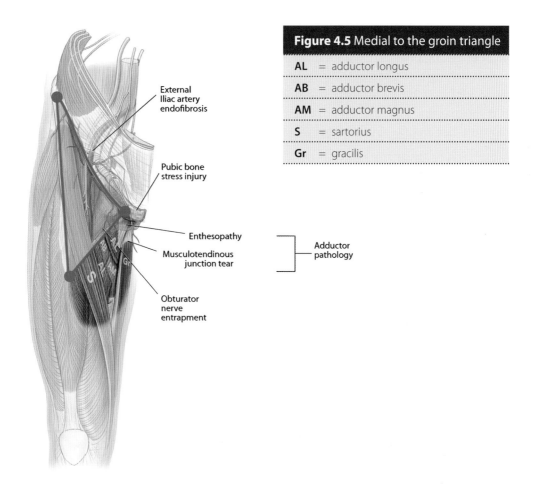

External
Iliac artery
endofibrosis

Pubic bone
stress injury

Enthesopathy

Musculotendinous
junction tear

Obturator
nerve
entrapment

Adductor
pathology

Figure 4.5 Medial to the groin triangle

AL	=	adductor longus
AB	=	adductor brevis
AM	=	adductor magnus
S	=	sartorius
Gr	=	gracilis

Differentiation of enthesis-related problems from those at the musculo-tendinous junction is important in terms of management and rehabilitation. A more aggressive rehabilitation program is warranted in the latter. The abnormal mechanics which arise due to adductor dysfunction play a critical role in the generation of a chronic pain/dysfunction cycle in the area.

Stress fracture of the inferior pubic ramus should be considered in those involved in long-distance endurance events, high-frequency training, and those who have significantly increased their workload. It is appreciated as exercise-related groin pain, often felt medial to the triangle.

Less common pathologies such as neuropathy and endofibrosis of the internal iliac artery must also be considered, although they are rare.

Obturator nerve entrapment has been described by Bradshaw et al.;[42] a number of potential sites for entrapment are described, but a surgical release of the fascia beneath the adductor longus is an effective treatment.

External iliac artery endofibrosis arises from the bifurcation of the common iliac artery. It passes downward and obliquely along the medial aspect of the psoas major, to the mid-point of the inguinal ligament (midway between the ASIS and the pubic symphysis). Here it enters the thigh, and becomes the femoral artery. Endofibrotic lesions occur within the first few centimeters of the external iliac, and manifest as thickening of the wall of the vessel. It is thought that a genetic predisposition may exist, but certainly the mechanical strain of repetitive flexion (it is almost exclusively seen in professional cyclists) plays a role.

Table 4.4 Patho-anatomical approach; medial to the groin triangle				
Define and align	**Pathology**	**Listen and localize**	**Palpate and recreate**	**Alleviate and investigate**
Medial to triangle	Adductor/gracilis enthesopathy	Insidious onset, diminished performance, warms up	Proximal adductor pain, at enthesis. Guarding, weakness[24, 25]	MRI[26]
	Adductor longus pathology at musculotendinous junction	Acute onset, worse during exercise	Pain in proximal adductor[25] (2–4 cm distal to enthesis), guarding, weakness[24, 25]	MRI[26]
	Pubic bone stress injury	Pain primarily at pubis radiating to proximal thigh	Bone tenderness, lack of point muscular tenderness	MRI[26, 43]
	Stress fracture inferior pubic ramus	Insidious onset, heavy training load	Hop test,[44] associated deep buttock pain	Plain x-ray, MRI[45]
	Nerve entrapment: > Obturator nerve > Ilioinguinal nerve > Genitofemoral nerve (genital branch)	Claudicant-type pain of medial thigh which settles on resting[42]	Exercise-related adductor weakness, superficial dysesthesia of mid-medial thigh[46]	Electromyography of adductor longus[47] Guided local anesthetic injection to obturator foramen[48]
		Altered skin sensation. Post-inguinal surgery?	Dysesthesia/ hyperesthesia over area of skin supplied by nerve in question[36, 37]	Relief of pain by ultrasound-guided local anesthetic infiltration[38] Nerve conduction studies[12]
	External iliac artery endofibrosis	Thigh discomfort post high-intensity exercise, mainly in cyclists	Exercise-related lower limb weakness. Exercise-altered bruit and ankle/brachial index[49]	Doppler ultrasound.[50] Angiography[51]

Superior to the triangle

The **rectus abdominis** inserts to the pubic tubercle and the superior aspect of the pubic bone. The rectus sheath attaches to the body of the pubis, just medial to the pubic tubercle, blending with the joint capsule of the pubic symphysis, passing over the tubercle to merge with the aponeurosis of the adductor longus.[19] The medial head of the rectus abdominis attaches to the pubis, just lateral to the symphysis. The lateral head of the rectus abdominis is, confusingly, posterior to both of these, attaching to the pubic body at its posterior lip.

The **superficial inguinal ring** is located superomedially to the pubic tubercle. As an opening in the external oblique aponeurosis, it transmits the cremasteric vessels, the vas deferens, and the testicular vessels in men, or the round ligament in women. The neural structures encountered include the genital branch of the genitofemoral nerve, and the ilioinguinal nerve.

The anatomy of the inguinal canal points to the areas where problems may arise. The oblique nature of both the deep and superficial inguinal rings means that the integrity of the inguinal canal depends on the strength of the anterior wall laterally, and the posterior wall medially. The weakness in the abdominal wall at the deep ring is the site of the direct inguinal hernia.

The **conjoint tendon** (a conglomeration of the transversalis fascia and the internal oblique fascia) sits posterior to the superficial inguinal ring, and resists the extrusion of the peritoneum and the bowel when abdominal pressure is raised.

To view the abdominal musculature and their respective fascias as merely the walls of the abdomen is to underestimate their function. The external oblique rotates the trunk to the opposite side. Together with the internal oblique and transversus abdominis muscles, the external oblique raises the pressure within the abdominal cavity and pelvis.[52]

The bodily region bounded by the abdominal wall, the pelvis, the lower back, and the diaphragm is known as "the **core**", probably due to its role in stabilizing the body during movement. The main muscles involved include the transversus abdominis, the internal and external obliques, the quadratus labarum, and the diaphragm. The core acts as an anatomical base for the motion of the distal segments. This can be considered "proximal stability for distal mobility" for throwing, kicking, or running activities.[53] Contraction of the abdominal muscles is vital to the stability of the lumbar spine – by forming a rigid cylinder, they enhance its stiffness.[54] The rectus abdominis and oblique abdominals are activated in direction-specific patterns with respect to limb movements, thus providing postural support before limb movements.[55] Contractions which increase intra-abdominal pressure occur before the initiation of large-segment movement of the upper limbs.[56] In this manner, the spine (and core of the body) are stabilized before limb movements occur, to allow the limbs to have a stable base for motion, and muscle activation.[52]

The inguinal canal represents a point of weakness in the lower abdominal musculature and its fascia, and, bearing in mind the stresses through the area (particularly during athletic activity), it is prone to injury.

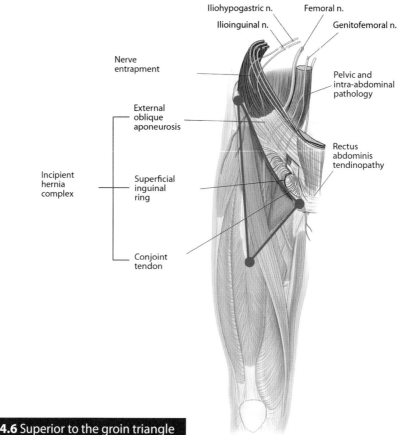

Figure 4.6 Superior to the groin triangle

Lateral to the groin triangle

As a cause of recalcitrant groin pain, the **pathology of the femoro-acetabular joint** should not be underestimated. The joint is prone to degenerative, inflammatory, and infective processes. The long-term contribution of acute or repetitive trauma to the development of degenerative conditions, such as osteoarthritis, is of particular concern in the sports setting. Pain from a degenerative femoro-acetabular joint may be appreciated anywhere from the lateral leg to the groin and the knee. The anatomy of the structures encountered lateral to the triangle is discussed in more detail in Chapter 5.

The **trochanteric bursa** presents with maximal pain on palpation over the greater trochanter of the hip. It is very painful to lie on, and comparatively unaffected by movements of the hip.[58] Ultrasound is a useful means of confirming what is essentially a clinical diagnosis. Infiltration with local anesthetic and corticosteroid may be done at ultrasound. Clinicians palpating and injecting the point of maximal tenderness often perform this procedure blind (unguided).

The tensor fasciae latae assists in the flexion, abduction, and medial rotation of the hip joint, and the extension of the knee joint. Through these actions, the tensor fasciae latae aids

Table 4.5 Patho-anatomical approach; superior to the groin triangle				
Define and align	**Pathology**	**Listen and localize**	**Palpate and recreate**	**Alleviate and investigate**
Superior to base	Rectus abdominis Tendinopathy	Well localized to insertion, acute or insidious onset	Pain from resisted sit-up.[6, 25] Pubic clock; 12	MRI[26]
	Incipient hernia; conjoint tendon tear	Insidious onset, diminished performance, warms up	Pain on resisted "torsion" of trunk "ipsilateral direction".[31] Pubic clock; 11	Ultrasound.[32] MRI[33] Confirmation by direct vision at arthroscopy[22, 34, 35]
	Incipient hernia; external oblique aponeurosis tear	Acute onset, related to sport specific movement e.g. "slap shot"[21]	Pain on resisted "torsion" of trunk "contralateral direction"[31] Tenderness and dilation of superficial inguinal ring on invagination of scrotum.[20] Pubic clock; 12–1	
	Inguinal hernia	Pain on Valsalva maneuver	Cough impulse, palpable mass at deep inguinal ring (direct), in inguinal canal/scrotum (indirect)	Ultrasound[32] Herniography[57] Laparoscopy
	Nerve entrapment: > Ilioinguinal nerve > Iliohypogastric nerve > Genitofemoral nerve (genital branch) > Lateral femoral cutaneous nerve	Altered skin sensation	Dysesthesia/ hyperesthesia over area of skin supplied by nerve in question[12, 15]	Relief of pain by ultrasound-guided local anesthetic infiltration[38] Nerve conduction studies[12]

in the stabilization of the pelvis on the head of the femur, and of the condyles of the femur on the tibial condyles. **Iliotibial band syndrome** typically occurs when repetitive knee flexion is necessary, such as in runners or cyclists.[59] Some patients have pain predominantly in the knee (approximately 2 cm proximal to the lateral femoral condyle), but others feel that the hip is dislocating, popping, or snapping even during normal ambulation. Localized tenderness over the greater trochanter is the most useful sign. There may also be a feeling of a band rolling over the greater trochanter.

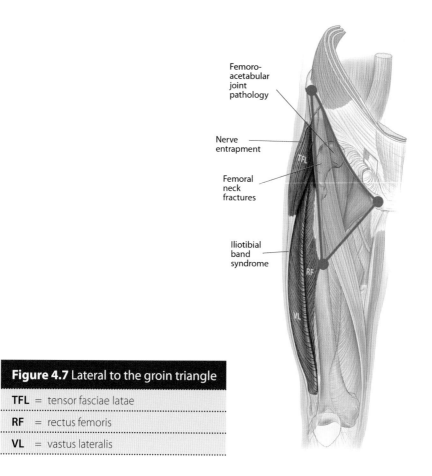

Femoro-
acetabular
joint
pathology

Nerve
entrapment

Femoral
neck
fractures

Iliotibial
band
syndrome

TFL

RF

VL

Figure 4.7 Lateral to the groin triangle

TFL	=	tensor fasciae latae
RF	=	rectus femoris
VL	=	vastus lateralis

Entrapment of the lateral femoral cutaneous nerve or meralgia paresthetica may result from damage or compression of the nerve as it passes inferior to the inguinal ligament. It causes dysesthesia in its myotome.

Within the triangle

Within the triangle, the iliopsoas may be palpated. As a sole diagnosis or part of a collection of symptoms, **iliopsoas pathology** is a common cause of chronic groin and hip pain. Iliopsoas bursitis and tendinosis may cause groin pain, but are relatively uncommon. Much more common is contracture, or tightness, of the muscle. This condition is of multifactorial etiology, and may relate to muscular, fascial, or even neural tension; as such, we refer to it as "neuromyofascial tension".

The iliopsoas is active in walking, running, and kicking; however, the primary role of the iliopsoas is as a postural muscle (maintaining posture while standing), which alludes to its structure and fiber content. This fiber content is dominated by slow-twitch, red, type-1 muscle fibers. Muscle of this type is susceptible to contracture (pathological shortening), especially when inactive or injured, and requires regular stretching to maintain normal tone. Such contracture shortens the distance from the lumbar spine to the hip, and can lead to increased anterior pelvic

Table 4.6 Patho-anatomical approach; lateral to the groin triangle				
Define and align	**Pathology**	**Listen and localize**	**Palpate and recreate**	**Alleviate and investigate**
Lateral to triangle	Impingement/labral pathology, femoro-acetabular joint	Mechanical signs, clicking in joint and/or catching	Impingement test[60]	MRI[61]
	Osteoarthritis/chondral damage, femoro-acetabular joint	History of traumatic/congenital insult. Older age group	Limited range of movement,[62] pain on weight bearing	Plain film x-ray, MRI[45]
	Stress fracture neck of femur	Heavy training load, biomechanical/gait abnormality	Hop test,[63] fulcrum test[64]	Plain-film x-ray, MRI[45]
	Trochanteric bursitis	Persistent lateral hip pain worse on lying on affected side	Pain on transition between lying/standing[65]	Ultrasound,[66] relief of pain by ultrasound-guided local anesthetic injection
	Iliotibial band friction syndrome	External "snapping" and/or lateral knee pain	Recreate snapping,[67] Ober's test[44]	Ultrasound[66]
	Nerve entrapment: lateral cutaneous femoral nerve/meralgia paresthetica	Exercise-induced, obesity[68]	Reproduction of symptoms on pressure inferior to anterior superior iliac spine[68]	Nerve conduction studies[12]

tilt, lumbar lordosis, and limitation of hip extension. When this occurs, tension in the muscle may manifest as a palpable "snap" as the tendon runs over the iliopectineal eminence on the ilium.

Palpation of the iliopsoas is easiest distally, where it may be palpated lateral to the femoral pulse, medial to the sartorius, and below the inguinal ligament (this is facilitated by passive flexion of the hip).[69] Pain on resisted flexion of the affected hip from the Thomas test position is, however, quite specific for this condition.

Due to its proximity to the hip joint, differentiation between iliopsoas and femoro-acetabular pathology may be difficult to differentiate. This is discussed fully in Chapter 5 on the greater trochanter. Indeed, it should be borne in mind that the iliopsoas bursa is often in direct continuation with the hip joint capsule.

The **rectus femoris** arises via two heads, the direct head from the anterior inferior iliac spine, and the reflected head from the lip of the acetabulum. Both heads unite, to form an aponeurosis (flat tendon). The muscle fibers arise from this. The aponeurosis continues along the anterior surface of the muscle, to insert into the patella. The rectus femoris therefore differs from other hip flexors, in that it also extends the knee. As the rectus femoris spans both the hip and the knee, increased muscle tension due to hip extension will exacerbate signs, not

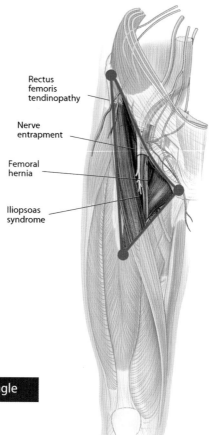

Rectus
femoris
tendinopathy

Nerve
entrapment

Femoral
hernia

Iliopsoas
syndrome

Figure 4.8 Within the groin triangle

seen in the vasti, which originate on the shaft of the femur. Similarly, differentiation from the iliopsoas may be made, as this spans the hip joint alone.

Femoral hernia, although classically inferior to the inguinal ligament and medial to the tubercle, is often indistinguishable from an inguinal hernia.[70] The cough impulse is less readily identifiable; the aperture is usually smaller, although a mass in the anteromedial thigh is sometimes appreciated.

The area of skin within the triangle is generally supplied superiorly by the femoral branch of the genitofemoral nerve, and inferiorly by the medial femoral cutaneous nerve. A history of lower abdominal or inguinal surgery should alert the examiner. Physically, the absence of muscle weakness, and the abolition of symptoms following local anesthetic injection, are helpful.

Intra-abdominal pathology

Pain arising from gastrointestinal and genitourinary pathology may mask itself as groin discomfort or pain. Key discriminating symptoms may be signs of systemic illness, systemic inflammatory

Table 4.7 Patho-anatomical approach; within the groin triangle				
Define and align	**Pathology**	**Listen and localize**	**Palpate and recreate**	**Alleviate and investigate**
Within the triangle	Iliopsoas syndrome	Pain above and below inguinal ligament. Associated snapping at hip joint	Thomas test, modified[44]	Ultrasound scan, dynamic view of snapping[66] ± injection[71] MRI
	Rectus femoris tendinopathy/ apophysitis	Does knee movement affect pain?	Rectus femoris contracture test[72]	Plain-film x-ray. Ultrasound scan[66] MRI
	Femoral hernia	Painful lump inferomedial to pubic tubercle	Minimal relationship to exercise	Ultrasound scan,[32] herniography[57]
	Nerve entrapment: > Genitofemoral nerve (femoral branch) > Medial femoral cutaneous nerve	Altered skin sensation	Dysesthesia/ hyperesthesia over area of skin supplied by nerve in question[9]	Relief of pain by local anesthetic infiltration[38] Nerve conduction studies[12]

response, and no correlation between exercise and symptoms or signs. Any of these, in conjunction with a negative musculoskeletal examination, serve to alert the examining physician to focus their examinations beyond the musculoskeletal system.

Intra-abdominal pathologies that may refer to the area of the groin triangle are shown in Table 4.8.

Table 4.8 Visceral referred pain in the groin triangle	
Listen and localize	Structure
Superior to the triangle	Urinary bladder
	Colon
	Appendix (right side)
Medial to the triangle	Ureter

Summary

Securing a diagnosis is the obvious first step in the treatment of any problem. Groin pain is often insidious in onset, so it is generally chronic when the athlete presents. An anatomically crowded area can make differentiation between structures difficult. This can be further complicated by an overload pattern, forcing other structures to bear more than their normal workload. They will, if the underlying cause is not addressed, become inflamed and painful.

Do not be afraid to consider a number of pathologies as the causal agent in chronic groin pain. The greater the chronicity, the more likely multiple pathologies are. As is illustrated in case 3, we must be prepared to revisit the diagnosis, and shape our differential diagnosis according to the symptoms and signs which become apparent.

Case histories

Case 1

A 35-year-old woman presents with a three-month history of groin pain. She is not usually active but joined a "boot camp" to lose some weight prior to her symptom onset. She first noticed the pain after a particularly heavy session, which involved performing weighted sit-ups. She developed a sharp pain in her groin. This was extremely sore, but settled somewhat, so she was able to resume some training after a number of days. At this point, her symptoms gradually worsened, and now she is unable to do any abdominal work and even running hurts.

This is a presentation of groin pain. As such, proceed to step 1, define and align the groin triangle.

Step 1: Define and align

Expose the patient properly; a pair of sports shorts will allow physical access and aid visibility.

Define the triangle: locate the anterior superior iliac spine (ASIS), locate the pubic symphysis, and mark the mid-point of the line between the ASIS and the superior pole of the patella (3G point).

Align the patient's pain on the triangle. Here the pain is quite specific: the patient points to the area just above her pubic bone.

The patient has localized the pain to the area "superior to the triangle". From here on, we recommend that the reader attempts to exclude the potential pathologies. From Table 4.5, the potential causal structures are:

Differential diagnosis
> rectus abdominis tendinopathy
> incipient hernia
> external oblique aponeurosis tear
> conjoint tendon tear
> inguinal hernia
> nerve entrapment
> ilioinguinal nerve
> iliohypogastric nerve
> genitofemoral nerve (genital branch)
> lateral femoral cutaneous nerve

We proceed to differentiate between these structures, step 2.

Step 2: Listen and localize

Addressing the rectus abdominis muscle we ask:

Q *Is the pain well localized to above the pubic bone (demonstrate where you mean)?*

A Yes.

Addressing an incipient hernia we ask:

Q *Does the pain have an insidious onset; does it occur during and post exercise?*

A No, it began severely but it does occur during exercise, and stops a while after.

Addressing an inguinal hernia we ask:

Q *Do you experience pain when you "bear down", for example, straining at stool, or lifting a heavy object?*

A Not initially, but I have noticed I do have pain when I lift heavy things now.

Addressing neuropathy we ask:

Q *Have you noticed any abnormal sensation of the skin in the area?*

A No.

This will narrow our differential diagnosis somewhat, and we proceed to examination to narrow it further. By palpating painful structures, and recreating the pain through diagnostic maneuvers, we move toward a diagnosis, step 3.

Differential diagnosis

More likely:

> rectus abdominis tendinopathy

> incipient hernia

> external oblique aponeurosis tear

> conjoint tendon tear

> inguinal hernia

Less likely:

> nerve entrapment

> ilioinguinal nerve

> iliohypogastric nerve

> genitofemoral nerve (genital branch)

> lateral femoral cutaneous nerve

Step 3: Palpate and re-create

From the pubic clock, pain at and around the 12 o'clock position indicates pathology of the rectus abdominis muscle. Incipient hernia is extremely uncommon in women, but the external inguinal ring may be palpated superolateral to the pubic tubercle at the 11 o'clock position. A palpable mass in this area indicates a true inguinal hernia; here a cough impulse is helpful. Normal superficial sensation in the area makes neuropathy unlikely, but, if you are unsure, have the patient perform the aggravating activity and re-examine post.

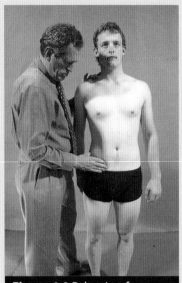

Figure 4.9 Palpating for a hernia mass

Differential diagnosis

More likely:
> rectus abdominis tendinopathy

Less likely:
> incipient hernia
> external oblique aponeurosis tear

> conjoint tendon tear
> inguinal hernia
> nerve entrapment
> ilioinguinal nerve
> iliohypogastric nerve
> genitofemoral nerve (genital branch)
> lateral femoral cutaneous nerve

Given step 2 and the results of our palpation, it is likely that this is a rectus abdominis enthesopathy/insertion tear. A test to recreate the pain is to have the patient sit up against resistance. Recreation of pain is a positive test.

Step 4: Alleviate and investigate

We may now proceed to step 4 to confirm our clinical suspicion via imaging. Ultrasonography is effective, but the most evidence-based test is MRI, with or without the use of gadolinium contrast.

Case 2

A 26-year-old soccer player presents with worsening groin pain over the previous five months. He first noticed pain when stretching for a ball in a tackle and felt pain both at the time and subsequently. Interventions included non-steroidal anti-inflammatory drugs, prolonged periods of rest, and simple analgesia. The pain tends to worsen with exercise and, when severe, lasts until the next day. Match situations are particularly aggravating. The player describes the pain as groin pain and points to the area on the inner thigh.

This is a presentation of groin pain. As such, proceed to step 1, define and align the groin triangle.

Step 1: Define and align

Expose the patient properly; a pair of sports shorts will allow physical access and aid visibility.

Define the triangle: locate the anterior superior iliac spine (ASIS), locate the pubic symphysis, and mark the mid-point of the line between the ASIS and the superior pole of the patella (3G point).

Align the patient's pain on the triangle: the patient localizes the pain to the area on the medial side of his leg, sometimes radiating toward the knee. This places the pain in the area medial to the triangle. From here on, we recommend that the reader attempts to exclude the potential pathologies that might be encountered in this region. From Table 4.4, the potential causal structures are:

Differential diagnosis
> adductor/gracilis enthesopathy
> adductor longus pathology at the musculotendinous junction
> pubic bone stress injury
> stress fracture of the inferior pubic ramus
> nerve entrapment
> obturator nerve
> ilioinguinal nerve
> genitofemoral nerve (genital branch)
> external iliac artery stenosis

We proceed to differentiate between these structures, step 2.

Step 2: Listen and localize
Addressing the adductor/gracilis muscle we ask:

Q *Did the pain come on gradually, and does it ease with warming up?*

A No.

Q *Did the pain come on suddenly, and is it worse on exercise?*

A Yes, that sounds right.

Addressing the pubic bone we ask:

Q *Has your training load increased over the last few months? Have you been doing more kicking than normal?*

A No, I have been at a two-week training camp, but that was no more intensive than my normal weekly training load.

Q *Is the pain at the pubic bone itself?*

A No; patient points to the lateral border of the pubis, radiating down the inside of the leg.

Addressing neuropathy we ask:

Q *Have you noticed any abnormal sensation of the skin in the area?*

A No.

Q *Have you had recent hernia or lower abdominal surgery?*

A No.

Q *Does the pain take the form of a gripping pain, settling with rest?*

A No.

Addressing the iliac artery we ask:

Q *Have you noticed the pain occurs particularly with intense exercise, and then eases with rest over 30 minutes or so?*

A No. The pain occurs with all activity.

This will narrow our differential diagnosis somewhat; nerve entrapment and external iliac artery fibrosis are very unlikely. We proceed to examination to narrow it further. By palpating painful structures, and recreating the pain through diagnostic maneuvers, we move toward a diagnosis, step 3.

Differential diagnosis

More likely:

> adductor/gracilis enthesopathy

> adductor longus pathology at the musculotendinous junction

> pubic bone stress injury

> stress fracture of the inferior pubic ramus

Less likely:

> nerve entrapment

> obturator nerve

> ilioinguinal nerve

> genitofemoral nerve (genital branch)

> external iliac artery stenosis

Step 3: Palpate and re-create

The most evidence-based test for adductor/gracilis enthesopathy is tenderness at the proximal enthesis of the adductors; this can be differentiated from adductor longus pathology at the musculoskeletal junction, as this is some 3–4 cm distal to the enthesopathy of insertion. Guarding and adduction weakness are seen with both pathologies.

Widespread bone tenderness over the pubic tubercle may indicate pubic bone stress injury. Symptomatically, this may be similar to a stress fracture (this is where the directed questioning should have hinted at stress fracture). The latter is, however, usually more inferior and posterior. An inferior ischial ramus fracture will usually have a positive Hop test – where the patient is asked to hop on one leg, and this exacerbates the pain with radiation to the buttock.

Palpation of the area indicates pain along the adductor longus muscle and tendon. The point of maximal tenderness is slightly distal to the enthesis, rather than directly at it.

Given our suspicion following questioning and findings on examination, we may proceed to step 4.

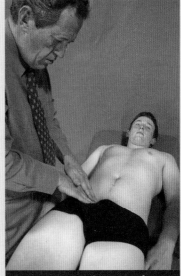

Figure 4.10 Palpation of inguinal and pubic areas

Differential diagnosis

More likely:

> adductor longus pathology at the musculotendinous junction

Less likely:

> adductor/gracilis enthesopathy

> pubic bone stress injury

> stress fracture of the inferior pubic ramus

> nerve entrapment

> obturator nerve

> ilioinguinal nerve

> genitofemoral nerve (genital branch)

> external iliac artery stenosis

Step 4: Alleviate and investigate

We may need no further investigation at this point, as it is very likely to be pathology involving the adductor longus musculotendinous junction. A careful rehabilitation program, with appropriate initial conservative management, should result in steady improvement, with a general and then sport-specific return to activity. If imaging confirmation were required, both ultrasound imaging and MRI would demonstrate the musculo-tendinous junction well.

Case 3

A 26-year-old field hockey player presents with worsening groin pain over the previous two years. Interventions included non-steroidal anti-inflammatory drugs and simple analgesia. Pain develops after 20–30 minutes of activity and, when severe, lasts until the next day. Heavy training and running, particularly game time, aggravate the pain. The player volunteers that rest is the only true relieving factor. The pain is a non-specific ache, but progresses to a sharp pinch when severe.

This is a presentation of groin pain; as such, proceed to step 1, define and align the groin triangle.

Step 1: Define and align

Expose the patient properly; a pair of sports shorts will allow physical access and aid visibility.

Define the triangle: locate the anterior superior iliac spine (ASIS), locate the pubic symphysis, and mark the mid-point of the line between the ASIS and the superior pole of the patella (3G point).

Align the patient's pain on the triangle: here it is a non-specific pain. In an effort to localize the pain, ask the patient to point to where the pain is with one finger.

The patient localizes the pain to within the triangle. From here on, we recommend that the reader attempts to exclude the potential pathologies. From Table 4.7, the potential causal structures are:

Differential diagnosis

> iliopsoas syndrome
> rectus femoris tendinopathy/apophysitis
> femoral hernia
> nerve entrapment
> genitofemoral nerve (femoral branch)
> medial femoral cutaneous nerve

We proceed to differentiate between these structures, step 2.

Step 2: Listen and localize

Addressing the psoas muscle we ask:

Q *Is there pain above and below the inguinal ligament?*

A Yes, there is.

Q *Is there associated snapping at the hip joint?*

A Maybe, it sometimes clicks a little.

Addressing rectus femoris tendinopathy/apophysitis we ask:

Q *Does knee movement affect the pain?*

A No.

This patient is too old for an apophysitis, but rectus femoris strain has to be differentiated from that of the iliopsoas, as they both act as hip flexors. Addressing femoral hernia we ask:

Q *Is there a painful lump inferomedial to the pubic tubercle?*

A No.

Addressing neuropathy we ask:

Q *Have you noticed any abnormal sensation of the skin in the area?*

A No.

This will narrow our differential diagnosis somewhat, and we proceed to examination to narrow it further. By palpating painful structures, and recreating the pain through diagnostic maneuvers, we move toward a diagnosis, step 3.

Differential diagnosis
More likely:
> iliopsoas syndrome
Less likely:
> rectus femoris tendinopathy/apophysitis
> femoral hernia
> nerve entrapment
> genitofemoral nerve (femoral branch)
> medial femoral cutaneous nerve

Step 3: Palpate and re-create

The most evidence-based test for iliopsoas strain is a modified Thomas test (Fig. 4.9). Stand a patient

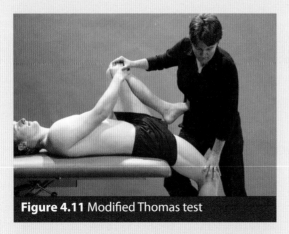

Figure 4.11 Modified Thomas test

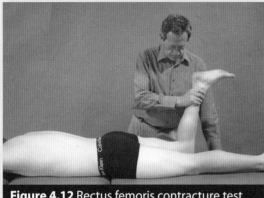

Figure 4.12 Rectus femoris contracture test

at the end of the examination table, so their buttocks are resting at its edge. They then take the knee off the unaffected leg in their hands, and lie back onto the table. The examiner ensures that the hip of the unaffected side is fully flexed, while extending the affected side. Pain is experienced above and below the inguinal ligament.

To differentiate from rectus femoris pathology, one must remember the anatomy of this muscle. Travelling from the AIIS (anterior inferior iliac spine) to the tibial tuberosity, it spans both the hip and the knee. If knee movement alters the pain at the hip, it suggests pathology of this muscle. This is best tested with the rectus femoris contracture test (Fig. 4.10). With the patient lying prone, the knee is fully flexed. Pathology of the rectus femoris will cause it to shorten; this is accommodated by involuntary flexion at the hip, indicating a positive test.

We find that there is some pain on Thomas and modified Thomas testing; however, the rectus femoris contracture test is negative. Palpation for any painful masses inferomedial to the pubic tubercle (femoral hernia) is negative, and sensation in the area is intact.

Returning to our anatomy, one structure that lies both within the triangle and lateral to it is the femoro-acetabular joint. This has been categorized as lateral to the triangle, to draw the reader to the greater trochanter triangle. This deals in depth with the hip joint, and the structures around it.

The proximity of the iliopsoas and the femoro-acetabular joint (remember the iliopsoas inserts into the lesser trochanter of the femur – Fig. 4.1) means that there may be co-existing hip/iliopsoas pathology.

Given the nature of the presentation to date and the findings on examination, we move to the lateral section of the triangle. The differential diagnosis is as follows:

Differential diagnosis

More likely:

> impingement/labral pathology, femoro-acetabular joint

> osteoarthritis/chondral damage, femoro-acetabular joint

Less likely:

> stress fracture neck of femur

> trochanteric bursitis

> iliotibial band friction syndrome

> nerve entrapment; lateral cutaneous femoral nerve/meralgia paresthetica

Given that the pain is within, rather than lateral to, the triangle, the pathologies responsible for the more lateral pain are less likely. A stress fracture of the femur would create the type of pain indicated, but is very unlikely in this situation.

A loss of range of movement at the hip may indicate femoro-acetabular pathology. In situations such as damage to the acetabular labrum, however, movement may be unaffected, and is an unreliable sign. Here the range of movement is normal, and we proceed to investigate the potential for impingement or labral pathology.

We ask the question:

Q *Have you noticed any clicking in your hip joint and/or catching?*

A Yes, I've noticed it clicks sometimes.

A discriminative test is the hip impingement test (Fig. 4.11). The hip is flexed fully, adducted, and internal rotation is added. This correlates very well with labral injury. At this point we may proceed to step 4.

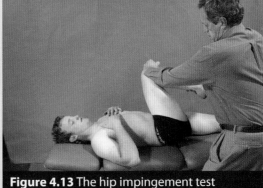

Figure 4.13 The hip impingement test

Step 4: Alleviate and investigate

A plain-film x-ray of the hip may identify some abnormal femoral head–neck offset or acetabular dysplasia, both indicating femoro-acetabular impingement. Where this is not present, we proceed to an MRI or MR arthrogram of the hip, to confirm our clinical suspicion of an acetabular labral injury.

References

1. Walden M, Hagglund M, Ekstrand J. Football injuries during European Championships 2004–2005. Knee Surg Sports Traumatol Arthrosc. 2007 Sep; 15(9):1155–62.

2. Orchard J, Seward H. Epidemiology of injuries in the Australian Football League, seasons 1997–2000. British Journal of Sports Medicine. 2002 Feb; 36(1):39–44.

3. Emery CA, Meeuwisse WH, Powell JW. Groin and abdominal strain injuries in the National Hockey League. Clin J Sport Med. 1999 Jul; 9(3):151–56.

4. Brooks JH, Fuller CW, Kemp SP, Reddin DB. Epidemiology of injuries in English professional rugby union: part 2 training injuries. British Journal of Sports Medicine. 2005 Oct; 39(10):767–75.

5. Brooks JH, Fuller CW, Kemp SP, Reddin DB. Epidemiology of injuries in English professional rugby union: part 1 match injuries. British Journal of Sports Medicine. 2005 Oct; 39(10):757–66.

6. Meyers WC, Foley DP, Garrett WE, Lohnes JH, Mandlebaum BR. Management of severe lower abdominal or inguinal pain in high-performance athletes. PAIN (Performing Athletes with Abdominal or Inguinal Neuromuscular Pain) Study Group. Am J Sports Med. 2000 Jan–Feb; 28(1):2–8.

7. Meyers WC, McKechnie A, Philippon MJ, Horner MA, Zoga AC, Devon ON. Experience with "sports hernia" spanning two decades. Annals of Surgery. 2008 Oct; 248(4):656–65.

8. Omar IM, Zoga AC, Kavanagh EC, Koulouris G, Bergin D, Gopez AG, et al. Athletic pubalgia and "sports hernia": optimal MR imaging technique and findings. Radiographics. 2008 Sep–Oct; 28(5):1415–38.

9. McCrory P, Bell S, Bradshaw C. Nerve entrapments of the lower leg, ankle and foot in sport. Sports Medicine (Auckland, NZ). 2002; 32(6):371–91.

10. Koliyadan SV, Narayan G, Balasekran P. Surface marking of the deep inguinal ring. Clinical Anatomy (New York, NY). 2004 Oct; 17(7):554–57.

11. Holmich P. Long-standing groin pain in sportspeople falls into three primary patterns, a "clinical entity" approach: a prospective study of 207 patients. British Journal of Sports Medicine. 2007 Apr; 41(4):247–52; discussion 52.

12. Rab M, Ebmer AJ, Dellon AL. Anatomic variability of the ilioinguinal and genitofemoral nerve: implications for the treatment of groin pain. Plastic and Reconstructive Surgery. 2001 Nov; 108(6):1618–23.

13. Tuite DJ, Finegan PJ, Saliaris AP, Renstrom PA, Donne B, O'Brien M. Anatomy of the proximal musculotendinous junction of the adductor longus muscle. Knee Surg Sports Traumatol Arthrosc. 1998; 6(2):134–37.

14. Krahenbuhl L, Striffeler H, Baer HU, Buchler MW. Retroperitoneal endoscopic neurectomy for nerve entrapment after hernia repair. British Journal of Surgery. 1997 Feb; 84(2):216–19.

15. Lee CH, Dellon AL. Surgical management of groin pain of neural origin. Journal of the American College of Surgeons. 2000 Aug; 191(2):137–42.

16. Morikawa R. Distribution and variations of the nerves deriving from the lumbar plexus and supplying the abdominal wall. Kaibogaku Zasshi. 1971 Oct; 46(5):312–38.

17. Starling JR, Harms BA. Diagnosis and treatment of genitofemoral and ilioinguinal neuralgia. World Journal of Surgery. 1989 Sep–Oct; 13(5):586–91.

18. Franklin–Miller A, Falvey EC, McCrory P, Briggs C. Landmarks for the 3G approach; Groin, gluteal, and greater trochanter triangles, a pathoanatomical method in sports medicine. Submitted. 2007.

19. Robinson P, Salehi F, Grainger A, Clemence M, Schilders E, O'Connor P, et al. Cadaveric and MRI study of the musculotendinous contributions to the capsule of the symphysis pubis. AJR. 2007 May; 188(5):W440–45.

20. Gilmore J. Groin pain in the soccer athlete: fact, fiction, and treatment. Clinics in Sports Medicine. 1998 Oct; 17(4):787–93, vii.

21. Irshad K, Feldman LS, Lavoie C, Lacroix VJ, Mulder DS, Brown RA. Operative management of "hockey groin syndrome": 12 years of experience in National Hockey League players. Surgery. 2001 Oct; 130(4):759–64; discussion 64–66.

22. Kluin J, den Hoed PT, van Linschoten R, JC IJ, van Steensel CJ. Endoscopic evaluation and treatment of groin pain in the athlete. Am J Sports Med. 2004 Jun; 32(4):944–49.

23. Lovell G. The diagnosis of chronic groin pain in athletes: a review of 189 cases. Australian Journal of Science and Medicine in Sport. 1995 Sep; 27(3):76–79.

24. Kendall FP, ME. Lower extremity muscles. In Kendall FP, ME, ed. Muscles – testing and function. Williams & Wilkins 1983:158–79.

25. Holmich P, Holmich LR, Bjerg AM. Clinical examination of athletes with groin pain: an intraobserver and interobserver reliability study. British Journal of Sports Medicine. 2004 Aug; 38(4):446–51.

26. Zoga AC, Kavanagh EC, Omar IM, Morrison WB, Koulouris G, Lopez H et al. Athletic pubalgia and the "sports hernia": MR imaging findings. Radiology. 2008 Jun; 247(3):797–807.

27. Lynch SA, Renstrom PA. Groin injuries in sport: treatment strategies. Sports Medicine (Auckland, NZ). 1999 Aug; 28(2):137–44.

28. Fricker PA, Taunton JE, Ammann W. Osteitis pubis in athletes. Infection, inflammation or injury? Sports Medicine (Auckland, NZ). 1991 Oct; 12(4):266–79.

29. Lovell G, Galloway H, Hopkins W, Harvey A. Osteitis pubis and assessment of bone marrow edema at the pubic symphysis with MRI in an elite junior male soccer squad. Clin J Sport Med. 2006 Mar; 16(2):117–22.

30. LaBan MM, Meerschaert JR, Taylor RS, Tabor HD. Symphyseal and sacroiliac joint pain associated with pubic symphysis instability. Archives of Physical Medicine and Rehabilitation. 1978 Oct; 59(10):470–72.

31. Kumar S. Ergonomics and biology of spinal rotation. Ergonomics. 2004 Mar 15; 47(4):370–415.

32. van den Berg JC, Rutten MJ, de Valois JC, Jansen JB, Rosenbusch G. Masses and pain in the groin: a review of imaging findings. European Radiology. 1998; 8(6):911–21.

33. Nelson EN, Kassarjian A, Palmer WE. MR imaging of sports-related groin pain. Magnetic Resonance Imaging Clinics of North America. 2005 Nov; 13(4):727–42.

34. Kumar A, Doran J, Batt ME, Nguyen-Van-Tam JS, Beckingham IJ. Results of inguinal canal repair in athletes with sports hernia. Journal of the Royal College of Surgeons of Edinburgh. 2002 Jun; 47(3):561–65.

35. Steele P, Annear P, Grove JR. Surgery for posterior inguinal wall deficiency in athletes. Journal of Science and Medicine in Sport/Sports Medicine Australia. 2004 Dec; 7(4):415–21; discussion 22–23.

36. Liszka TG, Dellon AL, Manson PN. Iliohypogastric nerve entrapment following abdominoplasty. Plastic and Reconstructive Surgery. 1994 Jan; 93(1):181–84.

37. Harms BA, DeHaas DR, Jr, Starling JR. Diagnosis and management of genitofemoral neuralgia. Arch Surg. 1984 Mar; 119(3):339–41.

38. Eichenberger U, Greher M, Kirchmair L, Curatolo M, Moriggl B. Ultrasound-guided blocks of the ilioinguinal and iliohypogastric nerve: accuracy of a selective new technique confirmed by anatomical dissection. British Journal of Anaesthesia. 2006 Aug; 97(2):238–43.

39. Kalebo P, Karlsson J, Sward L, Peterson L. Ultrasonography of chronic tendon injuries in the groin. Am J Sports Med. 1992 Nov–Dec; 20(6):634–39.

40. Martens MA, Hansen L, Mulier JC. Adductor tendinitis and musculus rectus abdominis tendopathy. Am J Sports Med. 1987 Jul–Aug; 15(4):353–56.

41. Orchard JW, Read JW, Neophyton J, Garlick D. Groin pain associated with ultrasound finding of inguinal canal posterior wall deficiency in Australian Rules footballers. British Journal of Sports Medicine. 1998 Jun; 32(2):134–39.

42. Bradshaw C, McCrory P, Bell S, Brukner P. Obturator nerve entrapment. A cause of groin pain in athletes. Am J Sports Med. 1997 May–Jun; 25(3):402–08.

43. Verrall GM, Slavotinek JP, Barnes PG, Fon GT, Esterman A. Assessment of physical examination and magnetic resonance imaging findings of hamstring injury as predictors for recurrent injury. Journal of Orthopaedic and Sports Physical Therapy. 2006 Apr; 36(4):215–24.

44. Malanga GA, Nadler SF. Physical examination of the hip. Musculoskeletal physical examination, an evidence-based approach. Philadelphia, PA: Elsevier Mosby 2006:251–79.

45. Berger FH, de Jonge MC, Maas M. Stress fractures in the lower extremity. The importance of increasing awareness amongst radiologists. European Journal of Radiology. 2007 Apr; 62(1):16–26.

46. Bradshaw C, McCrory P. Obturator nerve entrapment. Clin J Sport Med. 1997 Jul; 7(3):217–19.

47. Delagi E, Perotto A. Anatomic guide for the electromyographer. 2nd ed. Springfield: Charles C Thomas Publishers 1980.

48. Magora F, Rozin R, Ben-Menachem Y, Magora A. Obturator nerve block: an evaluation of technique. British Journal of Anaesthesia. 1969 Aug; 41(8):695–98.

49. Abraham P, Bickert S, Vielle B, Chevalier JM, Saumet JL. Pressure measurements at rest and after heavy exercise to detect moderate arterial lesions in athletes. J Vasc Surg. 2001 Apr; 33(4):721–27.

50. Abraham P, Leftheriotis G, Bourre Y, Chevalier JM, Saumet JL. Echography of external iliac artery endofibrosis in cyclists. Am J Sports Med. 1993 Nov–Dec; 21(6):861–63.

51. Abraham P, Chevalier JM, Saumet JL. External iliac artery endofibrosis: a 40-year course. Journal of Sports Medicine and Physical Fitness. 1997 Dec; 37(4):297–300.

52. Kibler WB, Press J, Sciascia A. The role of core stability in athletic function. Sports Medicine (Auckland, NZ). 2006; 36(3):189–98.

53. Putnam CA. Sequential motions of body segments in striking and throwing skills: descriptions and explanations. Journal of Biomechanics. 1993; 26 Suppl 1:125–35.

54. Cresswell AG, Oddsson L, Thorstensson A. The influence of sudden perturbations on trunk muscle activity and intra-abdominal pressure while standing. Experimental Brain Research. Experimentelle Hirnforschung. 1994; 98(2):336–41.

55. Aruin AS, Latash ML. Directional specificity of postural muscles in feed-forward postural reactions during fast voluntary arm movements. Experimental Brain Research. Experimentelle Hirnforschung. 1995; 103(2):323–32.

56. Hodges PW, Butler JE, McKenzie DK, Gandevia SC. Contraction of the human diaphragm during rapid postural adjustments. Journal of Physiology. 1997 Dec 1; 505(Pt 2):539–48.

57. Garner JP, Patel S, Glaves J, Ravi K. Is herniography useful? Hernia. 2006 Mar; 10(1):66–69.

58. Rowand M, Chambliss ML, Mackler L. Clinical inquiries. How should you treat trochanteric bursitis? Journal of Family Practice. 2009 Sep; 58(9):494–500.

59. Fredericson M, Cookingham CL, Chaudhari AM, Dowdell BC, Oestreicher N, Sahrmann SA. Hip abductor weakness in distance runners with iliotibial band syndrome. Clin J Sport Med. 2000 Jul; 10(3):169–75.

60. Ganz R, Parvizi J, Beck M, Leunig M, Notzli H, Siebenrock KA. Femoroacetabular impingement: a cause for osteoarthritis of the hip. Clinical Orthopaedics and Related Research. 2003 Dec; (417):112–20.

61. Leunig M, Podeszwa D, Beck M, Werlen S, Ganz R. Magnetic resonance arthrography of labral disorders in hips with dysplasia and impingement. Clinical Orthopaedics and Related Research. 2004 Jan; (418):74–80.

62. Birrell F, Croft P, Cooper C, Hosie G, Macfarlane G, Silman A. Predicting radiographic hip osteoarthritis from range of movement. Rheumatology (Oxford, England). 2001 May; 40(5):506–12.

63. Monteleone GP, Jr. Stress fractures in the athlete. Orthopedic Clinics of North America. 1995 Jul; 26(3):423–32.

64. Johnson AW, Weiss CB, Jr, Wheeler DL. Stress fractures of the femoral shaft in athletes – more common than expected. A new clinical test. Am J Sports Med. 1994 Mar–Apr; 22(2):248–56.

65. Bird PA, Oakley SP, Shnier R, Kirkham BW. Prospective evaluation of magnetic resonance imaging and physical examination findings in patients with greater trochanteric pain syndrome. Arthritis and Rheumatism. 2001 Sep; 44(9):2138–45.

66. Allen GM, Wilson DJ. Ultrasound in sports medicine – a critical evaluation. European Journal of Radiology. 2007 Apr; 62(1):79–85.

67. Brignall CG, Brown RM, Stainsby GD. Fibrosis of the gluteus maximus as a cause of snapping hip. A case report. J Bone Joint Surg Am. 1993 Jun; 75(6):909–10.

68. Seror P, Seror R. Meralgia paresthetica: clinical and electrophysiological diagnosis in 120 cases. Muscle & Nerve. 2006 May; 33(5):650–54.

69. Mitchell B. Hip joint injuries. In Brukner P, Khan K, eds. Clinical sports medicine. 3rd ed. Sydney: McGraw–Hill Professional 2006:399–403.

70. Rai S, Chandra SS, Smile SR. A study of the risk of strangulation and obstruction in groin hernias. Australian and New Zealand Journal of Surgery. 1998 Sep; 68(9):650–54.

71. Adler RS, Buly R, Ambrose R, Sculco T. Diagnostic and therapeutic use of sonography-guided iliopsoas peritendinous injections. AJR. 2005 Oct; 185(4):940–43.

72. Magee D. Orthopedic physical examination. 4th ed. Philadelphia: WB Saunders 2002.

The greater trochanter triangle

Introduction

Proximal lower limb pain is a cause of significant morbidity in athletes.[1-4] Trauma to the hip joint and bony structures of the hip may result in direct injury or chronic degenerative change.[5] Overload or overuse injury of muscle, tendon, ligament, or enthesis/apophysis at or around the femoro-acetabular joint may all result in chronic hip pain. The increasing popularity and availability of magnetic resonance imaging (MRI) and hip arthroscopy have both raised awareness, and offered therapeutic options for the management of hip and groin pain in the sports medicine community. Five to six percent of all adult athletic injuries, and 24% of all pediatric athletic injuries, relate to the hip joint.[6]

Pain localized to the lateral thigh may represent pathology within the femoro-acetabular joint,[7] or more superficial structures such as the iliotibial band[8] or trochanteric bursa. Differentiation of joint pathology from that of the structures responsible for its movement may be difficult, due to the complexity of movement at the joint. Radicular pain generated in the axial spine may also complicate an already busy area.[9]

The clinician must also bear in mind that pathology arising from the hip joint, and structures around it, may manifest as pain in the groin, buttock, and distal leg.[7] A thorough examination of the hip and will provide valuable information in the evaluation of any lower limb pathology.

The joint

The hip or femoro-acetabular joint is a ball-and-socket synovial joint (Fig. 5.1). Both the femoral head and the acetabulum of the pelvis are lined with articular hyaline cartilage. The union of the ischium, ilium, and pubis forms the cup-like acetabulum. They join at a Y-shaped growth plate – the triradiate cartilage which fuses at age 14–16 years. The acetabulum covers almost half of the femoral head, with the **acetabular labrum**, a fibrocartilaginous lip, extending this cover beyond the equator of the head.

The femoral head is attached to the shaft of the bone via the femoral neck. The concave nature of the head–neck junction allows the hip a range of motion second in the body only to the shoulder:

> lateral rotation: 30° with hip extended, 50° with hip flexed

> medial rotation: 40°

> extension: 20°

> flexion: 140°

> abduction: 50° with hip extended, 80° with hip flexed

> adduction: 30° with hip extended, 20° with hip flexed

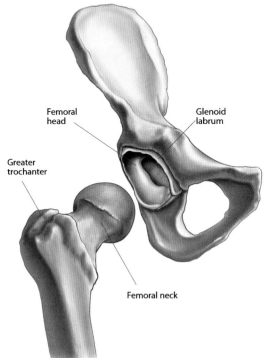

Femoral head

Glenoid labrum

Greater trochanter

Femoral neck

Figure 5.1 Anatomy of the hip

Despite this range of movement, the hip joint has sufficient stability to transmit the weight of the trunk, arms, and head. The strong but loose fibers of the hip capsule provide much of this stability. The capsule is attached to the acetabular rim, and on the femur midway along the femoral neck.

The hip capsule has fibers oriented in two directions:

> the circular fibers form a collar around the femoral neck called the zona orbicularis

> the longitudinal retinacular fibers travel along the neck, and carry blood vessels

Three ligaments are external to the capsule, and blend with it to reinforce the stability of the joint (Fig. 5.2).

The **iliofemoral ligament**, the strongest ligament in the body, is a broad, thick triangular band. It is attached proximally to the anterior inferior iliac spine and acetabular rim, and distally to the intertrochanteric line. The ligament is thicker toward the edges, and thinner in the middle. Its medial band is vertically orientated, and its lower end attaches to the medial end of the intertrochanteric line. The lateral band is obliquely orientated, and is attached to a tubercle at the upper lateral part of the intertrochanteric line. This is often considered an inverted Y- or V-shaped structure; the lateral band may then be referred to as the "iliotrochanteric ligament". It is taut in extension. In the upright position, it prevents the trunk from falling backward, without the need for muscular activity. In the sitting position, it becomes relaxed, thus permitting the pelvis to tilt backward into its sitting position.

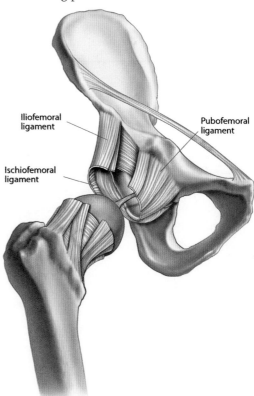

Iliofemoral
ligament

Pubofemoral
ligament

Ischiofemoral
ligament

Figure 5.2 Capsular ligaments of the
hip joint

The **pubofemoral ligament** is a triangular band. The base is attached to the iliopubic eminence, superior pubic ramus, and the pubic part of the acetabular rim. It passes distally to blend with the inferior aspect of the hip joint capsule, and underside of the femoral neck. Like the iliofemoral ligament, it is taut in extension, and restricts abduction in the hip joint.

The **ischiofemoral ligament** rises from the ischial component of the acetabulum, below and behind the hip joint. The fibers pass horizontally behind the joint, converging on the upper lateral aspect of the femoral neck, thereby preventing medial rotation.

The **ligamentum teres** arises from a depression in the acetabulum (the acetabular notch), and a depression on the femoral head (the fovea of the head). It is only stretched when the hip is dislocated, and may then prevent further displacement. It is less important in terms of stability than the other ligaments. As a conduit of a small artery, it may represent the only blood supply to the femoral head in the case of femoral neck fracture. Blood supply to the femoral head in early life is via the ligamentum teres, with the epiphyseal plate acting as a barrier to vessels entering from the femoral neck. This reverses between four and seven years of age, during which time the incidence of primary avascular necrosis (AVN), also known as Perthes' disease, increases.[10]

The blood supply

The hip joint is supplied with blood from the **arteria profunda femoris** (deep femoral) artery, via the **medial circumflex femoral**, and **lateral circumflex femoral** arteries. There are numerous variations, and one or both may also arise directly from the femoral artery.

The hip has two anatomically important anastomoses, the **cruciate**, and the **trochanteric anastomoses** (Fig. 5.3), the latter of which provides most of the blood to the head of the femur. These anastomoses exist between the femoral artery, or profunda femoris, and the gluteal vessels.

The arteria profunda femoris (deep femoral artery) is the largest branch of the femoral artery—supplying most of the muscles of the thigh (extensor and flexor). It arises from the lateral aspect of the femoral artery, about 3–4 cm below the inguinal ligament, medial to the greater trochanter triangle. The artery gives off three or four perforating arteries. These supply the muscles in the flexor and medial compartments of the thigh. Branches include the lateral circumflex femoral artery, and the medial circumflex femoral artery.

The femoral head and neck are supplied by an anastomotic ring of arteries found in the trochanteric fossa and around the neck of the femur. This anastomosis is called the trochanteric anastomosis, and is formed by the union of branches from:

1. the medial circumflex femoral artery
2. the ascending branch of the lateral circumflex femoral artery
3. the inferior gluteal artery
4. the superior gluteal artery

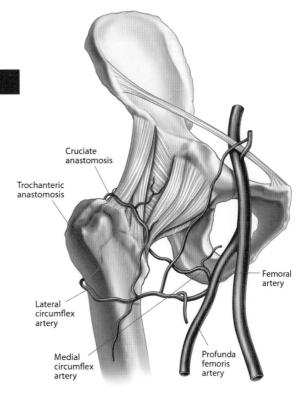

Figure 5.3 Blood supply to the hip

Cruciate anastomosis

Trochanteric anastomosis

Femoral artery

Lateral circumflex artery

Medial circumflex artery

Profunda femoris artery

The cruciate anastomosis is formed by a complex of arteries, which join together on the posterior aspect of the femoral shaft, distal to the greater trochanter. The main contributors to this anastomosis are:

1. the terminal part of the transverse branch of the lateral circumflex iliac artery
2. the terminal part of the transverse branch of the medial circumflex iliac artery
3. a branch of the inferior gluteal artery
4. a branch of the first perforating artery

The nerves

The **femoral nerve** (Fig. 5.4) arises from the dorsal divisions of the second, third, and fourth lumbar nerves. Formed within the fibers of the psoas major muscle, and emerging from the muscle at the lower part of its lateral border, the femoral nerve passes down between it and the iliacus (behind the iliac fascia). From there, it runs beneath the inguinal ligament, into the thigh, and splits into an anterior and a posterior division. Under the inguinal ligament, it lies lateral to the femoral artery. It is discussed further in Chapter 4.

The **lateral femoral cutaneous nerve** (Fig. 5.4) arises from the dorsal divisions of the second and third lumbar nerves. It emerges lateral to the psoas, running toward the anterior superior iliac spine, passing below the inguinal ligament, to supply the skin of the lateral thigh.

Figure 5.4 The greater trochanter triangle	
ASIS	= anterior superior iliac spine
3G	= the 3G point
G Max	= gluteus maximus
G Med	= gluteus medius
TFL	= tensor fascie late
Ilio Ps.	= Iliopsoas
RF	= rectus femoris
VL	= vastus lateralis
VM	= vastus medialis
n.	= nerve
a.	= artery
v.	= vein

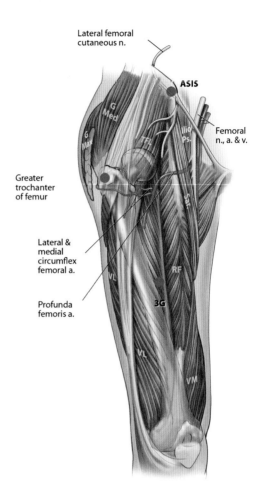

The **genitofemoral nerve** (Fig. 5.4) arises from the dorsal divisions of the first and second lumbar nerves, branching on the anterior aspect of the psoas into the genital and femoral branches.

The **genital** branch crosses the external iliac artery, passing through the deep inguinal ring supplying some of the skin of the scrotum or labia. This is discussed in Chapter 4.

The **femoral** branch passes beneath the inguinal ligament lateral to the external iliac artery, and pierces the femoral sheath, to provide the skin of the area anterior to the greater trochanter triangle.

Landmarks of the greater trochanter triangle

> greater trochanter of femur (GT)

> anterior superior iliac spine (ASIS)

> 3G point

The 3G point

From anthropometric measurements, the authors have defined a new reference point at the apex of the triangle. This point has been termed the "3G point" in reference to the three-dimensional pathology, and the groin, gluteal, and greater trochanteric regions. The relationship of this point in the anterior coronal plane is the mid-distance point between the ASIS and the superior pole of the patella, and in the posterior coronal plane, double the distance from the spinous process of the L5 lumbar vertebrae to the ischial tuberosity in the line of the femur.

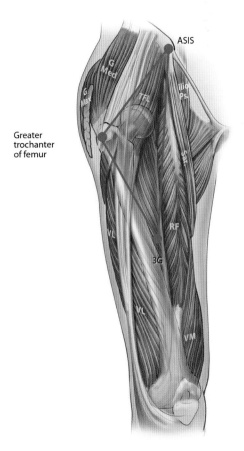

Figure 5.5 Greater trochanter triangle	
G Med	= Gluteus medius
G Max	= gluteus maximus
TFL	= tensor fasciae latae
Ilio Ps.	= Iliopsoas
Sar	= Sartorius
RF	= rectus femoris
VL	= vastus lateralis
VM	= vastus medialis

The **anterior superior iliac spine** (ASIS) is the salient physical landmark when the lower limb is viewed in the lateral decubitus position. From this position, it marks the most anterior projection of the structures responsible for abduction, extension, and lateral rotation of the hip, namely the gluteals, and tense fascia late. It is the origin of the sartorius, and the inguinal ligament. The iliac crest and the ASIS together act as anchor points for the thoracolumbar fascia, and its continuation, the fascia lata of the thigh. Just inferior to the ASIS lies the anterior inferior iliac spine (AIIS), the origin of the rectus femoris muscle. Inferior and medial to the ASIS, the lateral femoral cutaneous nerve may be compressed as it passes beneath the inguinal ligament.

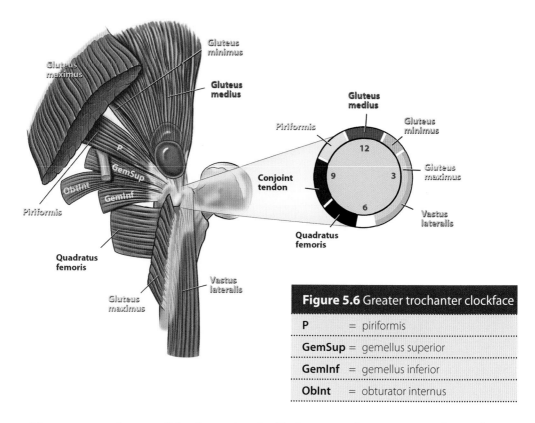

Figure 5.6 Greater trochanter clockface

P	= piriformis
GemSup	= gemellus superior
GemInf	= gemellus inferior
ObInt	= obturator internus

The **greater trochanter** of the femur is palpable in most subjects. Pain at the trochanter may be localized to one of the structures inserting into it. Palpatory anatomy of these structures is difficult, due to the overlying iliotibial band, and gluteus maximus. We present a schematic representation of these insertions in Figure 5.6. The authors recognize the variability of structures in this area, having based diagrams on cadaveric studies performed prior to this book.[II] Viewing the greater trochanter as a "clockface", the muscles insert as follows – the gluteus medius and its underlying bursa at 12 o'clock, the gluteus minimus and its underlying bursa at 1, the gluteus maximus overlaps the area, to insert from 2 to 6, with the vastus lateralis arising outside this. The quadratus femoris inserts between 7 and 8 o'clock, the conjoint tendon of the gemelli and obturator internus at 8–10, and the rounded tendon of the piriformis at 10–11.

Anatomical relations of the borders of the greater trochanter triangle

Superior border of the greater trochanter triangle

The line between the greater trochanter and the ASIS forms the superior border of the triangle (Fig. 5.5). Although the gluteus minimus is not palpable, the line runs parallel to the body of the muscle. This line transects the other gluteal muscles, and the tense fascia late (TFL).

Moving from the ASIS to the greater trochanter, the structures encountered are (Fig. 5.5, 5.6):

Superficial

> tensor fasciae latae (TFL)

> gluteus maximus

> gluteus medius

> gluteus minimus

Deep

> trochanteric bursae

> piriformis

> gemellus

  – superior

  – inferior

> obturator internus

The **tensor fasciae latae** (TFL) arises from the fascia lata (which arises along the full length of the rim of the ilium), just distal to the origin of the ITB, between the tubercle of the ileum, and the anterior superior iliac spine. It is supplied by superior gluteal nerve, and acts synergistically with the gluteus maximus to abduct the hip, and maintain the knee in extension.

The glutei

The **gluteus maximus** arises from the iliac wing behind the posterior gluteal line. This includes the iliac crest, from the posterior layer of the thoraco-lumbar fascia, the posterior surfaces of the sacrum, coccyx, and sacrotuberous ligament, and from the fascia covering the gluteus medius (the gluteal aponeurosis). It inserts into both the greater trochanter (2–6 o'clock), and the iliotibial band. Supplied by the inferior gluteal nerve, it is the largest muscle in the body. The portion (20%) inserting into the greater trochanter acts as a hip extensor, and lateral rotator. The part of the muscle inserting in the fascia lata and iliotibial band assists in adduction, and maintains knee extension.

The **gluteus medius** lies above the gluteus minimus, arising from the outer surface of the ilium, between the posterior and anterior gluteal lines. It inserts into the greater trochanter at 12 o'clock. Together with the gluteus minimus, it abducts and rotates internally or externally the hip joint, depending on the position of the femur, and which part of the muscle is active.[12, 13] Their anterior fibers, by drawing the greater trochanter forward, internally (medially) rotate the hip, in which action they are also assisted by the tense fascie late. When the hip is flexed to ninety degrees, however, the gluteus medius aids in externally (laterally) rotating the hip. Both muscles are fundamental in maintaining an upright trunk position when the contra-lateral foot is raised during walking. The superior gluteal nerve supplies the gluteus medius.

The **gluteus minimus** is the deepest and most lateral of the three gluteal muscles. It arises from the outer surface of the ilium, between the anterior and the inferior gluteal lines, inserting into the greater trochanter at 1 o'clock, as shown in Figure 5.6. The gluteus minimus is supplied by the superior gluteal nerve, like the gluteus medius, with which it works synergistically.

The **trochanteric bursae** are situated adjacent to the femur, between the insertion of the gluteus medius and gluteus minimus muscles, into the greater trochanter of the femur, and the femoral shaft. Their function, in common with other bursae, is as a shock absorber, and as a lubricant for the movement of the muscles adjacent to it.

The **piriformis** originates from the anterior aspect of the sacrum (costotransverse bars), and from the superior margin of the greater sciatic notch (as well as the sacroiliac joint capsule, and the sacrotuberous ligament). It exits the pelvis through the greater sciatic foramen, to insert on the greater trochanter of the femur at the 10–11 o'clock position. Its tendon sometimes joins the conjoined tendons of the superior gemellus, inferior gemellus, and obturator internus muscles, prior to insertion. The piriformis is supplied by the anterior primary rami of S1, S2, and it externally (laterally) rotates and stabilizes the hip joint. In 15% of the population, the sciatic nerve runs through the piriformis muscle.

The gemelli

The **gemelli** are two small muscular fasciculi, accessories to the tendon of the obturator internus, which is received into a groove between them. All three muscles form a conjoined tendon which inserts into the greater trochanter at 8–10 o'clock.

The **gemellus superior**, the smaller of the two, arises from the outer surface of the spine of the ischium, and blends with the upper part of the tendon of the obturator internus. It is supplied by the nerve to the obturator internus, and is sometimes absent.

The **gemellus inferior** arises from the upper part of the tuberosity of the ischium, immediately below the groove for the obturator internus tendon. It blends with the lower part of the tendon of the obturator internus. It is supplied by the nerve to the quadratus femoris, and, unlike its superior counterpart, it is rarely absent.

The **obturator internus** arises as a large fan-shaped muscle: (a) from the pelvic margins of the obturator foramen; (b) from the obturator membrane that fills it; and (c) from the anterolateral pelvic surface of the ilium. The muscle fibers converge, passing backward, to a groove on the lesser sciatic foramen. Here, its fibers make a right-angled turn, inferior to the ischial spine, to leave the pelvis. The groove is covered by hyaline cartilage, which is separated from the tendon of the obturator internus by a bursa, and is termed the "sciatic bursa of the obturator internus". The tendon usually fuses with the gemelli, to act as lateral (external) rotators of the hip. It is supplied by its own nerve.

Anterior border of the greater trochanter triangle

The anterior border of the triangle is the line from the ASIS to the apical point (Fig. 5.5). This corresponds to the force vector for abduction of the hip (the tense fascia late and gluteus maximus), and the manifestation of this force in the fascia late in the form of the iliotibial band (the anterior border of which is palpable on abduction of the hip). The rectus femoris arises via a direct head from the anterior inferior iliac spine, and via a reflected head from the superior acetabular rim and joint capsule.

Moving from lateral to medial, the structures encountered are (Fig. 5.5):

> tensor fasciae latae and iliotibial band

> iliopsoas

> vastus lateralis

> rectus femoris

The **iliotibial band** or tract (ITB) is a lateral thickening of the fascie late in the thigh. It is a continuation of the iliolumbar fascia, firmly attached to the rim of the ileum. Proximally, it splits into superficial and deep layers, enclosing the tensor fascie late, and anchoring this muscle to the iliac crest. This thickening probably reflects the force-load through the area during abduction, and when knee extension is maintained. The ITB inserts into Gerdy's tubercle but, as it crosses the lateral femoral condyle (LFC), thick fibrous attachments to the LFC are noted.[14]

The tensae fascica latae is described above.

The **iliopsoas** is a conjoint muscle of the psoas major, psoas minor, and iliacus.

The **psoas minor** arises as a series of slips, each of which arise from the adjacent margins of the vertebral bodies, and the intervening discs from the lower border of T12 and L1.

The **psoas major** arises from the transverse processes of L1–L5, the vertebral bodies of T12–L5, and the intervertebral discs below the bodies of T12–L4.

The **iliacus** arises from the upper two-thirds of the concavity of the iliac fossa and the inner lip of the iliac crest, as well as the ventral sacroiliac and iliolumbar ligaments, and the upper surface of the lateral part of the sacrum.

These muscles converge and pass downward and medially beneath the inguinal ligament, where they join, to pass over the hip joint, and into the lesser trochanter of the femur. The passage of this conjoined tendon over the hip joint is facilitated by the iliopsoas bursa, which is, in some cases, in direct communication with the hip joint. The iliopsoas is the primary hip flexor. The psoas minor and major are supplied by the anterior rami of the lumbar plexus L1, L2, L3, and the iliacus by the femoral nerve L2, L3.

The **vastus lateralis** forms part of the quadriceps femoris. It arises as a shared origin of the gluteus maximus at 2–6 on the greater trochanter clock by a broad aponeurosis. This passes in a line inferiorly to include the upper half of the lateral lip of the linea aspera, including the upper part of the intertrochanteric line, and the lateral lip of the gluteal tuberosity, and to the upper half of the lateral lip of the linea aspera. The aponeurosis covers the upper three-fourths of the muscle, and from its deep surface many fibers take origin. A number of fibers also arise from the lateral intermuscular septum, between the vastus lateralis and the short head of the biceps femoris. The tendinous insertion of the vastus lateralis is a broad flat aponeurosis, blending with the quadriceps femoris tendon, inserting into the superolateral patella; an expansion to the capsule of the knee joint is also seen. The vastus lateralis is innervated by the posterior division of the femoral nerve.

The **rectus femoris** forms part of the quadriceps femoris, arising by two tendons: the anterior head from the anterior inferior iliac spine (the reflected head from a groove above the brim of the acetabulum). Both heads unite to form an aponeurosis which is prolonged downward on the anterior surface of the muscle, and from this the muscular fibers arise. The muscle ends in a broad and thick aponeurosis, which occupies the lower two-thirds of its posterior surface, and, gradually becoming narrowed into a flattened tendon, is inserted into the base of the patella. Innervated by the posterior division of the femoral nerve, the rectus femoris is an extensor of the knee as part of the quadriceps, but, because of its origin above the hip joint, it is also a weak hip flexor. Both of the functions are affected by joint position. Thus when the knee is extended, the rectus femoris is a weak hip flexor, and when the hip is flexed, it is a weak knee extensor.

Posterior border of the greater trochanter triangle

The posterior border of the triangle is the line from the greater trochanter to the 3G/apical point (Fig. 5.5). Many of the structures encountered in this area are responsible for gluteal and posterior thigh pain. This pain is often ill defined, and the clinician should bear in mind the three-dimensional nature of the groin, hip, and gluteal areas. Pain localized to the lateral aspect of the triangle is dealt with comprehensively in Chapter 6. We will, however, discuss the structures encountered, in the order superior to inferior:

> gluteus maximus lies above the more proximal structures (Fig. 5.5 and 5.6)

> quadratus femoris

> adductor magnus

> vastus lateralis

> ischial tuberosity

> sciatic nerve

Quadratus femoris is the largest, and most inferior, of the small hip rotators. The muscle arises from the lateral aspect of the ischial tuberosity, anterior to the origin of the semimembranosus, passing superolaterally to a ridge on the intertrochanteric line (the quadrate tubercle). It passes inferior to the gemelli, and superior to the adductor magnus. Unsurprisingly, it acts as a lateral rotator, and adductor of the hip. It is supplied by the nerve to the quadratus femoris.

Adductor magnus is the most posterior, and lateral, of the adductors, the magnus arises from a curved origin, extending from the lateral inferior pubic ramus to the ischium, and the ischial tuberosity. It inserts into the femur inferomedially, to the gluteus maximus insertion, and as a linear aponeurosis, to the linea aspera, deep to the other adductors. A number of interruptions in the insertion allow the passage of vessels from the medial to posterior compartments. The most inferior of these is the adductor hiatus, through which the femoral vessels pass. The most inferior insertion of the aponeurosis is at the posterior aspect of the lateral femoral condyle. The most anterior component of the muscle behaves as an adductor (particularly with the hip extended), and is supplied by the posterior branch of the obturator nerve. The most posterior, and lateral, part of the muscle serves to extend the femur (in a similar way as a hamstring), and is supplied by the sciatic nerve.

The vastus lateralis is discussed in the section Anterior to the triangle (pg 196).

The largest nerve in the body, the **sciatic nerve** is a continuation of the upper band of the sacral plexus. Arising from the ventral rami of the fourth lumbar, to the third sacral spinal nerves L4, L5, S1, S2, S3, it consists of the medially placed tibial nerve, and the laterally placed common peroneal nerve. Leaving the pelvis through the greater sciatic foramen, the sciatic nerve passes below the piriformis muscle, and descends between the greater trochanter of the femur and the ischial tuberosity. Initially deep to the piriformis, the nerve runs inferiorly and laterally posterior to the ischium – crossing the obturator internus, gemelli, and quadratus femoris. The sciatic nerve supplies: (a) articular branches to the hip joint; and (b) muscular branches to the muscles of the posterior compartment of the thigh – the biceps femoris, semitendinosus and semimembranosus, and the most posterior portion (ischial head) of the adductor magnus.

The superior aspect of the **ischial tuberosity** gives rise to the hamstring group of muscles, semimembranosus, conjoint tendon of the semitendinosus, and long head of the biceps femoris. Inferior to this attachment, the adductor magnus arises laterally, and the sacrotuberous ligament arises medially. The individual anatomy of these structures is described in Chapter 6.

Within the greater trochanter triangle

Within the triangle, the main focus of our attention is the femoro-acetabular joint. This joint is not directly palpable within the triangle. It is projected medially and posteriorly from the palpable greater trochanter. When considering the pathology of the joint, we must consider not only the articular surfaces, but also the underlying bone, soft tissue structures (such as the synovium and acetabular labrum), and surrounding structures (such as the capsule, bursae, and muscles).

Internal (within the triangle)

Pathology of the hip joint often defies clinical distinction. The distance of the joint from the surface, the close proximity of the structures involved, and different conditions representing different stages in a clinical spectrum all help to explain why. In this section, discriminative signs are quite limited, so taking a thorough injury history, and performing an appropriate clinical examination may be even more important than usual.

Dividing patients according to adult and pediatric populations (Fig. 5.7) facilitates further stratification of the pathologies encountered within the triangle. The hip, be it adult or pediatric, is prone to inflammatory, infective, and degenerative processes. Degenerative changes, in particular, may be due to the large compressive loads transmitted through the hip's articular surfaces during ambulation.

Femoro-acetabular impingement

Irregular morphology of the acetabulum, or the femoral head/neck, may disrupt the labrum, resulting in pain, functional limitation, and, ultimately, joint degeneration. "Femoro-acetabular impingement" (FAI) is the collective term for this dysmotility. Where excessive

Table 5.1 Origins, insertions and nerve supply to the main movers of the hip joint				
Muscle	**Origin**	**Insertion**	**Nerve**	**Root**
Hip flexors				
Iliacus	Iliac fossa inner surface	Femur – lesser trochanter	Femoral nerve	L2, L3
Psoas major and minor	L1-L5 – transverse processes, T12-L5 – intervertebral discs	Femur – lesser trochanter	Lumbar plexus	L1, L2, L3
Rectus femoris	Anterior head – anterior inferior iliac spine Posterior head – supra acetabular groove	Tibia – tibial tuberosity	Femoral n.	L2, L3, L4
Sartorius	Ilium – anterior superior iliac spine	Tibia – proximal anteromedial tibia	Femoral n.	L2, L3
Glutei				
Gluteus minimus	Ilium – between anterior and inferior gluteal lines	Femur – greater trochanter (1–2 o'clock)	Superior gluteal n.	L4, L5, S1
Gluteus medius	Ilium – between posterior and anterior gluteal lines	Femur – greater trochanter (11–1 o'clock)	Superior gluteal n.	L4, L5, S1
Gluteus maximus	Ilium – posterior gluteal line, iliac crest posterior ⅓, lumbar fascia, lateral sacrum, coccyx, sacrotuberous ligament	Femur – greater trochanter (20%) Iliotibial band 80% (2–6 o'clock)	Inferior gluteal n.	L5, S1, S2
Tensor fasciae latae	Ilium – anterior superior iliac crest	Iliotibial band	Superior gluteal n.	L4, L5, S1
Lateral rotators				
Piriformis	Sacrum – anterior of costotransverse bars	Femur – greater trochanter (10–11 o'clock)	Anterior rami of S1, S2	S1, S2
Obturator internus	Pubis and ischium surrounding inner surface of obturator membrane	Femur – greater trochanter (8–10 o'clock)	Obturator internus n.	L3, L4
Obturator externus	Pubis and ischium surrounding outer surface of obturator membrane	Femur – greater trochanter (8–10 o'clock)	Obturator n., posterior division	L5, S1, S2
Gemellus inferior	Ischial tuberosity – upper border	Femur – greater trochanter (8–10 o'clock)	Quadratus femoris n.	L4, L5, S1
Gemellus superior	Ischium – spine	Femur – greater trochanter (8–10 o'clock)	Obturator internus n.	L5, S1, S2

Table 5.1 (continued)				
Muscle	**Origin**	**Insertion**	**Nerve**	**Root**
Quadratus femoris	Ischial tuberosity – lateral border	Femur – greater trochanter (6–8 o'clock)	Quadratus femoris n.	L4, L5, S1
Adductors				
Pectineus	Pubis – superior pubic ramus – pectineal line	Femur – pectineal line	Femoral n. and/or obturator n.	L2, L3 and/or L2, L3, L4
Adductor longus	Pubis – pubic tubercle (6–7 o'clock)	Femur – linea aspera middle ⅓	Obturator n.	L2, L3, L4
Adductor brevis	Pubis – body and inferior pubic ramus	Femur – linea aspera proximal ⅓	Obturator n.	L2, L3, L4
Adductor magnus	Anterior head – inferior pubic ramus and ischial ramus Posterior head – ischial tuberosity	Anterior head – linea aspera inferior ⅓ Posterior head – adductor tubercle of femur	Anterior – obturator n. Posterior – sciatic n.	L2, L3, L4 and L4, L5
Gracilis	Pubis – body and inferior pubic ramus	Tibia – anteromedial (pes anserinus)	Obturator nerve	L2, L3, L4

Table 5.2 Muscles responsible for the movements of the hip joint						
Movement	**Hip flexor**	**Lateral (external) rotation**	**Medial (internal) rotation**	**Adduction**	**Abduction**	**Hip extension**
Major	Iliopsoas	Gluteus maximus	Gluteus medius	Adductor longus	Gluteus medius	Gluteus maximus
	Rectus femoris		Gluteus minimus	Adductor brevis	Gluteus minimus	Adductor magnus (lower portion)
				Adductor magnus (upper portion)		
Minor	Pectineus	Piriformis	tensor fasciae latae	Pectineus		
	Adductor longus	Obturator (ext and int)	Adductor brevis	Gracilis		
	Adductor brevis	Gemelli (sup and inf)	Adductor longus			
	Adductor magnus	Quadratus femoris	Adductor magnus – superior portion			
	tensor fasciae latae					

coverage of the femoral head by the acetabulum occurs, this is termed a "pincer deformity". Where an abnormal femoral head–neck junction is present, this is deemed a "cam deformity". Osteoarthritis, often seen as a complication of old age, may be the natural progression of FAI. Where joint deformity causes damage to the smooth articular hyaline cartilage, even the hips of younger athletes may show signs of degenerative change.

Femoral stress fracture is sometimes seen in healthy athletes, and is associated with excessive loading of the area. More often, however, it is related to underlying nutritional and endocrine disturbance related to overtraining or the "female athletic triad" – severe dietary restriction, amenorrhoea, and osteoporosis.[15] Fractures of the femoral neck may be compression or tension fractures, depending on whether they occur on the inferior or superior aspect of the femoral neck.[16]

Non-traumatic disorders, such as septic arthritis, avascular necrosis of the head of the femur, tumor and inflammatory conditions, are also seen in the hip. Limitation of the range of movement of the hip, with associated systemic symptoms such as fever, weight loss, and night sweats, should flag further investigation to ensure that these serious, albeit rare, conditions are excluded.

Epiphyseal pathology

The presence of the femoral epiphysis, and the numerous secondary ossification centers in and around the hip, make the diagnosis and treatment of the pediatric and adolescent hip dissimilar to those of the adult (Fig. 5.7). A slipped upper femoral epiphysis, if untreated, has a high probability of being problematic later in life. The limping child or adolescent must be fully investigated.

Acute transient synovitis is the most common cause of hip pain in children up to the age of ten years.[28] Most often unilateral, this may be preceded by a viral illness, and presents as a mildly limited hip range of motion. The patient is very rarely unwell. Prognosis is good, and a full recovery is usually anticipated; recurrence is seen in up to 15% of cases. Although a benign condition, a thorough examination and investigation are mandatory, in order to exclude a toxic synovitis.

Apophysitis/avulsion fracture is seen in multiple sites around the hip:

> iliac crest

> anterior superior iliac spine

> anterior inferior iliac spine

> ischial tuberosity

> femoral greater trochanter

> femoral lesser trochanter

Within the greater trochanter triangle, apophysitis of the origin of the rectus femoris muscle may present as hip pain. Classically seen with explosive activity, such as kicking a ball from the ground or sprinting, this is often mistaken for a muscle tear.

Table 5.3 Patho-anatomic approach; within the greater trochanter triangle (adult), (diagnoses appear in order of frequency in an athletic population)				
Define and align	**Pathology**	**Listen and localize**	**Palpate and recreate**	**Alleviate and investigate**
Within the triangle (adult)	Femoro-acetabular impingement Labral injury	Mechanical symptoms, clicking ± locking	Impingement test[7]	Plain film x-ray, MRI ± arthrogram[17]
	Osteoarthritis	Insidious onset, night pain	Limited ROM, especially internal rotation[18]	Plain film x-ray
	Femoral stress fracture Neck	Groin pain, recent increase in activity levels	Hop test[19]	Plain film x-ray, isotope bone scans, MRI
	Shaft	Proximal thigh/knee pain, recent increase in activity levels	Fulcrum test[20]	Plain film x-ray, isotope bone scan, MRI
	Inflammatory conditions	Features of systemic inflammation	Systemic manifestations of particular condition[21]	Plain film x-ray, ultrasound-guided joint aspiration
	Septic arthritis	Systemic inflammatory response	Inability to weight bear, limited range of motion, ± sepsis[22]	Plain film x-ray, fluoroscopically/ ultrasound-guided joint aspiration
	Avascular necrosis of femoral head	Mechanical symptoms more prominent than functional limitation	Limited ROM[23]	Plain film x-ray, MRI
	Tumor	Systemic "red flags", absence of appropriate physical stressors[24]	May mimic stress fracture[24]	Plain film x-ray, computerised tomography (CT)/ MRI,[25] biopsy
	Transient osteoporosis of the hip	Women 3rd trimester of pregnancy, men 40–70, hip and groin pain, varied onset[26]	Pain on weight bearing and torsion, positive impingement test[26]	Plain film x-ray, MRI[27]

Perthes' disease is seen when there is osteonecrosis of the proximal femoral epiphysis (interrupted blood flow, thought to be causal). This is most often self-limiting, but pain and joint derangement are seen while remodeling occurs. Age is a critical factor in the outcome of this condition. When presenting prior to six years of age, the outcome is usually good. After this time, conservative measures are aimed at maintenance of the joint range of movement, and containment of the femoral head through the evolution of healing of the epiphysis. After age nine, conservative management is often unsuccessful.[29]

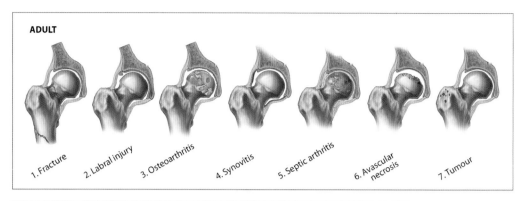

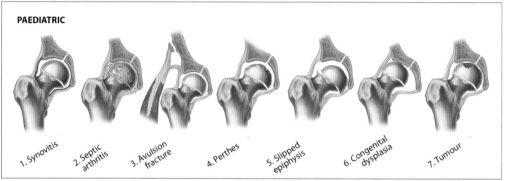

Figure 5.7 Within the greater trochanter triangle (adult and pediatric)

Slipped upper/capital femoral epiphysis (SUFE/SCFE) tends to occur in older children, possibly due to changes in the positioning of the joint, and resultant forces on the growth plate. Bilateral involvement occurs in almost one-third of cases – usually within six months of contralateral presentation.[30] The presentations of Perthes' disease and SUFE may be similar, and the clinician must bear them both in mind.

Septic arthritis is an emergency presentation. Delay in diagnosis increases the chance of joint-surface destruction, but may also endanger the health of the patient. Systemic signs of sepsis may be subtle; beware of the immunosuppressed (medications, illness, age) patient.

Congenital dysplasia, if severe, may be picked up at antenatal screening. However, undiagnosed acetabular dysplasia may be subclinical in terms of symptoms, and may present late in terms of joint destruction.

As part of every screen for joint pain and pathology, a thorough history, to exclude **red flags** such as weight loss and illness, must be completed. As a general, rule investigation of a painful joint where red flags may be present should include a plain film x-ray.[25]

Superior to the triangle

The iliac crest, and the muscle and fascia which arise from it, all lie superior to the line drawn between the GT and ASIS. The most common presentation of pain in this region is that of

Table 5.4 Patho-anatomic approach; within the greater trochanter triangle (pediatric), (diagnoses appear in order of frequency in an athletic population)					
Define and align	**Pathology**	**Listen and localize**	**Age group**	**Palpate and recreate**	**Alleviate and investigate**
Within the triangle (pediatric)	Acute transient synovitis	Males, refusal to weight-bear, poorly localized pain, viral precipitant	3–6 yrs	Well, non-toxic, variable range of motion	Diagnosis of exclusion, to be monitored to exclude septic arthritis[28]
	Apophysitis/ avulsion fracture	Associated injury/event	<18 yrs[31]	Point tenderness[32]	Plain film x-ray,[33] computerised tomography (CT)[34]
	Perthes' disease	Males (M:F = 4:1), limp, associated knee pain	4–9 yrs	Decreased range of movement of hip, abduction and internal rotation ↓ Joint effusion[35]	Plain film x-ray, antero/posterior (AP), lateral, and comparative views[35]
	Slipped capital femoral epiphysis	Overweight males, bilateral in 30% cases[30]	12–15 yrs	Decreased range of motion of hip, abduction and internal rotation ↓ Limb shortening, external rotation of hip[36]	Plain film x-ray, antero/posterior (AP), lateral, and comparative views
	Septic arthritis	Refusal to weight-bear, systemically unwell	All	Unwell, toxic, variable range of motion	Temp >38.5, CRP >20, ESR >40, refusal to weight-bear, leukocytosis >12[28] Plain film x-ray, joint aspiration, isotope bone scan
	Congenital dysplasia	Delayed mobilizing/ limp, walking on tiptoe[37]	All	Limb length discrepancy, unilateral symptoms, limitation of abduction[37]	Ultrasound, x-ray
	Tumor	Night pain, systemic "red flags", absence of appropriate physical stressors[24]	All	Systemic features, may mimic stress fracture[24]	Plain film x-ray, MRI[25]

myofascial trigger points. These are amenable to dry-needling or transverse friction myotherapy. It should be acknowledged that this pain may be the result of a problem elsewhere. The trigger points may lie superficially in the gluteus maximus or tense fascie late, or deeper in the gluteus medius and gluteus minimus.

"**Greater trochanter pain syndrome**" is an umbrella term for the pathology involving the insertion of the gluteus medius into the greater trochanter and the bursae which separate the gluteal tendons from each other and the underlying bone. Traditionally this was diagnosed as trochanteric bursitis, and, while a classical bursitis is often present, pathology of the gluteus medius tendon must be excluded as, if left untreated, symptoms will persist despite treatment of bursitis (traditionally corticosteroid injection[38]). Pain tends to be persistent at a low grade, but is aggravated by activity; when sore, it is worsened by movements which move a flexed hip into extension, such as rising from a chair or climbing stairs.

The iliotibial band receives 70% of the fibers of the gluteus maximus, and passes directly over the greater trochanter, where excessive tension may cause a palpable and/or audible capping or clicking; this is the so-called external snapping hip (*coxa saltans externa*), and proximal **iliotibial band friction**. This is seen more often in women than men,[39] and most often in an athletic population.[40] The click or snap is often easily recreated by the patient, and needs to be differentiated from the internal snapping hip seen when the iliopsoas tendon moves over the iliopectineal eminence (where the pubis and ilium join).

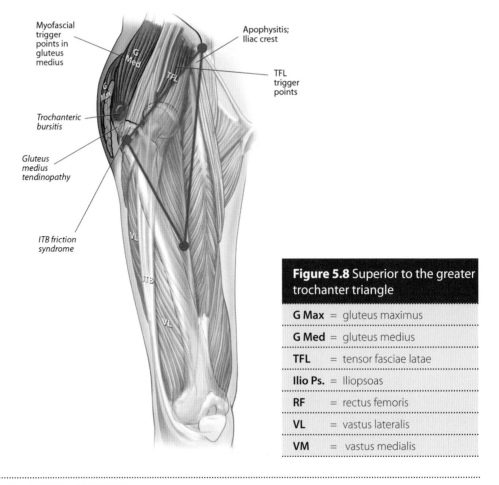

Myofascial trigger points in gluteus medius

Apophysitis; Iliac crest

TFL trigger points

Trochanteric bursitis

Gluteus medius tendinopathy

ITB friction syndrome

Figure 5.8 Superior to the greater trochanter triangle

G Max	= gluteus maximus
G Med	= gluteus medius
TFL	= tensor fasciae latae
Ilio Ps.	= Iliopsoas
RF	= rectus femoris
VL	= vastus lateralis
VM	= vastus medialis

Define and align	Pathology	Listen and localize	Palpate and recreate	Alleviate and investigate
Superior to the triangle	Myofascial trigger points in gluteus medius and tensor fasciae latae	Gluteal and lateral leg tightness and discomfort ± accompanying lateral knee pain	Restricted movement/strength in affected muscle.[41] Tender "trigger" points palpable within muscle[42, 43]	Dry-needling effective in relieving trigger points[42]
	Greater trochanter pain syndrome Gluteus medius tendinopathy	Weakness in stance phase of walking and/or running, climbing stairs[44]	Trendelenberg test 72% sensitive, 76% specificity[45]	Ultrasound[46]
	Trochanteric bursitis	Boggy feel and swelling	Pain on rising/ standing[45]	Ultrasound, relief of pain by local anesthetic injection[47]
	Iliotibial band friction syndrome	Snapping at hip joint associated lateral knee pain Women 15–40, athletic population, particularly ballet[39]	Ober's test,[48] patient voluntarily reproduces snap [39]	Ultrasound, dynamic view[46]
	Apophysitis; iliac crest	Age group (13–25 yrs),[31] activity load	Point tenderness,[32] painful Trendelenberg[4]	Plain film x-ray,[33] Computerised Tomography (CT)[34]

Table 5.5 Patho-anatomic approach; superior to the greater trochanter triangle (diagnoses appear in order of frequency in an athletic population)

Apophysitis, as elsewhere in the hip, is a load-related pathology occurring at the site of a growth plate – superior to the triangle, this may be seen at the iliac crest. Traction of the insertion of the oblique muscles superiorly, and the origin of tense fascia late and the gluteal muscles inferiorly, may cause pain, and loss of function at this site.

Posterior to the triangle

Beyond the posterior border of the triangle, in the gluteal area, poorly differentiated pain is common. The complex anatomy around the greater trochanter, the most superior point of this region, highlights the complexity of the area. The small muscles of the gluteal area (the piriformis, gemelli, and obturator internus) all insert here, and, due to their depth below the gluteal muscles, differentiation between them is problematic.

More medially, the ischial tuberosity is often the site of pain in the athlete. Pain caused by **hamstring tendinopathy** is anticipated in this area. It may be extremely difficult to differentiate from ischial bursitis, or even irritation of the sciatic nerve, which passes in close proximity to the hamstring origin.

Hamstring tendinopathy may be of sudden or insidious origin. Pain is felt high up at the ischial tuberosity, but may be felt to radiate down the hamstring. Typically worsened by activity or hamstring loading, hamstring tendinopathy may significantly impact on athletic performance.

Referred pain form the lumbar and sacral spine may cause pain posterior to the triangle. The exiting nerve root may be compressed in the neural foramen by disc material, facet joint hypertrophy, or be mechanically irritated due to muscle spasm. More distally, entrapment or irritation of the sciatic nerve may also cause buttock pain. This is discussed in depth in Chapter 6.

Ischial tuberosity apophysitis, or avulsion injuries, represent a spectrum of injury seen depending on patient age. The physis (growth plate) is far more vulnerable than a muscle or tendon, and is prone to avulsion. This may occur after a sharp hamstring contraction, or forced knee extension. The physis fuses at age 25, at which point bone avulsion is possible.[49]

Piriformis tendinopathy tends to be of more insidious onset than the nearby hamstring tendinopathy. There is a good deal of debate regarding the possibility of sciatic nerve involvement, and the direct etiology of piriformis-related pain[50]. This is discussed in Chapter 6.

Table 5.6 Patho-anatomic approach; posterior to the triangle (diagnoses appear in order of frequency in an athletic population)				
Define and align	Pathology	Listen and localize	Palpate and recreate	Alleviate and investigate
Medial to the triangle	Hamstring tendinopathy	Sudden pain in buttock/posterior thigh, walking painful[51]	Pain localized to ischial tuberosity/common origin, on resisted or eccentric contraction of hamstring	MRI[51], association between proximity of muscle defect to ischial tuberosity and recovery[52]
	Referred pain	Diffuse ache, may not have back pain	Lasègue straight leg raise (sensitivity 72–97%, specificity 11–66%)[48] Braggard's sign (94% +ve)[53]	Response to lumbar mobilization,[54] guided nerve root injection,[55] MRI
	Ischial tuberosity apophysitis/avulsion	Age-group (15–25 yrs),[31] shooting pain following high-energy kick or change of direction	Pain standing on one leg and Hop test,[48] associated deep buttock pain	Plan film x-ray, MRI[56]
	Piriformis tendinopathy	Hamstring origin pain with gradual rather than sudden onset and/or sciatic referred pain	Tenderness over sciatic notch and aggravated by flexion, adduction, and internal rotation (Lasègue sign) of the hip,[57] also FAIR test,[58] Pace test[48]	Ultrasound-guided injection[59]

Anterior to the triangle

The area anterior to the greater trochanter triangle is discussed in full in Chapter 4, the groin triangle. We consider here only the structures which need to be differentiated from femoro-acetabular pathology.

The origin of the rectus femoris at the anterior inferior iliac spine, and reflected head at the upper border of the acetabulum and joint capsule itself, mean that pathology at the muscle/tendon enthesis is easily mistaken for joint pathology.

The insertion of the conjoint tendon of the iliopsoas at the lesser tuberosity, having passed over the hip joint, provides the intimate relationship responsible for iliopsoas syndrome, internal snapping hip, and iliopsoas bursitis. The iliopsoas bursa is often continuous with the joint capsule.

Entrapment of the lateral femoral cutaneous nerve, or *meralgia paresthetica*, may result from damage or compression of the nerve as it passes inferior to the inguinal ligament. It causes dysesthesia in its myotome.

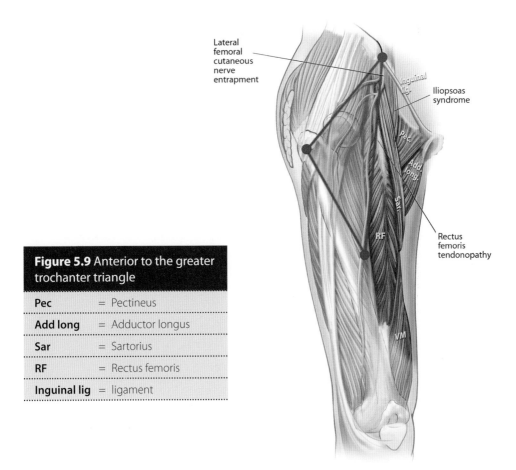

Lateral femoral cutaneous nerve entrapment

Iliopsoas syndrome

Rectus femoris tendonopathy

Figure 5.9 Anterior to the greater trochanter triangle

Pec	= Pectineus
Add long	= Adductor longus
Sar	= Sartorius
RF	= Rectus femoris
Inguinal lig	= ligament

Table 5.7 Patho-anatomic approach; anterior to the greater trochanter triangle (diagnoses appear in order of frequency in an athletic population)				
Define and align	**Pathology**	**Listen and localize**	**Palpate and recreate**	**Alleviate and investigate**
Anterior to the triangle	Iliopsoas syndrome	Pain on forced hip extension, unrelated to knee position. Pain above and below inguinal ligament	Thomas test[60]	Ultrasound ± guided local anesthetic injection,[61] MRI[62]
	Rectus femoris tendinopathy Apophysitis/avulsion	Pain in hip flexion worse with knee flexion. Sharp pain after explosive activity i.e. kick	Flexion contracture test[60] Modified Thomas test	MRI[62] Plain film x-ray
	Neuropathy, lateral femoral cutaneous nerve	Altered skin sensation	Paresthesia/dysesthesia over superficial area of lateral thigh	Local anesthetic infiltration to anterior iliac superior spine Nerve conduction studies[63]

Summary

The deep position of the hip joint makes diagnosis of pathology difficult. The close proximity of the lumbar spine, buttock, and groin, and the propensity of hip pain to radiate elsewhere, mean the clinician must consider not only the hip, but those structures around it. The authors particularly acknowledge the link between the buttock, hip, and groin presenting pathologies as the "3G" series.

Case histories

Case 1

A 40-year-old male golfer presents with a six-month history of worsening right hip pain. He is a professional golfer, and has been struggling with his game due to the pain. He particularly notices pain when practicing his drive at the driving range – when he feels a sharp pinch in his hip at the end of his backswing, after he has hit at least 30 balls. On playing a round of golf, he gets tired and sore by the end of his round. He used to jog three times a week for fitness, but has stopped this due to the pain.

To diagnose the cause of this presentation of hip pain, proceed to step 1, define and align the greater trochanter triangle.

Step 1: Define and align

Expose the patient properly; a pair of shorts and t-shirt allow an adequate view of the proximal lower limb. Initially, the patient should be examined while standing, and then lying comfortably.

Define the triangle: locate the greater trochanter (GT) of the femur, the anterior superior iliac spine (ASIS), and the 3G point (the mid-point between the ASIS and the superior pole of the patella).

Align the patient's pain on the triangle. Here the pain is non-specific. The patient points to the anterior aspect of the thigh, and the area within the greater trochanter triangle.

The patient has localized the pain to the area "within the triangle". From this point, we recommend that the reader attempt to exclude the potential pathologies. From Table 5.3, the potential causal structures are:

Differential diagnosis
> femoro-acetabular impingement (± labral injury)
> osteoarthritis
> femoral stress fracture (neck/shaft)
> inflammatory conditions
> septic arthritis
> avascular necrosis of femoral head
> tumor
> transient osteoporosis of the hip

We proceed to differentiate between these structures, step 2.

Step 2: Listen and localize

Addressing femoro-acetabular impingement with labral injury we ask:
Q *Is the pain associated with any clicking or locking?*
A Yes, it occasionally clicks if I rotate my hip.

Addressing osteoarthritis we ask:
Q *Is the pain persistently worse, particularly at night?*
A No, it really tends to be only after activity, but if I do a lot, it can be sore at night too.

Addressing femoral neck stress fracture we ask:
Q *Have you recently increased your amount of training – such as running?*
A No, I have now stopped but, prior to this, I always ran for 25–30 minutes three times a week.

Addressing inflammatory joint pathology we ask:
Q *Have you been unwell lately; have you had aches and pain in any other parts of your body; have you suffered form any rash, or skin irritation; have you had uveitis/iritis, or penile discharge (urethritis)?*
A No, I am actually very well.

Addressing septic arthritis we ask:
Q *Have you had a temperature, fever, or sweating?*
A No.

Addressing avascular necrosis of the head of the femur we ask:
Q *Is the clicking you mentioned more prominent than the pain you feel?*
A No. I don't mind the click, it doesn't always happen. The pain is the problem.

Addressing a tumor of the femur we ask:
Q *Have you noticed any weight loss or fevers recently?*
A No.

Addressing transient osteoporosis of the hip we ask (the patient cannot be pregnant, but may be in the male age category):
Q *Do you have much pain on walking normally?*
A No. Just after a full round of golf, or after a run.

This will narrow our differential diagnosis somewhat, and we proceed to examination to narrow it further. By palpating painful structures, and recreating the pain through diagnostic maneuvers, we move toward a diagnosis, step 3.

Differential diagnosis

More likely

> femoro-acetabular impingement (± labral injury)

> osteoarthritis

Less likely

> femoral stress fracture (neck/shaft)

> inflammatory conditions

> septic arthritis

> avascular necrosis of femoral head

> tumor

> transient osteoporosis of the hip

Step 3: Palpate and re-create

The hip joint lies deep to a significant muscle mass, the greater trochanter and the anterior inferior iliac spine, and may be palpated. Beyond these structures, however, much of the information to be gained about the joint is gained through assessment of the range of movement and pain-provoking maneuvers.

Given the presence of septic arthritis, a set of observations should be performed to include blood pressure, temperature, and oxygen saturation.

In this case, there is a full range of flexion and extension. Lateral rotation is normal (50°), but medial rotation is limited at 20°. Pain is reproduced on placing the patient in the impingement position; the patient lies supine, the hip and knee are flexed, the hip is adducted, and then medially rotated. Performing the Thomas and modified Thomas test helps to differentiate extra-articular causes, such as iliopsoas and rectus femoris pathology (examinations discussed in Chapter 4).

In the absence of any red flags in the history or examination, we must differentiate between two causes of degenerative change in the hip – osteoarthritis, or femoro-acetabular impingement. Given the history, stress fracture or transient osteoporosis are unlikely.

Step 4: Alleviate and investigate

We may now proceed to step 4 to confirm our clinical suspicion via imaging. Plain film AP and lateral views of the hip will demonstrate the loss of joint space seen in osteoarthritis; this will also show any abnormalities in bone density. It is possible to comment on acetabular osteophyte formation, and femoral head coverage, which is reduced in dysplasia. Where doubt remains, or to further clarify chondral pathology, MRI may be indicated.

Case 2

A five-year-old little-league baseball player attends the ED with a limp, and has difficulty running. He had been sent home from practice 24 hours earlier, as he was unable to run properly. Overnight he was well, but his mother became worried the next morning when he limped badly at breakfast. Of note, he had suffered sinusitis and a sore throat five days prior.

To diagnose the cause of this presentation of hip pain, proceed to step 1, define and align the greater trochanter triangle.

Step 1: Define and align

Expose the patient properly; a pair of shorts and t-shirt allow an adequate view of the proximal lower limb. Initially, the patient should be examined while standing, and then lying comfortably.

Define the triangle: locate the greater trochanter of the femur (GT), the anterior superior iliac spine (ASIS), and the 3G point (the mid-point between the ASIS and the superior pole of the patella).

Align the patient's pain on the triangle. Here the pain is located on the anterior thigh, in the area within the greater trochanter triangle (Paediatric).

From this point we recommend that the reader attempt to exclude the potential pathologies. From Table 5.4, the potential causal structures are:

Differential diagnosis
> acute transient synovitis
> apophysitis/avulsion fracture
> Perthes' disease
> slipped capital femoral epiphysis
> septic arthritis
> congenital dysplasia
> tumor

We proceed to differentiate between these structures, step 2.

Step 2: Listen and localize

Addressing acute transient synovitis, we note difficulty weight-bearing and preceding viral illness, so we ask:

Q *I know you have pain in your leg. Is it in your hip?*
A It's at the top of my leg.
Q *Could you stand on that leg only?*
A No, ouch!

Addressing apophysitis/avulsion fracture we ask:

Q *Was there any injury. Did you fall or trip?*

A No.

Addressing femoral Perthes' disease we ask:

Q *Do you have any knee pain?*

A I don't know. All of my leg is sore.

Addressing slipped capital femoral epiphysis (SCFE) we ask:

Q *Do you have any pain on the other side?*

A No. My other side is fine

Addressing septic arthritis we ask:

Q *Have you had a temperature, fever, or sweating?*

A No.

Addressing congenital dysplasia of the acetabulum we ask:

Q *Do you have any history of limping, or hip pain as a younger child?*

A No (patient's mother confirms this).

Addressing a tumor of the femur we ask:

Q *Have you noticed any weight loss or fevers recently?*

A No.

This will narrow our differential diagnosis somewhat, but we still have a relatively broad differential diagnosis. We proceed to examination to narrow it further. By palpating painful structures, and recreating the pain through diagnostic maneuvers, we move toward a diagnosis, step 3.

Differential diagnosis

More likely

> acute transient synovitis

> Perthes' disease

> slipped capital femoral epiphysis

> congenital dysplasia

Less likely

> tumor

> apophysitis/avulsion fracture

> septic arthritis

Step 3: Palpate and re-create

The hip joint lies deep to a significant muscle mass, the greater trochanter and the anterior inferior iliac spine, and may be palpated. Beyond these structures, however, much of the information to be gained about the joint is gained through assessment of the range of movement and pain-provoking maneuvers.

Given the fact there is a potential for septic arthritis, a set of observations should be performed to include blood pressure, temperature, and oxygen saturation. These are normal: temperature 37°C/98.6°F, pulse 88 bpm, BP 90/62 mmHg, O_2 sats 99% on room air. The patient is well.

In this case, there was no injury. The pathologies within the joint, such as synovitis, septic arthritis, and Perthes' disease, must be considered. Slipped capital femoral epiphysis (SCFE) is unlikely, due to the age profile.

Palpation is negative for any site of tenderness.

Active movement of the joint is painful. Passive flexion (70°), internal rotation (20°), and external rotation (40°) are all limited and painful. Pain is reproduced on placing the patient in the impingement position. The Thomas and modified Thomas test are both painful.

Globally, the limited range of motion requires the exclusion of articular pathology.

Step 4: Alleviate and investigate

We may now proceed to step 4 to confirm our clinical suspicion via imaging. Plain film AP and lateral and comparative views of the hip exclude apophysitis, congenital dysplasia, Perthes', and SCFE. Serology returns with a normal white-cell count, and sedimentation rate of 18 mm, effectively excluding septic arthritis. A diagnosis of exclusion of acute transient synovitis is made.

Case 3

A 14-year-old female soccer goalkeeper presents with a history of acute hip pain following a kick in the second half of a game, 72 hours earlier. She had been very well before the injury. She describes a sharp pain as she kicked the ball, and felt something snap in her hips. She developed immediate swelling on the anterior thigh, and has been finding walking and sitting up from lying painful. She has not tried to play football since. She points to the anterior thigh, and has marked swelling and ecchymosis in the area.

To diagnose the cause of this presentation of hip pain, proceed to step 1, define and align the greater trochanter triangle.

Step 1: Define and align

Expose the patient properly; a pair of shorts and t-shirt allow an adequate view of the proximal lower limb. The patient should be examined while standing initially, and then lying comfortably.

Define the triangle: locate the greater trochanter of the femur (GT), the anterior superior iliac spine (ASIS), and the 3G point (the mid-point between the ASIS and the superior pole of the patella).

Align the patient's pain on the triangle. Here the pain is non-specific; the patient points to the anterior aspect of the thigh, and the area within the greater trochanter triangle.

The patient has localized the pain to the area "anterior to the triangle". From this point, we recommend that the reader attempt to exclude the potential pathologies. From Table 5.7, the potential causal structures are:

Differential diagnosis

> iliopsoas syndrome

> iliotibial band friction syndrome

> rectus femoris tendinopathy

> apophysitis/avulsion

> neuropathy, lateral femoral cutaneous nerve

We proceed to differentiate between these structures, step 2.

Step 2: Listen and localize

Addressing iliopsoas syndrome we ask:

Q *Is the pain also felt in the lower abdomen?*

A Yes.

Q *Does bringing your knee up to your chest worsen the pain?*

A Yes.

Addressing iliotibial band friction syndrome we ask:

Q *Have you noticed a clicking or snapping at the edge of your hip?*

A No.

Q *Have you noticed any knee pain?*

A No.

Addressing rectus femoris pathology we ask:

Q *Did your pain commence immediately on kicking the ball; was your kick weak after the injury?*

A Yes! I fell to the ground and couldn't kick again.

Addressing neuropathy, lateral femoral cutaneous nerve we ask:

Q *Have you noticed any change in the feeling of your leg?*

A No.

This will narrow our differential diagnosis somewhat, and we proceed to examination to narrow it further. By palpating painful structures, and recreating the pain through diagnostic maneuvers, we move toward a diagnosis, step 3.

Differential diagnosis

More likely

> rectus femoris tendinopathy

> apophysitis/avulsion

> iliopsoas syndrome

Less likely

> iliotibial band friction syndrome

> neuropathy, lateral femoral cutaneous nerve

Step 3: Palpate and re-create

The obvious injury history, and limitation and pain of movement, particularly hip flexion, make hip flexor (iliopsoas, rectus femoris) pathology likely.

In this case, there is a full range of motion of the hip. There is no evidence of any external snapping or pain associated with the iliotibial band. The Thomas test is positive; here the patient is positioned supine at the end of the examination couch, with the painful hip extended, and the contralateral side flexed. This indicates pathology of either hip flexor. The addition of knee flexion (the modified Thomas test) fully recreates the patient's pain, as it engages the rectus femoris primarily due to knee movement.

Step 4: Alleviate and investigate

We may now proceed to step 4 to confirm our clinical suspicion via imaging. Plain film AP and lateral views of the hip may demonstrate avulsion of the physis at the AIIS. Where doubt remains, or to further clarify musculotendinous injury, MRI may be indicated.

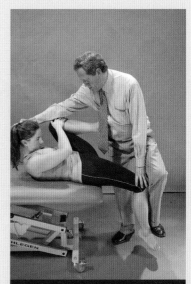

Figure 5.10 Modified Thomas test

References

1. Brooks JH, Fuller CW, Kemp SP, Reddin DB. Epidemiology of injuries in English professional rugby union: part 2 training injuries. British Journal of Sports Medicine. 2005 Oct; 39(10):767–75.
2. Orchard J, Seward H. Epidemiology of injuries in the Australian Football League, seasons 1997–2000. British Journal of Sports Medicine. 2002 Feb; 36(1):39–44.
3. Walden M, Hagglund M, Ekstrand J. Football injuries during European Championships 2004–2005. Knee Surg Sports Traumatol Arthrosc. 2007 Sep; 15(9):1155–62.
4. Paluska SA. An overview of hip injuries in running. Sports Medicine (Auckland, NZ). 2005; 35(11):991–1014.
5. Reginster JY. The prevalence and burden of arthritis. Rheumatology (Oxford, England). 2002 Apr; 41(Supp 1):3–6.
6. Bharam S. Labral tears, extra-articular injuries, and hip arthroscopy in the athlete. Clinics in Sports Medicine. 2006 Apr; 25(2):279–92, ix.
7. Ganz R, Parvizi J, Beck M, Leunig M, Notzli H, Siebenrock KA. Femoroacetabular impingement: a cause for osteoarthritis of the hip. Clinical Orthopedics and Related Research. 2003 Dec; (417):112–20.
8. Fredericson M, Weir A. Practical management of iliotibial band friction syndrome in runners. Clin J Sport Med. 2006 May; 16(3):261–68.
9. Brukner P, Khan K. Buttock pain. In: Brukner P, Khan K, eds. Clinical sports medicine. 3rd ed. Sydney: McGraw Hill 2006.
10. Anderson IA, Read JW. The pelvis, hip and thigh. Atlas of imaging in sports medicine. Sydney: McGraw-Hill Australia 2008:285–390.
11. Franklin-Miller A, Falvey EC, McCrory P, Briggs C. Landmarks for the 3G approach; groin, gluteal, and greater trochanter triangles, a pathoanatomical method in sports medicine. Submitted. 2007.
12. Beck M, Sledge JB, Gautier E, Dora CF, Ganz R. The anatomy and function of the gluteus minimus muscle. The Journal of Bone and Joint Surgery. 2000 Apr; 82(3):358–63.
13. Fredericson M, Cookingham CL, Chaudhari AM, Dowdell BC, Oestreicher N, Sahrmann SA. Hip abductor weakness in distance runners with iliotibial band syndrome. Clin J Sport Med. 2000 Jul; 10(3):169–75.
14. Fairclough J, Hayashi K, Toumi H, Lyons K, Bydder G, Phillips N, et al. The functional anatomy of the iliotibial band during flexion and extension of the knee: implications for understanding iliotibial band syndrome. Journal of Anatomy. 2006 Mar; 208(3):309–16.
15. Benjamin HJ. The female adolescent athlete: specific concerns. Pediatric Annals. 2007 Nov; 36(11):719–26.
16. DeFranco MJ, Recht M, Schils J, Parker RD. Stress fractures of the femur in athletes. Clinics in Sports Medicine. 2006 Jan; 25(1):89–103, ix.
17. Leunig M, Podeszwa D, Beck M, Werlen S, Ganz R. Magnetic resonance arthrography of labral disorders in hips with dysplasia and impingement. Clinical Orthopedics and Related Research. 2004 Jan; (418):74–80.
18. Birrell F, Croft P, Cooper C, Hosie G, Macfarlane G, Silman A. Predicting radiographic hip osteoarthritis from range of movement. Rheumatology (Oxford, England). 2001 May; 40(5):506–12.
19. Monteleone GP, Jr. Stress fractures in the athlete. The Orthopedic Clinics of North America. 1995 Jul; 26(3): 423–32.
20. Johnson AW, Weiss CB, Jr, Wheeler DL. Stress fractures of the femoral shaft in athletes – more common than expected. A new clinical test. Am J Sports Med. 1994 Mar–Apr; 22(2):248–56.
21. Izenberg DA, Maddison PJ, Woo P, Glass D, Breedveld FC. Oxford textbook of rheumatology. 3rd ed. Oxford University Press 2004.
22. Margaretten ME, Kohlwes J, Moore D, Bent S. Does this adult patient have septic arthritis? JAMA. 2007 Apr 4; 297(13):1478–88.
23. Steinberg ME. Osteonecrosis of the hip: summary and conclusions. Seminars in Arthroplasty. 1991 Jul; 2(3): 241–49.
24. Kumar V, Abbas A, Fausto N. Bones, joints and soft tissue tumors. In: Kumar V, Abbas A, Fausto N, eds. Robbins and Cotran pathologic basis of disease. 7th ed. Saunders Elsevier 2007:1273–325.
25. Reeder J. Hip. In: Edelman R, Hesselink J, Zlatkin M, Crues J, eds. Clinical magnetic resonance imaging. Philadelphia: Saunders Elsevier 2006:3366–99.
26. Ritchie JR. Orthopedic considerations during pregnancy. Clinical Obstetrics and Gynecology. 2003 Jun; 46(2):456–66.

27. Takatori Y, Kokubo T, Ninomiya S, Nakamura T, Okutsu I, Kamogawa M. Transient osteoporosis of the hip. Magnetic resonance imaging. Clinical Orthopedics and Related Research. 1991 Oct; (271):190–94.
28. Caird MS, Flynn JM, Leung YL, Millman JE, D'Italia JG, Dormans JP. Factors distinguishing septic arthritis from transient synovitis of the hip in children. A prospective study. J Bone Joint Surg Am. 2006 Jun; 88(6):1251–57.
29. Thompson GH, Price CT, Roy D, Meehan PL, Richards BS. Legg-Calve-Perthes disease: current concepts. Instructional Course Lectures. 2002; 51:367–84.
30. Kocher MS, Tucker R. Pediatric athlete hip disorders. Clinics in Sports Medicine. 2006 Apr; 25(2):241–53, viii.
31. Paletta GA, Jr., Andrish JT. Injuries about the hip and pelvis in the young athlete. Clinics in Sports Medicine. 1995 Jul; 14(3):591–628.
32. Dalton SE. Overuse injuries in adolescent athletes. Sports Medicine (Auckland, NZ). 1992 Jan; 13(1):58–70.
33. Scopp JM, Moorman CT, 3rd ed. The assessment of athletic hip injury. Clinics in Sports Medicine. 2001 Oct; 20(4):647–59.
34. Bencardino JT, Palmer WE. Imaging of hip disorders in athletes. Radiologic Clinics of North America. 2002 Mar; 40(2):267–87, vi–vii.
35. Catterall A. The natural history of Perthes' disease. The Journal of Bone and Joint Surgery. 1971 Feb; 53(1):37–53.
36. Reynolds RA. Diagnosis and treatment of slipped capital femoral epiphysis. Current Opinion in Pediatrics. 1999 Feb; 11(1):80–83.
37. Dezateux C, Rosendahl K. Developmental dysplasia of the hip. Lancet. 2007 May 5; 369(9572):1541–52.
38. Rowand M, Chambliss ML, Mackler L. Clinical inquiries. How should you treat trochanteric bursitis? The Journal of Family Practice. 2009 Sep; 58(9):494–500.
39. Winston P, Awan R, Cassidy JD, Bleakney RK. Clinical examination and ultrasound of self-reported snapping hip syndrome in elite ballet dancers. Am J Sports Med. 2007 Jan; 35(1):118–26.
40. Teitz CC, Garrett WE, Jr, Miniaci A, Lee MH, Mann RA. Tendon problems in athletic individuals. Instructional Course Lectures. 1997; 46:569–82.
41. Travell JG, Simons DG. Myofascial pain and dysfunction. The trigger point manual. Philadelphia: Lippincott Williams & Wilkins 1993.
42. Lavelle ED, Lavelle W, Smith HS. Myofascial trigger points. Med Clin North Am. 2007 Mar; 91(2):229–39.
43. Njoo KH, Van der Does E. The occurrence and inter-rater reliability of myofascial trigger points in the quadratus lumborum and gluteus medius: a prospective study in non-specific low back pain patients and controls in general practice. Pain. 1994 Sep; 58(3):317–23.
44. Ozcakar L, Erol O, Kaymak B, Aydemir N. An underdiagnosed hip pathology: apropos of two cases with gluteus medius tendon tears. Clinical Rheumatology. 2004 Oct; 23(5):464–66.
45. Bird PA, Oakley SP, Shnier R, Kirkham BW. Prospective evaluation of magnetic resonance imaging and physical examination findings in patients with greater trochanteric pain syndrome. Arthritis and Rheumatism. 2001 Sep; 44(9):2138–45.
46. Allen GM, Wilson DJ. Ultrasound in sports medicine – a critical evaluation. European Journal of Radiology. 2007 Apr; 62(1):79–85.
47. Walker P, Kannangara S, Bruce WJ, Michel D, Van der Wall H. Lateral hip pain: does imaging predict response to localized injection? Clinical Orthopedics and Related Research. 2007 Apr; 457:144–49.
48. Malanga GA, Nadler SF. Physical examination of the hip. Musculoskeletal physical examination, an evidence-based approach. Philedlphia, PA: Elsevier Mosby 2006:251–79.
49. Hamada G, Rida A. Ischial apophysiolysis (IAL). Report of a case and review of the literature. Clinical Orthopedics and Related Research. 1963; 31:117–30.
50. McCrory P. The "piriformis syndrome" – myth or reality? British Journal of Sports Medicine. 2001 Aug; 35(4):209–10.
51. Verrall GM, Slavotinek JP, Barnes PG, Fon GT. Diagnostic and prognostic value of clinical findings in 83 athletes with posterior thigh injury: comparison of clinical findings with magnetic resonance imaging documentation of hamstring muscle strain. Am J Sports Med. 2003 Nov–Dec; 31(6):969–73.
52. Askling CM, Tengvar M, Saartok T, Thorstensson A. Acute first-time hamstring strains during high-speed running: a longitudinal study including clinical and magnetic resonance imaging findings. Am J Sports Med. 2007 Feb; 35(2):197–206.
53. Stankovic R, Johnell O, Maly P, Willner S. Use of lumbar extension, slump test, physical and neurological examination in the evaluation of patients with suspected herniated nucleus pulposus. A prospective clinical study. Manual Therapy. 1999 Feb; 4(1):25–32.

54. Brukner PD, Khan K. Buttock pain. In: Brukner PD, Khan K, eds. Clinical sports medicine. Sydney: McGraw Hill 2006.

55. Manchikanti L, Cash KA, Pampati V, McManus CD, Damron KS. Evaluation of fluoroscopically guided caudal epidural injections. Pain Physician. 2004 Jan; 7(1):81–92.

56. Berger FH, de Jonge MC, Maas M. Stress fractures in the lower extremity. The importance of increasing awareness amongst radiologists. European Journal of Radiology. 2007 Apr; 62(1):16–26.

57. Beatty RA. The piriformis muscle syndrome: a simple diagnostic maneuver. Neurosurgery. 1994 Mar; 34(3): 512–14; discussion 14.

58. Solheim LF, Siewers P, Paus B. The piriformis muscle syndrome. Sciatic nerve entrapment treated with section of the piriformis muscle. Acta Orthopedica Scandinavica. 1981 Feb; 52(1):73–75.

59. Smith J, Hurdle MF, Locketz AJ, Wisniewski SJ. Ultrasound-guided piriformis injection: technique description and verification. Archives of Physical Medicine and Rehabilitation. 2006 Dec; 87(12):1664–67.

60. Magee D. Orthopedic physical examination. 4th ed. Philedelphia: WB Saunders 2002.

61. Adler RS, Buly R, Ambrose R, Sculco T. Diagnostic and therapeutic use of sonography-guided iliopsoas peritendinous injections. AJR. 2005 Oct; 185(4):940–43.

62. Shellock FG, Fleckenstein JL. Muscle physiology and pathophysiology: magnetic resonance imaging evaluation. Seminars in Musculoskeletal Radiology. 2000; 4(4):459–79.

63. Seror P, Seror R. Meralgia paresthetica: clinical and electrophysiological diagnosis in 120 cases. Muscle & Nerve. 2006 May; 33(5):650–54.

6

The gluteal triangle

Introduction

O veruse of the gluteal muscles is common; a long cycle ride can elicit signs of this, but does not always result in pain, There are, however, many potential diagnoses and, while one commonly thinks of hamstring-origin pain, a range of less common sources of pain exist. The area is complex, with many structures lying deep to each other, and difficult to palpate or test independently. The area is also a common source of radicular or referred pain[1]. The musculoskeletal presentation of systemic disease can commonly present as sacroiliac joint pathology, or non-specific buttock pain, but also as more acute on-track or on-field injuries.

The presentations of gluteal strains, hamstring tears, and sacroiliac joint pathology are similar and, for the clinician, eliciting the significant signs in order to differentiate the diagnosis requires inherent understanding of the anatomy. This chapter aims to clearly delineate those anatomical structures of the area, and divide the more common from the less common diagnoses. This will enable the clinician to discriminate more easily between pathological conditions, and to target their management to specific diagnoses.

The gluteal triangle contains the hip joint. While this is also a source of some of the pathologies encountered in this region, the hip is covered comprehensively in Chapter 5 on the greater trochanter, although there is some crossover in these chapters, As the reader will see, the common anatomical landmark, the 3G point, is used to highlight the co-pathology in this region, and the three chapters 4, 5, and 6 comprehensively cover the region.

Learning objectives

The landmarks of the gluteal triangle

The pain-generating structures of the region

Significant joints, ligaments, and muscle actions and properties

The presenting symptoms of pathology of each of these structures, to allow differentiation between them

Discriminative examinations and maneuvers to alter (reduce/increase) the presenting pain

Evidence-based examinations to confirm the clinical diagnosis

The region

The gluteal region is made up of the lumbar spine, sacrum, sacroiliac joints, and hip joint from the posterior approach. It is important to understand the bony anatomy, before trying to appreciate the overlying tissues, and we focus here on the construction of the posterior pelvis.

Lumbar spine

The lumbar spine is made up of five vertebrae. Each has a vertebral rounded body, with a vertebral arch posteriorly. The arch forms within itself the vertebral foramen, through which the spinal cord runs. The vertebral arch is made up of two identical pedicles, and two lamine, which make up the arch laterally and posteriorly. The vertebral arch gives rise to a posterior, spinous process formed by the junction of the two lamine, and two lateral transverse processes, which arise from the junction of the lamine and the pedicles.

The articular surface of the intervertebral joints are both superior and inferior, and are cartilaginous joints, the superior surface of one vertebra corresponding to the posterior surface of the superior vertebral body. On either side of the space between the intervertebral joint is the foramen, through which passes the spinal nerve root and associated vessels.

The nerve roots passing through the lumbar vertebrae foramina contribute to form the lumbar plexus. Between the lumbar vertebrae lies the intervertebral disc, described in detail in Chapter 9 on the spine.

Sacroiliac joint

The sacroiliac joint is a large, part-synovial joint between the sacrum and the ilium. It is synovial in its anterior third, and the remainder is formed by ligamentous attachments. It is subject to significant vertical shear forces, dependent on the anatomical variation of length and angulation. It aims to restrict movement in all directions, but itself is the cause of much pathology.

The **interosseous sacroiliac ligament** is a dense collection of fibers connecting the surface of the sacrum to the ilium. The ligament lies the full length of the narrow space between the two bones, and locks the interconnecting surfaces together.

The **sacrotuberous ligament** runs from the posterior superior and inferior iliac spine, and the posterior surface of the sacrum, and merges with the long posterior sacroiliac ligaments; the fibers from these origins twist as they travel down to attach to the medial aspect of the ischial tuberosity and ischial ramus.

The **sacrospinal ligament** arises from a broad base at the lateral edge of the sacrum, and runs forward to the iliac spine. Together with the sacrotuberous ligament, it prevents caudal tilt of the anterior pelvis, by anchoring it to the sacrum. The coccygeus runs anterior to this ligament.

The **anterior sacroiliac ligament** covers the ventral portion of the sacroiliac joint. Long fibers extend transversely from the anterior surface of the sacrum to the anterior surface of the ilium. The fibers span a large distance either side of the joint, and aim to stabilize and prevent the anterior diastasis of the joint.

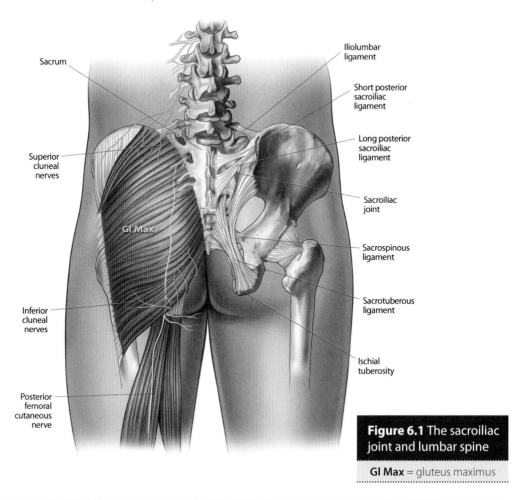

Sacrum

Superior cluneal nerves

Gl Max

Inferior cluneal nerves

Posterior femoral cutaneous nerve

Iliolumbar ligament

Short posterior sacroiliac ligament

Long posterior sacroiliac ligament

Sacroiliac joint

Sacrospinous ligament

Sacrotuberous ligament

Ischial tuberosity

Figure 6.1 The sacroiliac joint and lumbar spine

Gl Max = gluteus maximus

The **posterior sacroiliac ligament** lies deep to the interosseus ligament, connecting the lateral crest of the sacrum to the posterior superior iliac sine of the iliac crest. The fibers from the S3/S4 segments are the longest, and give the descriptive name of the long posterior sacroiliac ligament, whereas the short posterior sacroiliac ligament arises from the interosseus ligament and first to sacral segments.

The hip joint

The hip joint is a synovial joint formed between the acetabulum, at the union of the ischium, pubic bone, and ilium. This, a joint in itself, fuses at 14–16 years of age, and is termed the "triradiate cartilage". The acetabulum is surrounded by the acetabular cartilaginous labrum, which acts like a suction cup to the rounded, ball-like head of the femur, securing it to form the articular joint. The joint is capsular, and the capsule is strengthened by the extracapsular ligaments: the ilio-, ishio-, and pubofemoral ligaments. The ligamentum teres is the intracapsular ligament, supplying along its course the arterial supply to the femoral head. Detailed descriptions of these ligaments are covered in Chapter 5.

The lumbosacral plexus

A comprehensive understanding of the lumbosacral plexus is requisite in order to appreciate the effect of nerve entrapments, not only in the gluteal region, but also in the whole lower limb.

The sacral plexus lies on the back of the pelvis, between the piriformis and the pelvic fascia. Anterior to it run the internal iliac artery and vein, accompanied by the ureter and colon. The superior gluteal artery and vein divide the lumbosacral trunk, and the first sacral nerve, as seen in Figure 6.2, and the inferior gluteal artery and vein lie between the second and third sacral nerves.

The anterior divisions of the lumbar nerves form the lumbar plexus, where they are joined proximally by the rami communicantes, from the lumbar ganglia of the sympathetic trunk. These rami accompany the lumbar arteries around the vertebral bodies, deep to the psoas major. Although not reliable in terms of anatomy, the nerves usually pass obliquely deep to the psoas major, distributing filaments to the quadratus lumborum, while forming the lumbar plexus.

Unlike the brachial plexus, several nerves of distribution arise from one or more of the spinal nerves (Fig. 9.4): the first lumbar nerve, commonly joined by divisions from the last thoracic, splits into upper and lower branches; the upper and larger branch divides into the iliohypogastric and ilioinguinal nerves; and the lower and smaller branch unites with a branch of the second lumbar, to form the genitofemoral nerve. The remainder of the second nerve, and the third and fourth nerves, divide into ventral and dorsal divisions. These can be seen above in Figure 6.2. The ventral division of the second nerve unites with the ventral divisions of the third and fourth nerves, to form the obturator nerve. The dorsal divisions of the second and third nerves divide into two branches, a smaller branch from each uniting to form the lateral femoral cutaneous nerve, and a larger branch from each

Figure 6.2 The lumbar and sacral plexus

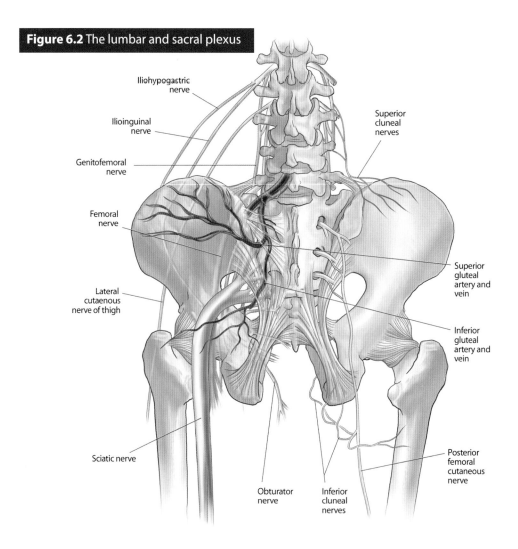

Iliohypogastric nerve

Ilioinguinal nerve

Genitofemoral nerve

Femoral nerve

Lateral cutaenous nerve of thigh

Sciatic nerve

Obturator nerve

Inferior cluneal nerves

Superior cluneal nerves

Superior gluteal artery and vein

Inferior gluteal artery and vein

Posterior femoral cutaneous nerve

joining with the dorsal division of the fourth nerve to form the femoral nerve. The union of two small branches from the third and fourth nerves forms the accessory obturator, where it exists.

The gluteal triangle

The 3G point

From anthropometric measurements in cadaveric dissection studies,[2] the authors have defined a new reference point at the apex of the triangle. This point has been termed the "3G point" in reference to the three-dimensional pathology, and the **g**roin, **g**luteal and **g**reater trochanteric regions. The relationship of this point in the posterior coronal plane is double the distance

Table 6.1 Abbreviated muscle attachments and innervations				
Muscle	**Origin**	**Insertion**	**Nerve**	**Root**
Gluteus maximus	Posterior iliac crest, sacrum, coccyx, and sacrotuberous ligament, along with contralateral and ipsilateral lumbar fascia	Upper ¾ into iliotibial tract and gluteal tuberosity of femur	Inferior gluteal nerve	L5, S1, S2
Gluteus medius	Outer surface of ilium between anterior and posterior gluteal lines	Superior and lateral trochanter	Superior gluteal nerve	L4, L5, S1
Gluteus minimus	Outer surface of ilium between anterior and inferior gluteal lines	Anterior surface of greater trochanter	Superior gluteal nerve	L4, L5, S1
Piriformis	Anterior sacrum and sacrotuberous ligament	Superior medial surface of greater trochanter	Nerve to piriformis	L5, S1, S2
Superior gemellus	Ischial spine	Medial surface of greater trochanter	Nerve to obturator internus	L5, S1, S2
Inferior gemellus	Superior aspect of ischial tuberosity	Medial surface of greater trochanter	Nerve to obturator internus	L5, S1, S2
Obturator internus	Obturator foramen and obturator membrane (posterior surface)	Medial surface of greater trochanter	Nerve to obturator internus	L5, S1, S2
Obturator externus	Obturator foramen and obturator membrane (anterior surface)	Medial aspect of greater trochanter	Nerve to obturator internus	L5, S1, S2
Quadratus femoris	Ischial tuberosity	Intertrochanteric crest of femur	Nerve to quadratus femoris	L4, L5, S1
Tense fascia late	Anterior superior iliac spine	Iliotibial thickening of fascia	Superior gluteal nerve	L4, L5, S1
Semitendinosus	Ischial tuberosity	Proximal anterior medial tibia	Sciatic nerve, tibial part	L5, S1, S2
Semimembranosus	Ischial tuberosity	Medial tibial condyle	Sciatic nerve – tibial part	L5, S1, S2
Biceps femoris	Long head – ischial tuberosity Short head – lateral lip of linea aspera	Head of fibula and lateral tibial condyle	Sciatic nerve (long head – tibia part, short head common peroneal)	Long – L5, S1, S2 Short S1, S2

Table 6.1 Abbreviated muscle attachments and innervations *(continued)*				
Muscle	**Origin**	**Insertion**	**Nerve**	**Root**
Vastus lateralis	Lateral lip of linea aspera, intertrochanteric line, and lateral intermuscular septum	Tibial tuberosity via quadriceps tendon and patellar ligament	Femoral nerve	L2, L3, L4
Adductor magnus	Posterior – ischial tuberosity	Anterior – linea aspera	Anterior – obturator nerve	Anterior L2, L3, L4
	Anterior – inferior pubic ramus and ischial ramus	Posterior – adductor tubercle of femur	Posterior – sciatic nerve	Posterior L4, L5
Gracilis	Body and inferior ramus of pubis	Proximal anterior medial tibia	Obturator nerve	L2, L3, L4

Table 6.2 Prime movers of key movements				
Adduction of hip	**Extension of hip**	**Abduction of hip**	**Lateral rotation**	**Internal rotation**
Adductor magnus	Gluteus maximus	Gluteus medius	Gemelli	Gluteus medius
Gracilis	Gemelli	Gluteus minimus	Quadratus femoris	Gluteus minimus
Adductor longus		Tensor fasciae latae	Piriformis	

from the spinous process of the L5 lumbar vertebra to the ischial tuberosity, as a continuation of that line to the femur.

The specific anatomical landmarks and borders of the gluteal triangle are set out in Figure 6.3:

> spinous process of L5 lumbar vertebra

> lateral edge of greater trochanter

> 3G point

The **spinous process of the L5 lumbar vertebra** is a readily identifiable landmark. It lies below the level of the iliac crests, which usually allows us to demarcate the spinous process of L4; inferiorly, the next spinous process is that of the fifth.

The **lateral edge of the greater trochanter** in the femur is a palpable reference point, in all but the most obese of patients. A clear image of the insertions is shown in Chapter 5, in order to familiarise the reader with the palpable structures.

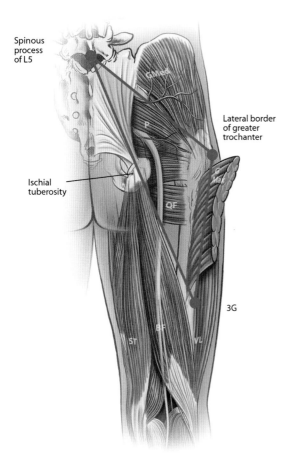

Spinous
process
of L5

Lateral border
of greater
trochanter

Ischial
tuberosity

3G

Figure 6.3 The gluteal triangle	
G Med	= gluteus medius
P	= piriformis
QF	= quadratus femoris
G Max	= gluteus maximus
ST	= semitendinosus
VL	= vastus lateralis
BF	= biceps femoris
3G	= the 3G point

The **3G point**, common to the groin, greater trochanter and gluteal triangles, is located posteriorly by palpating the spinous process of the L5 lumbar vertebra and the ischial tuberosity, and a similar distance again inferiorly to the posterior thigh.

Anatomical relationships of the borders of the gluteal triangle

Superficially, in all cases the skin provides the surface covering, with epidermis and dermis, with underlying superficial fat superficial to the fascia.[3] The fascia overlying the gluteal triangle is a continuation of the posterior lumbar fascia, in which the gluteus maximus is embedded, then extending to join the tensor fascie late and form the iliotibial band, with a slip insertion into the greater trochanter. This gives rise to a continuous layer of fascia, which plays a significant role in the pathology of the lower limb. As clearly seen in Chapter 7 on the knee, the fascia envelops the whole of the lower limb, and is not a discrete band running down the lateral thigh, although the fascia is at its thickest here, and is commonly referred to as the "iliotibial band".

Superior border of the gluteal triangle

> iliolumbar ligament and fascia

> gluteus maximus

> gluteus medius

> gluteus minimus

The spinous process of the L5 lumbar vertebra is an easily palpable reference point located at the midline, at a level just below a line drawn between the posterior iliac crests. The posterior layer of the thoracolumbar fascia makes a major contribution to the supraspinous and interspinous ligaments in the lower thoracic spine. The multifidus combines with the thoracolumbar fascia, to form the lumbar supraspinous and interspinous ligaments. The spinal attachments of these ligaments form a dense connective tissue, and support the composition by both muscle tendon and aponeurosis along the length of the lumbar spine. Specific attachments at the L5 spinous process are difficult to differentiate on palpation. The supraspinous ligament is the deepest structure, with the proximal insertion of the multifidus, erector spine, and thoracolumbar fascia more superficially.

The line between the L5 and the greater trochanter forms the superior border of the triangle, which corresponds to the medial border of the gluteus medius muscle.[2] This fan-shaped muscle arises from the outer surface of the ilium, between the posterior and anterior gluteal lines, and converges to form a tendon; this is attached to the oblique ridge sloping downward and forward on the lateral surface of the greater trochanter. The posterior border of the gluteus medius may merge with the piriformis at its insertion.

The **gluteus maximus** overlies the medius, and is transected by the superior border of the triangle. This is usually the largest muscle of the body, and acts to externally rotate and extend the hip joint. It arises from the ilium, behind the posterior gluteal line, iliac crest, thoracolumbar fascia, and posterior surfaces of the sacrum, coccyx, and sacrotuberous ligament, and from the fascia covering the gluteus medius. The fibers descend inferolaterally, the deeper fibers inserting into the greater trochanter between the 2 and 6 o'clock positions, while the superficial fibers and the upper part of the muscle end in a tendinous band, passing laterally to the greater trochanter and inserting into the iliotibial band.

The **iliolumbar ligament** runs form the transverse process of the L5 to the medial aspect of the anterior iliac crest.

The **gluteus medius** lies deep to the gluteus maximus, and runs almost caudally from the outer ilium, between the anterior and posterior gluteal lines, to insert into the superior and lateral surface of the greater trochanter at the 1 o'clock position. The muscle plays an important role in the stability of the pelvis. When performing the Trendelenburg test, the gluteus medius contracts, to stabilize the pelvis, and prevent a drop of the contralateral side. It is vital to have good neuromuscular control of this muscle in all dynamic sports, as it is commonly a site of breakdown. It acts in conjunction with the gluteus minimus to abduct and internally rotate the hip, unless in full flexion, where it acts to externally rotate.

The **gluteus minimus** is the smallest of the gluteal muscles, deep to the medius and maximus. It arises in the outer ilium between the anterior and inferior gluteal lines, and runs vertically inferiorly to insert into the anterior part of the greater trochanter at the 1 o'clock position. The muscle has been described as having two parts, although this was not seen in the authors' recent cadaveric work. It does on occasion form a conjoint tendon with the piriformis, to insert into the same location.

Medial border of the gluteal triangle

> L5 lumbar vertebra

> gluteus maximus

> sacroiliac joint

> sacrotuberous ligament

> ischial tuberosity and common hamstring origin

> semimembranosus origin

> gemellus superior, inferior

The medial border runs from the 3G point on the femur to the spinous process of the L5. The mid-point of this line is the ischial tuberosity, which allows for its easy location. The ischial tuberosity marks the lateral boundary of the pelvic outlet, but also is found at the mid-point of the medial border of the gluteal triangle.

Inferiorly, the medial border of the triangle transects the posterior compartment. The bellies of the semimembranosus and semitendinosus, along with the biceps femoris, are palpable when working from medial to lateral. Superiorly, the border follows the line of the sacrotuberous ligament, with the gluteus maximus palpable superficially. The medial line of the triangle also serves to remind us of the vector of referred pain from the sciatic nerve, which is an important differential diagnosis in the buttock.

The L5 lumbar vertebra – the lumbar vertebrae – are described extensively in Chapter 9, and will not be addressed here.

The **gluteus maximus** is the prime mover of the standing position. It is the first structure encountered medially, due to its bulk; it is slow to fatigue, and commonly has a widespread origin, which is discussed in detail above.

The **sacroiliac joint** is an important cause of gluteal pathology, which is discussed in detail earlier in this chapter and seen in Figure 6.1.

The **sacrotuberous ligament** runs from the posterior inferior superior iliac spine to the ischial tuberosity (Figs 6.1 and 6.4), and is critical in maintaining the strength and stability of the pelvis.

The **ischial tuberosity** is the bony protuberance of the posterior inferior part of the pelvis. The importance of palpable knowledge here is critical. From a posterior view of the right buttock, in the 2 o'clock position, is palpable the origin of the semimembranosus and, from the 4 o'clock position around to 7 o'clock, the combined tendinous insertion of the long head of the biceps femoris and semitendinosus. The sacrotuberous ligament at 10 o'clock is palpable at the 8 o'clock position, and the origin of the gemellus at the 7 o'clock position.

The **semimembranosus** is the largest of the hamstring muscles. It is a long muscle arising from the 2 o'clock position of the ischial tuberosity, and running deep to the semitendinosus. The muscle runs down the posterior thigh, to insert into a horizontal groove at the posterior medial tibial condyle. A number of fibers diverge to insert into the medial meniscus.

The **semitendinosus** arises from the 4–7 o'clock position, along with the common tendon of the biceps femoris, at the ischial tuberosity. The muscle runs superficial to the semimembranosus, and inserts into the anterior part of the medial tibia, as part of the pes anserine complex, where the tendons of the gracilis and sartorius join to form a common insertion surrounded by a complex bursa.

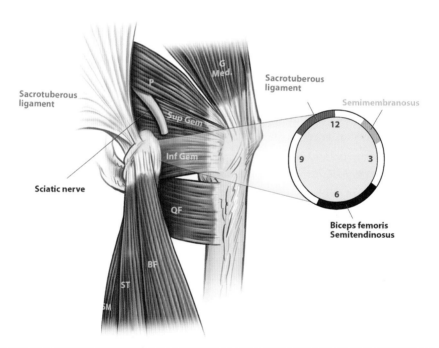

Figure 6.4 The ischial clock						
G Med	= gluteus medius	**QF**	= quadratus femoris	**VL**	= vastus lateralis
P	= piriformis	**G Max**	= gluteus maximus	**BF**	= biceps femoris
Sup Gem	= superior gemelli	**ST**	= semitendinosus	**3G**	= the 3G point
Inf Gem	= inferior gemelli	**SM**	= semimembranosus		

The **gemellus** is divided into superior and inferior muscle bellies. The superior muscle originates from the ischial spine, and inserts into the medial surface of the greater trochanter. Its action is as a deep external rotator, and commonly fibers merge at the insertion with those of the inferior belly and obturator internus. The inferior belly runs from the ischial tuberosity at the 7 o'clock position, and inserts at the same location.

Lateral border of the gluteal triangle

> tensor fascie late

> iliotibial band

> vastus lateralis

> biceps femoris

The lateral border of the triangle is marked from the greater trochanter (GT), along the shaft of the femur, to the 3G point. The iliotibial band runs parallel to this border. It blends with the capsule of the knee joint, to attach to the lateral femoral condyle, Gerdy's tubercle, and the head of the fibula.[4] The vastus lateralis and biceps femoris form the bulk of this muscular compartment, with the bellies of these muscles the only palpable structures. The apex of the triangle is at the 3G point, which lies in line with the femur at a point double the distance from the spinous process of L5 to the ischial tuberosity.

The **tensor fasciae latae (TFL)** is encapsulated within the deep fascia of the leg. It originates at the anterior superior iliac spine, and inserts into the fascia of the leg in the line of the iliotibial tract. Its action is multiple and it abducts, flexes, and internally rotates the hip joint. The iliotibial tract inserts in the line of tension from the pull of the TFL into Gerdy's tubercle on the tibia.

The **iliotibial band** was once thought of as a discrete entity. The authors have performed extensive work to delineate this structure.[5] We now believe it to be part of a complex "rigging" structure of force transmission across the lower limb, and part of the lower limb fascia.

The **vastus lateralis** is part of the quadriceps group, and originates from the lip of the linea aspera on the greater trochanteric line, and the intermuscular septum of the lateral compartment. It runs inferiorly to insert as part of the quadriceps tendon, via the patellar tendon, into the tibial tuberosity.

The **biceps femoris** usually has two heads. The long head originates, along with the semitendinosus, between the 4 and 7 o'clock positions on the ischial tuberosity, and the short head arises from the linea lateral lip of the linea aspera. The two bellies merge to form a common insertion into the head of the fibula.

Within the gluteal triangle

> gluteus maximus

> piriformis

> sciatic nerve

The structures contained within the gluteal triangle are the causal agents in much gluteal pathology; however, they lie deep to the gluteus maximus, and are palpable, at best, at their insertion to the greater trochanter.

The **sciatic nerve** arises from the ventral rami of the fourth lumbar to the third sacral spinal nerves, and exits the pelvis through the greater sciatic foramen, deep to the piriformis, and descends between the greater trochanter of the femur and the ischial tuberosity. The sciatic nerve is sandwiched on its exit between the greater sciatic foramen by the piriformis muscle superiorly, and the gemellus inferiorly,[6] and there has been much variation in anatomy described, potentially infringing on the nerve on its extra-pelvic course.

The **piriformis** arises from the anterior aspect of the sacrum, between and lateral to the sacral foramina. As the muscle leaves the pelvis, some slips arise from the pelvic surface of the sacrotuberous ligament. The muscle passes out of the pelvis through the greater sciatic foramen. Its rounded tendon is attached to the upper border and medial aspect of the greater trochanter, close to the insertion of the obturator internus and the gemellus, with which it may be partially conjoined. Occasionally the sciatic nerve can pierce the belly of the piriformis, or indeed it can be composed of two bellies. The contribution of this anatomical variant to pathologies is often discussed, and it can be considered a possible cause of gluteal pain.

The diagnostic triangle

The step-wise approach using the gluteal triangle is summarized in Tables 6.3–6.7. This gives the clinician a guide to the diagnostic process and pathological causes of chronic gluteal pain in relation to the triangle. Each table shows the differential diagnosis for conditions presenting within that anatomical area, and the combined sieve represents a comprehensive assessment of the region. Prior to each table, the most common diagnosis is drawn out, but the reader is directed to the table for a comprehensive differential.

It is recognized that some argue the discriminatory nature of clinical tests[7] but, where appropriate, the evidence-based examination of choice is given.[8] Some tests are widely utilized in clinical practise with limited or conflicting evidence, as the best available, and in this case these are included.

Medial to the gluteal triangle

The area lying medial to the line from the spinous process of the L5 vertebra to the apical point of the gluteal triangle highlights the sacroiliac joint (SIJ), and the most common presentation within this region of the triangle is that of sacroiliac pain. The SIJ is a joint with limited mobility, acting as a force transducer, and a shock absorber. This is affected as part of three closed, kinematic chains involving the lumbar spine, sacrum, pelvic girdle, and lower extremities. This is a significant area, as it contains the sacroiliac joint.

A source of musculoskeletal pain on its own, the cause of pain in **sacroiliac joint dysfunction** is not clear. The joint is a synovial joint, which suggests that the pain may come from inflammation of the synovium, either through asymmetric repetitive movement, such as with limb length discrepancy, or poor footwear, or through recovery from injury causing an altered gait pattern; the joint can also be inflamed following trauma. We know that pregnancy can disrupt the joint, and certainly it is a common cause of pain in pregnant women. The joint is increasingly the site at which the spondyloarthritidies are diagnosed and confirmed; a recent paper by Bennett et al.[9] illustrates the diagnostic ability of MRI, in conjunction with inflammatory hematological markers, and this is highlighted in recent summaries.[10, 11]

The **spondyloarthritidies** include ankylosing spondylolitis, alongside Reiter's syndrome, psoriatic arthropathy, and many other HLA B27-negative arthropathies. They are characterized by pain and inflammation of the joints, commonly the spine, and can be associated with systemic disease. Reiter's is commonly overlooked in the athlete, where the triad of iritis, arthritis, and urethitis is seen usually post-infection, and presents as a painful joint.

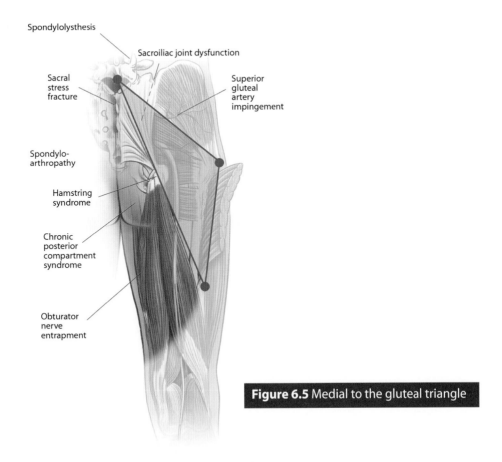

Spondylolysthesis

Sacroiliac joint dysfunction

Sacral stress fracture

Superior gluteal artery impingement

Spondylo-arthropathy

Hamstring syndrome

Chronic posterior compartment syndrome

Obturator nerve entrapment

Figure 6.5 Medial to the gluteal triangle

Spondylolysis is the most common stress fracture of the lumbar spine. An isolated unilateral fracture of the pars interarticularis (Figure 9.1 from the spine chapter) is responsible for a proportion of pain in this area, and a recent systematic review examined the evidence available on diagnosis and management, concluding that STIR or fat-suppressed T2-weighted MRI were the best evidence-based investigations. This can progress to bilateral fractures, in which case the term "spondylolisthesis" is used to delineate any degree of forward or backward slippage of one vertebral body on the next.

Rarer conditions, including posterior compartment syndrome, gluteal artery entrapment, and **obturator nerve entrapment** are also present as pain in this area. **Hamstring syndrome** is rather more controversial. Described by Orava[34] as adhesions restricting the sciatic nerve,

Table 6.3 Patho-anatomic approach; medial to the gluteal triangle				
Define and align	**Pathology**	**Listen and localize**	**Palpate and recreate**	**Alleviate and investigate**
Medial to triangle	Sacroiliac joint (SIJ) pain	Pain in lumbar spine and gluteal region	Axial femoral compression test with sustained pressure[12] has highest specificity,[13] but thigh thrust greater inter-tester reliability[8]	Plain film, guided local anesthetic injection to SIJ,[14] Computerised tomography
	Spondyloarthritides	Systemic symptoms include morning stiffness, mechanical back pain for > 3m, improvement with moderate activity, diffuse buttock pain. Past medical history i.e. psoriasis, ASAS, ESSG criteria[16]	Limited range of movement, general tenderness to palpation. Asymmetrical poly-arthropathy with tendency toward axial spine and large joints	HLA-B27, CRP,[16] Plain x-rays, MRI scan back, bone scan
	Sacral stress fracture	Vague incapacitating gluteal pain, pelvic anteversion, insufficiency vs fatigue, leg length discrepancy	Tests poorly discriminative. Pain on percussion,[17] FABER, Genslen's[18] and Spring tests[14] for SIJ dysfunction all may be +ve	Plain film, bone scan,[19] MRI[20]
	Spondylolisthesis	Unilateral back pain, exacerbated in extension	Single leg extension, Michelis' or Stork test[21]	Lateral plain film, MRI[22] followed by CT if unclear[23]
	Obturator nerve entrapment	Medial thigh pain on exercise relieved by rest	Adductor weakness, superficial dysesthesia/ hyperesthesia of mid-medial thigh[24]	EMG of obturator innervated muscles,[25] guided local anesthetic injection to obturator foramen[26]

Table 6.3 Patho-anatomic approach; medial to the gluteal triangle (*continued*)				
Define and align	Pathology	Listen and localize	Palpate and recreate	Alleviate and investigate
	Posterior compartment syndrome I. acute II. chronic	Associated with avulsion fracture. Sudden tearing pain gradual worsening over 24 hrs	Tense swelling and firm feel to posterior compartment of thigh, tender ischial tuberosity[27, 28]	Compartment pressure studies usual, but MRI[30, 31] better in this area
		Insidious onset prevents completion of training with relief with rest		
	Superior gluteal artery entrapment/ endo fibrosis	Claudicant gluteal pain on exercise relieved by rest, smoking	Exercise-related gluteal pain[31]	Pre/post exercise ankle-brachial index, duplex ultrasound scan /angiography[32]
	Hamstring syndrome	Pain worse on sitting and localized to ischial tuberosity during and after exercise	Tenderness over ischial tuberosity, Puranen-Orava test[33]	MRI[34]

CRP	=	C reactive protein
MRI	=	magnetic resonance imaging
FABER	=	flexion, abduction, and external rotation test of the hip
EMG	=	electromyographic muscle testing

caused by trauma to the hamstring group origin, there is much crossover with the etiology purported to be behind piriformis syndrome and that of proximal hamstring tear, but we include it for completeness.

Superior to the gluteal triangle

The area lying superior to the line from the spinous process of the L5 vertebra to the greater trochanter transects the postural and locomotor muscles of the gluteals, of which the muscle bellies and insertions are the cause of much pathology located in this area.

The **fascia** is currently attracting increasing attention in the sports medicine world, both as a structure which can be injured,[35] and also in understanding of its possible functions. In the transverse fascia of patients with inguinal hernias, Klinge[36] identified an increased disordering of collagen fibers and increased vascularity, alongside a change in the proportion of Type I and Type III collagen, suggesting this might be responsible for fascial weakness.

There are many theories as to fascial function. A tension or rigging effect has been demonstrated in the lumbar fascia,[44, 45] but no similar proposal has been made in the lower

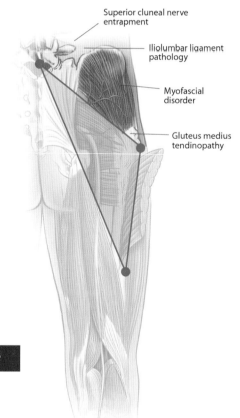

Superior cluneal nerve
entrapment

Iliolumbar ligament
pathology

Myofascial
disorder

Gluteus medius
tendinopathy

Figure 6.6 Superior to the gluteal triangle

Table 6.4 Patho-anatomic approach; superior to the gluteal triangle				
Define and align	Pathology	Listen and localize	Palpate and recreate	Alleviate and investigate
Superior to triangle	Myofascial pain	Hamstring/gluteal tightness, poorly localized pain	Tender "trigger" points palpable within muscle[37, 38]	Dry-needling effective in relieving trigger points[37]
	Gluteus medius tendinopathy	Weakness or pain in stance phase of walking and/or running[39]	Trendelenburg test 72% sensitive, 76% specific[40]	Ultrasound scan,[41] MRI
	Iliolumbar ligament pain	Lumbar ache, worse on exercise	Due to anatomy, may mimic SIJ pain[42, 43] may have trigger points	Responds to dry-needling if palpable trigger points[37]

limb. Alternatively, the crossover of fascial force transmission to contralateral limbs has been proposed by Vleming,[46] and has the fiber orientation of the fascia in its support. The hydraulic amplifier effect[47] of longitudinal muscle tension is increasingly seen as a means by which the fascial role in muscle function can be identified. These all contribute to the manual therapy and dry-needling roles in the management of this condition.

The gluteus medius is the prime abductor of the hip, and **Gluteus medius tendinopathy** is commonly an overuse condition in the detrained athlete, or in one changing discipline, or increasing workload. It is equally common in the recreational athlete and, in particular, given that the muscle stabilizes the pelvis when running, in those training for their first marathon. Commonly misdiagnosed, it can be associated with some numbness in the cutaneous distribution of the lateral cutaneous nerve of the thigh.

The iliolumbar ligament is commonly ascribed as a source of pain in this area, but the authors believe it is more often associated with SIJ dysfunction than as an independent source of pathology.

Lateral to the gluteal triangle

The area lying lateral to the line from the greater trochanter to the 3G point on the shaft of the femur highlights the hip and structures around it as potential origins of pathology, in particular, the acetabulum. The pathology of this region is best considered in conjunction with Chapter 5.

There are two bursae adjacent to the greater trochanter; the gluteus medius bursa lies deep to the tendon of the gluteus medius as it inserts, and the trochanteric bursa is superficial to the greater trochanter but in turn deep to the tense fascia late.

The Tensor fasciae latae (TFL) is intrinsically linked to the pathologies not only of itself, but also the dysfunction of the iliotibial tensioning line of the deep fascia of the leg. Snapping characteristically highlights this tension, and can be relieved commonly by the treatment of trigger points in the TFL. Femoro-acetabular pathologies are covered in great depth in Chapter 5, and will not be covered further specifically here.

The **cluneal nerve** is often overlooked as a source of pain in this region, often attributed to facet joint pain. The superior cluneal nerve runs in a tunnel between the posterior iliac crest and the thoracolumbar fascia, as the nerve passes over the iliac crest some 7–8 cm lateral to the midline, superolateral to the posterior superior iliac spine.[48] By flexing the hip, and applying pressure over the location of this tunnel, one can often alleviate the symptoms, and hence make a diagnosis.[49] The medial cluneal branches perforate the gluteus maximus, and originate from the dorsal branches of S1–S3, and innervate the skin over the gluteus maximus; entrapment can be relieved by myofascial release, and mimics gluteus maximus pain. The inferior branches originate from the posterior femoral cutaneous nerve and sacral plexus, and emerge from under the gluteus maximus to supply some of the perineum and posterior thigh. Possible decompression surgery is an option, if it is not responding to myofascial techniques.[50]

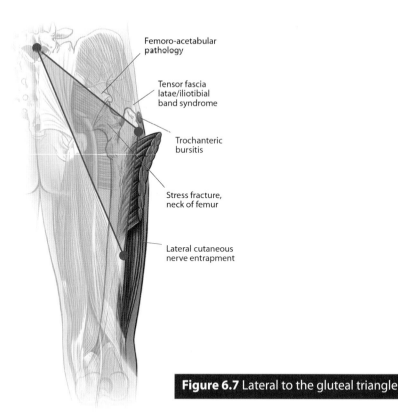

Femoro-acetabular
pathology

Tensor fascia
latae/iliotibial
band syndrome

Trochanteric
bursitis

Stress fracture,
neck of femur

Lateral cutaneous
nerve entrapment

Figure 6.7 Lateral to the gluteal triangle

Within the gluteal triangle

Within the space marked by the lines described above are contained the lateral rotators of the hip, which sit deep to the gluteal muscles, in particular the piriformis, but this region is also divided by the sciatic nerve, an important cause of referred pain.

Lower-back pain is common in both the athletic and non-athletic populations. When found presenting within the triangle, it is often radicular. There are numerous causes of radicular pain, including **intervertebral disc herniation**, foraminal stenosis, and spinal canal stenosis, but radiating pain can also be more mechanical, from facet or apophyseal joints. The table below highlights some of the discriminatory maneuvers available on examination.

Piriformis syndrome[51] also presents in this area. It is again often mistaken for more common conditions, such as facet joint arthropathy, sacroiliitis, lumbar disc, and radiculopathy.[52] It is by no means certain that piriformis syndrome is a distinct clinical entity, or whether it involves pain from entrapment of the sciatic nerve as it abuts the piriformis muscle, or myofascial pain from a tight, hypertrophic, and tender piriformis muscle without nerve entrapment.[53, 54] Some are using botulinum toxin to confirm this diagnosis, by releasing myofascial tension and subsequent tethering.[55]

Table 6.5 Patho-anatomic approach; lateral to the gluteal triangle				
Define and align	**Pathology**	**Listen and localize**	**Palpate and recreate**	**Alleviate and investigate**
Lateral to triangle	Trochanteric bursitis	Pain getting up off bed or painful lying on floor[56]	Tenderness directly superior and over greater trochanter	Ultrasound scan +/– local anesthetic injection[57]
	Tensor fascie late/ iliotibial band syndrome	"Snapping" of hip, sharp burning pain in lateral thigh worsens with exercise	Recreate snapping,[58] Ober's test[59]	Ultrasound scan[41]
	Femoral-acetabular I. acetabular/labral II. degenerative	Mechanical symptoms, clicking ± locking	Impingement test[60]	Magnetic resonance imaging, arthrogram[61]
		Night pain, restriction in daily living	Limited range of movement,[62] pain on weight-bearing	Plain film x-ray, MRI[21]
	Stress fracture neck of femur	Female, change in volume of training, osteopenia	Hop test,[63] Fulcrum test[64]	Plain film bone scan,[20] MRI[21]
	Lateral cutaneous nerve entrapment	Exercise induced para/hyperesthesia	Reproduction of symptoms on pressure inferior to ASIS[65]	Relief of pain by local anesthetic,[66] nerve conduction studies
	Cluneal nerve entrapment	Deep pain localized to gluteus maximus, but can present as lumbar back pain	Myofascial release technique of direct pressure over iliac crest and hip flexion to release compression	Local anesthetic injection, myofascial release, or surgery if persistent[67]

Table 6.6 Patho-anatomic approach; within the gluteal triangle				
Define and align	**Pathology**	**Listen and localize**	**Palpate and recreate**	**Alleviate and investigate**
Within the triangle	Acute disc prolapse	Lumbar back pain, +/– radiation to back of leg	Lasègue straight leg raise (sensitivity 72–97%, specificity 11–66%),[73] Braggard's sign (94% +ve)[74]	Fluoroscopic guided nerve root injection,[75] MRI
	Lumbar facet joint	Revels criteria,[76] lumbar back pain, radiation to buttock	Pain on palpation of facet joint and worse in extension[8]	Fluoroscopic guided facet joint injection[76]

Define and align	Pathology	Listen and localize	Palpate and recreate	Alleviate and Investigate
	Piriformis tendinopathy	Hamstring origin pain with gradual rather than sudden onset and/or sciatic referred pain	Tenderness over sciatic notch and aggravated by flexion, adduction, and internal rotation (Lasègue sign) of the hip,[77] also FAIR test,[78] Pace test[8]	Ultrasound scan[65]
	Pelvic floor dysfunction	Post pregnancy, perineal trauma, cyclists	Coccygeus and levator ani, along with conjoint bellies of pubococcygeus, often ignored attachments to pelvis can give cause to gluteal pain[79]	Urine examination, pelvic manometry, MRI of pelvic floor musculature, EMG
	Circumflex femoral vein thrombosis	Hamstring origin pain with gradual onset and deep vein thrombosis risk factors	Tenderness and pain on resisted flexion[80] without muscle weakness	Venography, duplex ultrasound/MRI
	Posterior femoral cutaneous nerve entrapment	Mimics hamstring injury with sudden onset, can be localized below gluteal fold	Pain on stretching, can mimic weakness in bridging and opposed knee flexion[71]	Exclude hamstring injury by MRI and then myofascial release techniques

Table 6.6 Patho-anatomic approach; within the gluteal triangle (*continued*)

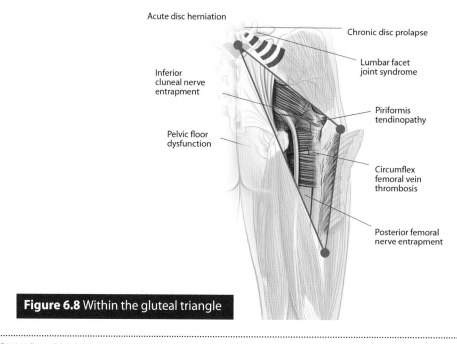

Figure 6.8 Within the gluteal triangle

CLINICAL SPORTS ANATOMY

Pelvic floor dysfunction is often overlooked; indeed, the authors, while researching the connections for groin pain, found that the pelvic floor muscles have a strong role to play, not only in women post-childbirth. A variety of syndromes masquerade here, including levator ani syndrome, prostadynia, and pudendal neuralgia. Levator ani syndrome is possibly more common, often presenting with pelvic and gluteal pain.[68] Few treatment options have truly been evaluated, but encouraging results have been seen with botulinum toxin injections, which serve to confirm the diagnosis by preventing the spasm, and hence the cause of the pain.[69]

Circumflex femoral vein thrombosis has been described by Papasterigou et al.[70] as presenting in the same way as an acute hamstring tear. The circumflex femoral vein joins the femoral vein before it drains into the saphenous vein, near the faossa ovalis. It is a rare cause, but venous doppler ultrasound should make an accurate diagnosis, and local trauma such as a kick or tackle is the precipitant.

The **posterior femoral cutaneous nerve** passes through the sciatic notch, and usually inferior to the piriformis, before emerging between the inferior border of the gluteus maximus, to run down the posterior thigh. It does have perforating branches through the posterior fascia and, where the fascia is tethered to the skin, it appears that these are associated with the inferior cluneal nerve and the femoral cutaneous nerve. Isolated lesions are rare,[71] and compression may occur within the pelvis itself,[72] or from direct pressure when sitting in the saddle, or may occur where the nerve perforates through the posterior fascia, occurring secondary to myofascial injury.

Ischial tuberosity

The significant point at the midline of the medial triangle is the ischial tuberosity. The anatomy of the insertions and relations here has been discussed above, but is highlighted again in the associated Figure 6.9. The high incidence of hamstring strains, their causation by long periods of absence from sport, and frequent recurrence rates, make them particularly significant in causes of gluteal pain.[81]

As previously described, the multiple attachments of the biceps femoris, semimembranosus, and semitendinosus allow the group to act to flex and extend the knee, and extend and rotate the hip, along with pelvic tilting.

Hamstring injury recurrence makes it particularly common in sports presentations,[82] and the site of injury can depend very much on the age of the participant. Youth and adolescents whose epiphysis has yet to fuse, between 15 and 17 years old, can rupture the apophyseal origin and, at the older end of the spectrum, the insertion tendons are more prone to rupture. Otherwise, the proximal third of the muscle appears slower to recovery.[83] Diagnosis of hamstring strain can be made clinically, although increasingly trackside ultrasound imaging and rapid MRI are being used to confirm the diagnosis.[84–86]

Grading of hamstring injury

Increasingly MRI reports will grade the hamstring tear, so as to offer a guide to prognosis. It is included here as it will often be relevant in terms of investigations.

Figure 6.9 The ischial tuberosity

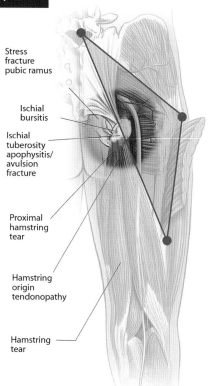

Stress
fracture
pubic ramus

Ischial
bursitis

Ischial
tuberosity
apophysitis/
avulsion
fracture

Proximal
hamstring
tear

Hamstring
origin
tendonopathy

Hamstring
tear

Grade 1 tears are often referred to as "microtears" or "strains". MRI commonly reports edema and fascial line fluid, but no disruption to the muscle belly, or hematoma. Prognosis suggests recovery within 7–10 days.

Grade 2 tears always involve some macroscopic damage to the muscle, and MRI commonly demonstrates perimuscular and intramuscular spaces and hematoma, along with vertical splits in muscle fibers. Prognosis of up to two months is anticipated.

Grade 3 tears are defined by tendon separation, and complete disruption of the muscle. These often require significant rehabilitation periods, to achieve pre-injury fitness levels.

Hamstring origin tendinopathy occurs at the ischial tuberosity, or in the proximal tendinous attachment; given the arrangement at the origin (Fig. 6.4), one can see it is likely that the semimembranosus is more likely to be affected biomechanically. It presents with pain at the ischial tuberosity on active stretching. A single study has looked at histological specimens,[87] and seen some degenerative change; here a surgical repair is more likely, but conservative management can be successful.

Hamstring tears are frequently distal musculo-tendinous junction or muscle belly tears, more distal to the origin. On occasion, more proximal muscle tears occur at the proximal musculo-tendinous junction,[88] and these present with sudden-onset, sharp, high posterior thigh pain; acutely this is unmistakable as a hamstring tear, but as the time from injury to presentation increases, care must be taken to exclude this as a diagnosis. It may result in an ischial bursitis as a concurrent injury, or ischial bursitis can present independently. The ischial bursa lies superficial to the tuberosity and its attachments, but deep to the gluteus maximus, which it serves by providing a low-friction buffer to its contraction. When inflamed, the bursa and hence the tuberosity are tender, and this can be caused primarily by prolonged sitting, direct falls on the tuberosity, or occasionally concurrently with hamstring injury.

Ischial tuberosity apophysitis and tuberosity avulsion fracture are probably part of the same continuum. The apophysitis is an overuse condition often seen in younger athletes in kicking sports, who present with pain at the ischial tuberosity.[89] It may be a result of poor pelvic stability, and biomechanical analysis will improve this, but to diagnose the condition, there must be no trauma at the onset. Avulsion fracture, however, typically occurs with an explosive action; given that the apophysis does not fuse until the age of 17 years or so, it is at risk of avulsion should it contact hard against resisistance. These are often missed, and plain x-ray can detect the lesion, but not at the time of onset.

Stress fractures of the pubic rami are rare, but have been seen in the female military soldier, and also in endurance athletes.[91] There is also an association with connective tissue

Table 6.7 Patho-anatomic approach; ischial tuberosity				
Define and align	**Pathology**	**Listen and localize**	**Palpate and recreate**	**Alleviate and investigate**
Ischial tuberosity	Hamstring origin tendinopathy	Sudden pain in buttock/ posterior thigh, walking painful[81]	Tenderness of muscle belly, or tendon from common origin	Magnetic resonance imaging[81, 83]
	Proximal hamstring tear	Sudden pain on acceleration or deceleration, localized to hamstring muscle belly, weakness, stiffness	Tenderness, palpable hematoma, or defect in muscle	Ultrasound scan,[41] MRI[81]
	Ischial bursitis	Pain on sitting, worsens on movement, likely to be co-existent injury with hamstring injury	Tenderness of ischial tuberosity[56]	Ultrasound scan,[51] guided local anesthetic injection[41]
	Ischial tuberosity apophysitis/ avulsion fracture	Shooting pain following high-energy kick or change of direction	Bogginess of ischial tuberosity, tenderness to palpation[90]	Plain film[93]
	Stress fracture of pubic ramus	Gradual onset, change in training load	Pain standing on one leg and Hop test,[59] associated deep buttock pain	Plain film, bone scan,[20] MRI[21]

disorders.[92] Biomechanical causes are likely, with osteopenia, nutrition, and gait abnormality all causative factors. The military subjects in the reference above all altered their stride pattern, to adjust to squad running with men, and put unacceptable load moments on their rami. This reiterates the need for a careful history to be taken, and biomechanical assessment.

Intra-abdominal pathology

A type of gluteal pain which has not been discussed so far is intra-abdominal causes. Endometriosis is known to widely radiate pain, and the gluteal region is not immune. Vascular causes, such as abdominal aortic aneurysm, can present as gluteal pain, alongside rarer vascular insufficiencies, such as Leriche's syndrome, or common iliac stenosis.[94] Colorectal pathology can present with referred pain, and inflammatory bowel disease is seen in association with the spondyloarthritidies. Malignancy, either of the pelvis or of soft tissues, cannot be ignored and must be excluded, but is beyond the scope of this diagnostic sieve, which restricts itself necessarily to musculoskeletal diagnoses.

Malignancy

Both bone and muscle malignancy can present in the gluteal region. Leiomyosarcoma should always be considered in the slowly recovering muscle strain, out of proportion to the mechanism and in the adolescent. Neuroblastoma, although thankfully rare, is known to commonly[95] mimic lower back, buttock, and hip pain, and care should be taken to always look for systemic signs in the slowly resolving or otherwise fit patient.

Primary bone tumors, such as osteosarcoma, and chondrosarcoma, are rare, but frequently present with bone pain in the lower back/buttock. Many can be seen on plain film radiographs and, with the advent of rapid MRI and advice to avoid spinal plain films when possible, one must consider the differential diagnosis at all times.

Summary

This chapter has covered the wide-ranging differential diagnoses of the gluteal region. One can see the significant crossover with the groin and greater trochanter chapters, and the authors encourage the reader to treat the area as a three-dimensional joint, with the 3G point at the apex. The divison of the diagnosis is based on the presentations, and the reader is reminded to consider systemic disease carefully in this area.

Case histories

Case 1

A 29-year-old fitness trainer presents with a four-week history of right-sided right-buttock pain. It has stopped him working, as he finds it difficult to bend, or even walk. He has had this pain before, and put it down to heavy training sessions, which triggered it. He tells you he has seen his family doctor regarding the pain, which on occasions has extended down his right leg. He has had six episodes in the last five years.

Step 1: Define and align

Expose the patient properly. It may be necessary to undress the patient to a pair of swim shorts, to allow inspection and effective palpation. It is impossible to examine the gluteal region through clothing.

Define the triangle: locate the L5 spinous process, the 3G point, and the greater trochanter.

Align the patient's pain. Here the pain is located "medial to the triangle".

From this point we recommend that the reader attempt to exclude potential pathologies. From Table 6.3, the potential differential diagnoses include:

differential diagnosis
> sacroiliac joint pain
> spondyloarthritides
> sacral stress fracture
> spondylolisthesis
> obturator nerve entrapment
> posterior compartment syndrome
> superior gluteal artery entrapment
> hamstring syndrome

We proceed to differentiate between these structures, step 2.

Step 2: Listen and localize

Addressing the question of sacroiliac joint pain we ask:

Q *Is the pain localized to one side?*

A Yes, it is localized to the right side.

Q *Do you think the following applies to you: Do you have a deep pain which makes climbing stairs and rolling over in bed difficult?*

A Not really, my pain makes everything difficult.

Addressing the spondyloarthritides we ask:

Q *Are you worse on waking?*

A Yes, my butt gets better by mid-morning, but worsens then through the day.

Q *Have you had any eye irritation or GU infections?*

A Yes, I went to the GU clinic about three years ago, and was treated with my partner for chlamydia.

Q *Do you have any other joints which cause you pain?*

A Yes, I used to suffer from a painful right shoulder at the time of the chlamydia infection, but it has not come back. (MRI showed no injury.)

Addressing sacral stress fracture we ask:

Q *Is the pain made worse by weight-bearing exercise?*

A No, the pain is there at rest, and with exercise.

Addressing spondylolisthesis we ask:

Q *Is the pain made worse by extending your back, or long periods sitting?*

A No, extending my back relieves the pain a little; long periods sitting do make it worse though.

Addressing obturator nerve entrapment we ask:

Q *Do you get any pain in the inner aspect of your thigh?*

A No.

Addressing posterior compartment syndrome we ask:

Q *Does the pain in the back of your thigh feel like a tight, numbing pressure?*

A No, it is more electrical when it happens.

Addressing the entrapments of artery and nerve we ask:

Q *Do you get pain when you sit down localized to one spot?*

A No, it is more lower back/butt pain on sitting, and it does not go away with rest.

Differential diagnosis

More likely
> SIJ pain
> spondyloarhthrities including Reiter's
> spondylolisthesis

Less likely
> sacral stress fracture
> obturator nerve entrapment
> posterior compartment syndrome
> superior gluteal artery entrapment
> hamstring syndrome

This narrows our diagnostic sieve a little; by palpating and examining the structures, we can further exclude confounding conditions from the history. We are still concerned by SIJ pain and spondyloarthritides, including Reiter's, and possible spondylolisthesis.

Step 3: Palpate and re-create

On examination of the lumbar spine, we find that Schober's test is restricted to 1 cm of movement in flexion, but extension is normal, along with quadrant signs and the Stork test.

He has no tenderness through palpation of the sacroiliac joints, and the shear test and vertical thrust tests are negative.

Step 4: Alleviate and investigate

This leads us to consider the spondyloarthritides; given the history of GU infection, it is possible that Reiter's is the diagnosis, but we need to exclude ankylosing spondyloarthritis. A plain film of the SIJ and CRP[96, 97] would be of use in confirming the diagnosis and referral to a rheumatologist, although current evidence[10, 11] suggests that an MRI may be of most usefulness. The Bath Ankylosing Spondylolysis Disease Activity Index can aid the making of a diagnosis of AS in the presence of HLA-B27 positivity, persistent buttock pain which resolves with exercise, and x-ray or MRI-evident involvement of the sacroiliac joints.

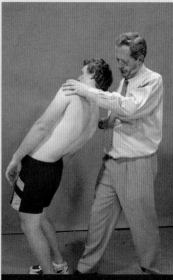

Figure 6.10 Quadrant test (combined extension, lateral flexion, and rotation)

Case 2

A 53-year-old women presents with gluteal pain. She has been running four kilometers a day in an attempt to get fit for a ten-kilometer fun run in two months' time. Previously she was a keen netballer, but over the last 20 years she has been quite inactive. The return to exercise has reawakened her competitive spirit, and she admits she has been going a bit hard. Her pain is in both gluteals.

Step 1: Define and align

Expose the patient properly. It may be necessary to undress the patient to a pair of swim shorts, to allow inspection and effective palpation. It is impossible to examine the gluteal region through clothing.

Define the triangle: locate the L5 spinous process, the 3G point, and the greater trochanter.

Align the patient's pain. Here the pain is located "superior to the triangle".

From this point we recommend that the reader attempt to exclude potential pathologies. From Table 6.4, the potential differential diagnoses include:

Differential diagnosis
> myofascial pain
> gluteus medius tendinopathy
> iliolumbar ligament pain

Step 2: Listen and localize

Addressing the question of myofascial pain we ask:

Q *Do you get any weakness or pain when you run?*

A Yes, the pain occurs each time I push off in the running stride, it feels high up in my gluts.

Q *Have you changed running shoes?*

A No, I'm using my old netball shoes.

Q *Have you had any other medical conditions, or are you on any medication?*

A No.

Addressing the question of gluteus medius tendinopathy we ask:

Q *Can you balance on one leg comfortably?*

A No, I'm struggling with a step out to my conservatory, when I have to lift my knee quite high.

Addressing the iliolumbar ligament we ask:

Q *Do you get any pain at night?*

A No, I get off to sleep okay; it is sore in the morning though when I go downstairs.

Differential diagnosis
More likely
> gluteus medius tendinopathy

Less likely
> myofascial pain
> iliolumbar ligament pathology

This focuses our attention on the gluteus medius in step 3.

Step 3: Palpate and re-create

On examining the patient's gluteals, we find a tight trigger spot in both the gluteus maximus, and deep in the gluteus medius. The Trendelenburg test is positive on the right, and weakly positive on left; she confirms the problem is worse on the right (she leads with her right leg when running).

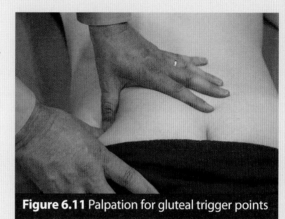

Figure 6.11 Palpation for gluteal trigger points

We could confirm the diagnosis here, without progressing on to step 4, although of course ultrasound examination of the muscle may reveal more than inflammation, so the authors would agree that, if she fails to respond to treatment, then an USS might be indicated.

Case 3

A 66-year-old tennis player presents with gluteal pain on the left side. She tells you that the pain started two weeks ago, came on gradually, and is a sharp pain, which seems to radiate down to her knee. She has never had the pain before. It is worse when she lunges for a low forehand, and is stopping her playing her best games.

Step 1: Define and align

Expose the patient properly. It may be necessary to undress the patient to a pair of swim shorts, to allow inspection and effective palpation. It is impossible to examine the gluteal region through clothing.

Define the triangle: locate the L5 spinous process, the 3G point, and the greater trochanter.

Align the patient's pain. Here the pain is located "lateral to the triangle".

From this point we recommend that the reader attempt to exclude potential pathologies. Table 6.5 is the relevant one; however, in this case we would also draw the reader to the greater trochanter

Chapter 6, as this much more comprehensively covers the differential diagnoses. For the purposes of completeness, we shall consider the following potential differential diagnosis here.

Differential diagnosis

> trochanteric bursitis

> tensor fascia late and iliotibial band syndrome

> femoro-acetabular – labral

> femoro-acetabular – degenerative

> stress fracture neck of femur

> lateral femoral cutaneous nerve entrapment

Step 2: Listen and localize

Addressing the possibility of trochanteric bursitis we ask:

Q *Does the pain affect you at night, when moving, or getting up after lying on the floor?*

A No, really the pain only affects me when playing tennis or running.

Q *Is there a tender spot?*

A All my gluteal muscles feel sore.

Q *Have you changed footwear recently?*

A Yes, I'm surprised, as this seemed to start after I bought new tennis shoes, which the store said would be better for my joints, but things seemed to get worse.

Addressing the possibility of iliotibial band syndrome we ask:

Q *Have you heard a snapping, or had a flicking sensation down at the knee?*

A Yes, I do occasionally feel a twinge and a click around my knee.

Q *Does the pain worsen the more you do?*

A Yes, it seems to get to a point where I can't continue.

Q *Have you increased the amount you are playing?*

A Yes, I've just started playing doubles with my women's group, as well as my weekly singles tournament.

Addressing the possibility of acetabular or labral pathology we ask:

Q *Do you get any locking or clicking within the hip?*

A Yes, on occasions I get a clicking, but my hips feel good to me, there is no pain when I wake up, and the clicking does not make me weak or give way.

Q *Do you get any pain sitting or standing?*

A No, really just when I'm playing tennis.

Addressing the degenerative hip we ask:

Q *Do you have symptoms on both sides?*

A No, it is mainly on the left.

Q *Do you suffer from pain in other joints?*

A No, I take glucosamine 1 gram daily, and my joints do not cause me any trouble.

Addressing the possibility of stress fracture of the neck of the femur we ask:

Q *Have you suffered any broken bones?*

A Not since I was seven, when I fell from a tree.

Q *Do you take any calcium supplements?*

A Yes, regular vitamins and calcium.

Q *Do you get the pain if you jump, or step down off a kerb or a train?*

A No, I do get impact pain when playing tennis, but not unless the pain has come on during a game.

Addressing the possibility of lateral femoral cutaneous nerve entrapment we ask:

Q *Do you notice any numbness or tingling over your thigh, or gluteals?*

A No, not at all, just a pain.

This all leads us to consider perhaps acetabular labral pathology, and that of iliotibial band syndrome.

Differential diagnosis
More likely
> acetabular and labral pathology
> iliotibial band syndrome
Less likely
> trochanteric bursitis
> stress fracture of neck of femur
> lateral femoral cutaneous nerve entrapment

Step 3: Palpate and re-create

On examination of her hips, the patient demonstrates a good bilateral, active range of movement; she does have some reduction in internal rotation, consistent with her age, but this did not reproduce her pain in FADIR (Flexion, Aduction, Internal Rotation) testing, although she did hold the hip slightly externally rotated. She was negative for a Hop test, and did not get any pain on pressure above her ASIS.

She did have gluteal trigger points, and was tender on the Ober's test, which in part reproduced her pain, but not absolutely.

As clinicians, we would want to examine the patient after a tennis game, so we could see if this is, as seems likely, overuse of the tensor fascia late. In her rested state, this was not possible to delineate, and so highlights the need for examination after the precipitating activity.

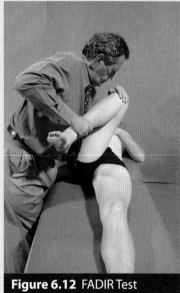

Figure 6.12 FADIR Test (Flexion, Adduction, and internal rotation of hip),

Step 4: Alleviate and investigate

Shoot-through plain films of her hips are likely to exclude a CAM lesion and, since her range of movement does not reproduce her pain, further imaging is unlikely to reveal more until a post-exercise examination.

Ultrasound examination may show damage to the tensor fascia late, if the overuse was significant enough, and may warrant a guided injection of local anesthesia as part of a diagnostic maneuver.

Case 4

A 23-year-old Australian Rules footballer presents with right gluteal pain. The pain came on acutely after training, and seems to radiate down his leg. He has no weakness, and did not feel anything give or pull. He had been completing a sprint session, and so was doing a heavy load of accelerating and decelerating. He has no previous injury on this side, nor any history of back pain.

Step 1: Define and align

Expose the patient properly. It may be necessary to undress the patient to a pair of swim shorts, to allow inspection and effective palpation. It is impossible to examine the gluteal region through clothing.

Define the triangle: locate the L5 spinous process, the 3G point, and the greater trochanter.

Align the patient's pain. Here the pain is located "within the triangle".

From this point we recommend that the reader attempt to exclude potential pathologies. From Table 6.6, the potential differential diagnoses include:

Differential diagnosis

> acute disc prolapse

> lumbar facet joint pain

> piriformis tendinopathy

> pelvic floor dysfunction

> circumflex femoral vein thrombosis

> posterior femoral cutaneous nerve entrapment

> cluneal nerve entrapment

Step 2: Listen and localize

Addressing the question of lumbar disc prolapse we ask:

Q *Does the pain radiate down the back of your leg, to the foot?*

A Yes, the pain is really focused at the lower edge of the gluts, and it does extend down to the top of my medial gastrocnemius.

Q *Do you have any back pain, or have you had any before this happened?*

A No, my back has been good. I increased my weight training in the pre-season, and this caused me some occasional pain after a heavy squatting session or dead lifts. But all is good at the moment.

Q *Is the pain electrical at all?*

A No, there is a sharp nagging pain in the one place.

Addressing the possibility of lumbar facet joint pain we ask:

Q *Is the pain worse if you turn in one direction?*

A No.

Q *Is the pain worse when you exercise?*

A Yes, it gets worse with impact and stopping suddenly.

Addressing the possibility of piriformis tendinopathy we ask:

Q *Did the pain come on gradually?*

A No, it came on suddenly at the end of training.

Addressing pelvic floor dysfunction we ask:

Q *Do you have any urinary problems, or pain opening your bowels?*

A No.

Addressing the thrombosis risk we ask:

Q *Have you had a deep vein thrombosis in the past, or do you have any of these risk factors: smoker, frequent long-haul travel, or recent surgery?*

A No. No other risk factors.

Addressing the risk of nerve entrapments we ask:

Q *Do you have any associated numbness on the back of your leg, or buttock?*

A There does seem to be a bit of numbness over the back of my calf, I think. I can still feel it, but it just feels a bit strange; I haven't noticed this.

Q *Does stretching make the pain worse?*

A Yes, stretching seems to send the pain up into my back.

This targeted questioning makes us focus our examination on the patient's back, to exclude an acute disc prolapse. We screen him at this stage for red flags, in particular any other illness, weight loss, or night sweats, or indeed night pain, bilateral numbness, or problems with opening bowels, or urinating – all of which are negative.

Differential diagnosis

More likely
> acute disc prolapse

Less likely
> lumbar facet joint pain
> piriformis tendinopathy
> pelvic floor dysfunction
> circumflex femoral vein thrombosis
> posterior femoral cutaneous nerve entrapment
> cluneal nerve entrapment

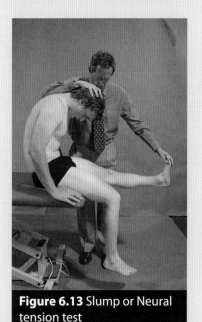

Figure 6.13 Slump or Neural tension test

Step 3: Palpate and re-create

On examination, we find that the patient is positive for a *slump test*, and does have some slight sensation deficiency in the L4 distribution. His lower limb strength, and hip strength are normal, and he has no irritation on FAIR testing, suggestive of piriformis irritability.

Step 4: Alleviate and investigate

Given his positive slump test and Braggard's sign, an MRI of the patient's lumbar spine would be an appropriate investigative test, although, given the acute nature of the symptoms, a trail of soft tissue therapy and analgesia, with a rehabilitation package, might be the most appropriate next step prior to imaging.

Case 5

A 34-year-old woman presents with acute-onset left-buttock pain. The pain started suddenly, after she climbed out of her car. She does not normally do much sport, but completed a multi-sport adventure race, as part of a team-building exercise at work, two weeks ago. She has no past medical history, and has a BMI of 22. The pain is quite severe at times, and her over-the-counter medication has not really worked.

Step 1: Define and align

Expose the patient properly. It may be necessary to undress the patient to a pair of swim shorts, to allow inspection and effective palpation. It is impossible to examine the gluteal region through clothing.

Define the triangle: locate the L5 spinous process, the 3G point, and the greater trochanter.

Align the patient's pain. Here the pain is located "within the triangle at the ischial tuberosity".

From this point we recommend that the reader attempt to exclude potential pathologies. From Table 6.7, the potential differential diagnoses include:

Differential diagnosis
> hamstring origin tendinopathy
> proximal hamstring tear
> ischiofemoral bursitis

> ischial tuberosity avulsion fracture
> stress fracture pubic ramus

Step 2: Listen and localize

Addressing hamstring origin tendinopathy we ask:

Q *Did the pain come on suddenly, and were you able to complete the exercise?*

A Yes, the pain came on suddenly, but not until about a week after the exercise. I didn't feel anything give or go, although I felt a hamstring twinge but no pain in the race.

Addressing a hamstring tear we ask:

Q *What were you doing when the pain came on?*

A I woke with the pain. It was a bit sore when I was going to bed, but in the morning it was very painful.

Addressing ischiofemoral bursitis we ask:

Q *Is the pain worse on sitting?*

A Yes, it is at its worst.

Q *Did you pull a hamstring during your race at all?*

A Yes, I think I tweaked the muscle in the back of my leg while getting out of the kayak; my leg was a bit numb while I was in the kayak as well, but I could move it ok when I got out.

Addressing the possibility of avulsion fracture, the patient's age rules her out as the ossification site is closed; however, to address the stress fracture risk we ask:

Q *Have you increased the amount of training you do recently?*

A No, I don't really train at all.

Q *Have you had any bone fractures, or a family history of osteoporosis?*

A Not that I know about.

Q *Have you started dieting, or lost weight recently?*

A No.

This focuses the examination in the next step to the ischial tuberosity, and the risk of bursitis.

Differential diagnosis

More likely
> ischial tuberosity avulsion fracture
> ischial bursitis

Less likely
> hamstring origin tendinopathy
> proximal hamstring tear

> ischiofemoral bursitis

> ischial tuberosity avulsion fracture

> stress fracture pubic ramus

On examination, we check Revel's criteria to exclude a facet joint problem, and all lumbar spine movements are pain-free. On palpation of the ischial tuberosity, we feel tenderness, which "is her pain". This is likely to be ischial bursitis; we go on to examine the hamstrings, as concomitant injury is often found, although in this case we can find no evidence of hamstring injury.

Step 3: Alleviate and investigate

If this was a younger patient, we would recommend of course a plain film, in order to exclude an avulsion fracture, as the two run in parallel. But in this patient, no further investigation is required at this stage.

Conclusion

In summary, the case histories have given portraits of the varied differential diagnoses, and methods for accurately assessing the gluteal region. As previously stated, there is significant overlap here with the groin and greater trochanter chapters and, if there is any doubt, the examination should always include these regions for completeness. The case histories are not intended to provide examples for every situation, but to be representative of the normal deductive process.

References

1. Lawrence JP, Greene HS, Grauer JN. Back pain in athletes. J Am Acad Orthop Surg. 2006 Dec; 14(13):726–35.
2. Franklyn-Miller A, Falvey E, McCrory P, Briggs CA. Landmarks for the 3G approach: groin, gluteal and greater trochanter triangles – a patho-anatomical method in sports medicine. Submitted.
3. Last R, Suinnatamby C. *Last's anatomy: regional and applied.* 10th ed. London: Churchill Livingstone; 1999.
4. Fairclough J, Hayashi K, Toumi H, Lyons K, Bydder G, Phillips N, et al. The functional anatomy of the iliotibial band during flexion and extension of the knee: implications for understanding iliotibial band syndrome. Journal of Anatomy. 2006 Mar; 208(3):309–16.
5. Falvey EC, Clark RA, Franklyn-Miller A, Bryant AL, Briggs C, McCrory PR. Iliotibial band syndrome: an examination of the evidence behind a number of treatment options. Scand J Med Sci Sports. 2009 Aug; 23.
6. Windisch G, Braun EM, Anderhuber F. Piriformis muscle: clinical anatomy and consideration of the piriformis syndrome. Surg Radiol Anat. 2007 Feb; 29(1):37–45.
7. Hancock MJ, Maher CG, Latimer J, Spindler MF, McAuley JH, Laslett M, et al. Systematic review of tests to identify the disc, SIJ or facet joint as the sorce of low back pain. Eur Spine J. 2007 Oct; 16(10):1539–50.
8. Malanga G, Nadler S. *Musculoskeletal physical examination: An evidence-based approach.* Philadelphia: Elsevier Mosby; 2006.
9. Bennett AN, Marzo-Ortega H, Emery P, McGonagle D. Diagnosing axial spondyloarthropathy. The new assessment in SpondyloArthritis International Society criteria: MRI entering center stage. Ann Rheum Dis. 2009 Jun; 68(6):765–67.
10. Sidiropoulos PI, Hatemi G, Song IH, Avouac J, Collantes E, Hamuryudan V, et al. Evidence-based recommendations for the management of ankylosing spondylitis: systematic literature search of the 3E initiative in rheumatology

involving a broad panel of experts and practising rheumatologists. Rheumatology (Oxford). 2008 Mar; 47(3): 355–61.

11. McVeigh CM, Cairns AP. Diagnosis and management of ankylosing spondylitis. BMJ (Clinical research ed). 2006 Sep 16; 333(7568):581–85.

12. Solonen KA. The sacroiliac joint in the light of anatomical, roentgenological and clinical studies. Acta Orthop Scand Suppl. 1957; 27:1–127.

13. Laslett M, Williams M. The reliability of selected pain provocation tests for sacroiliac joint pathology. Spine. 1994 Jun 1; 19(11):1243–49.

14. Boswell MV, Shah RV, Everett CR, Sehgal N, McKenzie Brown AM, Abdi S, et al. Interventional techniques in the management of chronic spinal pain: evidence-based practise guidelines. Pain Physician. 2005 Jan; 8(1):1–47.

15. Rudwaleit, editor. The majority of peripheral spondyloarthritis is "undifferentiated" at the time of diagnosis – lessons from the ASAS study on new classification criteria for peripheral spondyloarthritis. ACR 2009; Philaphedia, USA.

16. Warrell D, Cox TM, Firth J, Benz E, Isner-Horobeti M. *Oxford textbook of medicine*. Oxford University Press; 2004.

17. Lorie H. Spontaneous osteoporotic fracture of the sacrum. An unrecognized syndrome of the elderly. JAMA. 1982 Aug 13; 248(6):715–17.

18. Cattley P, Winyard J, Trevaskis J, Eaton S. Validity and reliability of clinical tests for the sacroiliac joint. A review of literature. Australas Chiropr Osteopathy. 2002 Nov; 10(2):73–80.

19. Ryan PJ, Fogelman I. The role of nuclear medicine in orthopedics. Nuclear Medicine Communications. 1994 May; 15(5):341–60.

20. Berger FH, de Jonge MC, Maas M. Stress fractures in the lower extremity. The importance of increasing awareness amongst radiologists. European Journal of Radiology. 2007 Apr; 62(1):16–26.

21. Brukner P, Khan KM. *Clinical sports medicine*. 3rd ed. Australia: McGraw-Hill; 2007.

22. Watters WC, 3rd, Bono CM, Gilbert TJ, Kreiner DS, Mazanec DJ, Shaffer WO, et al. An evidence-based clinical guideline for the diagnosis and treatment of degenerative lumbar spondylolisthesis. Spine. 2009 Jul; 9(7): 609–14.

23. Campbell RS, Grainger AJ, Hide IG, Papastefanou S, Greenough CG. Juvenile spondylolysis: a comparative analysis of CT, SPECT and MRI. Skeletal Radiol. 2005 Feb; 34(2):63–73.

24. Bradshaw C, McCrory P. Obturator nerve entrapment. Clin J Sport Med. 1997 Jul; 7(3):217–19.

25. Delagi EF PA. *Anatomic guide for the electromyographer*. 2nd ed. Springfield: Charles C Thomas Publishers; 1980.

26. Magora F, Rozin R, Ben-Menachem Y, Magora A. Obturator nerve block: an evaluation of technique. British Journal of Anaesthesia. 1969 Aug; 41(8):695–98.

27. Oseto MC, Edwards JZ, Acus RW, 3rd. Posterior thigh compartment syndrome associated with hamstring avulsion and chronic anticoagulation therapy. Orthopedics. 2004 Feb; 27(2):229–30.

28. Kwong Y, Patel J, Ramanathan EB. Spontaneous complete hamstring avulsion causing posterior thigh compartment syndrome. Br J Sports Med. 2006 Aug; 40(8):723–24; discussion 24.

29. Brandser EA, el-Khory GY, Kathol MH, Callaghan JJ, Tearse DS. Hamstring injuries: radiographic, conventional tomographic, CT, and MR imaging characteristics. Radiology. 1995 Oct; 197(1):257–62.

30. Orava S, Laakko E, Mattila K, Makinen L, Rantanen J, Kujala UM. Chronic compartment syndrome of the quadriceps femoris muscle in athletes. Diagnosis, imaging and treatment with fasciotomy. Ann Chir Gynecol. 1998; 87(1):53–58.

31. Batt M, Baque J, Bouillanne PJ, Hassen-Khodja R, Haudeborg P, Thevenin B. Percutaneous angioplasty of the superior gluteal artery for buttock claudication: a report of seven cases and literature review. J Vasc Surg. 2006 May; 43(5):987–91.

32. Berthelot JM, Pillet JC, Mitard D, Chevalet-Muller F, Planchon B, Maugars Y. Buttock claudication disclosing a thrombosis of the superior left gluteal artery. Report of a case diagnosed by a selective arteriography of the iliac artery, and cured by per-cutaneous stenting. Joint Bone Spine. 2007 May; 74(3):289–91.

33. Puranen J, Orava S. The hamstring syndrome. A new diagnosis of gluteal sciatic pain. The American Journal of Sports Medicine. 1988 Sep–Oct; 16(5):517–21.

34. Orava S. Hamstring syndrome. Operative Techniques in Sports Medicine. 1997; 5(3):143.

35. Franklyn-Miller A, Falvey E, McCrory P. Fasciitis first before tendinopathy; Does the anatomy hold the key? Br J Sports Med. 2009 Jan; 9.

36. Klinge U, Binnebosel M, Mertens PR. Are collagens the culprits in the development of incisional and inguinal hernia disease? Hernia. 2006 Dec; 10(6):472–77.

37. Lavelle ED, Lavelle W, Smith HS. Myofascial trigger points. Med Clin North Am. 2007 Mar; 91(2):229–39.

38. Njoo KH, Van der Does E. The occurrence and inter-rater reliability of myofascial trigger points in the quadratus lumborum and gluteus medius: a prospective study in non-specific low back pain patients and controls in general practice. Pain. 1994 Sep; 58(3):317–23.

39. Ozcakar L, Erol O, Kaymak B, Aydemir N. An underdiagnosed hip pathology: apropos of two cases with gluteus medius tendon tears. Clin Rheumatol. 2004 Oct; 23(5):464–66.

40. Bird P, Oakley S, Shnier R, Kirkham B. Prospective evaluation of magnetic resonance imaging and physical examination findings in patientiets with trochanteric pain syndrome. Arthritis Rheum. 2001; 44:2138–45.

41. Allen GM, Wilson DJ. Ultrasound in sports medicine – a critical evaluation. Eur J Radiol. 2007 Apr; 62(1):79–85.

42. Aihara T, Takahashi K, Yamagata M, Moriya H, Tamaki T. Biomechanical functions of the iliolumbar ligament in L5 spondylolysis. J Orthop Sci. 2000; 5(3):238–42.

43. Pool-Goudzwaard A, Hoek van Dijke G, Mulder P, Spoor C, Snijders C, Stoeckart R. The iliolumbar ligament: its influence on stability of the sacroiliac joint. Clinical Biomechanics (Bristol, Avon). 2003 Feb; 18(2):99–105.

44. Barker PJ, Briggs CA, Bogeski G. Tensile transmission across the lumbar fascie in unembalmed cadavers: effects of tension to various muscular attachments. Spine. 2004 Jan 15; 29(2):129–38.

45. Barker PJ, Guggenheimer KT, Grkovic I, Briggs CA, Jones DC, Thomas CD, et al. Effects of tensioning the lumbar fascie on segmental stiffness during flexion and extension: Young Investigator Award winner. Spine. 2006 Feb 15; 31(4):397–405.

46. Vleeming A, Pool-Goudzwaard AL, Stoeckart R, van Wingerden JP, Snijders CJ. The posterior layer of the thoracolumbar fascia. Its function in load transfer from spine to legs. Spine. 1995 Apr 1; 20(7):753–58.

47. Aspden RM. Review of the functional anatomy of the spinal ligaments and the lumbar erector spine muscles. Clinical Anatomy. 1992;(5):372–87.

48. Lu J, Ebraheim NA, Huntoon M, Heck BE, Yeasting RA. Anatomic considerations of superior cluneal nerve at posterior iliac crest region. Clin Orthop Relat Res. 1998 Feb; (347):224–28.

49. Maigne JY, Maigne R. Trigger point of the posterior iliac crest: painful iliolumbar ligament insertion or cutaneous dorsal ramus pain? An anatomic study. Arch Phys Med Rehabil. 1991 Sep; 72(10):734–37.

50. Filler AG. Piriformis and related entrapment syndromes: diagnosis & management. Neurosurg Clin N Am. 2008 Oct; 19(4):609–22, vii.

51. Robinson D. Piriformis syndrome in relation to sciatic pain. Am J Surg. 1947; 73:355–58.

52. Kirkaldy–Willis WH, Hill RJ. A more precise diagnosis for low-back pain. Spine (Philadelphia, PA). 1979 Mar–Apr; 4(2):102–09.

53. Smith J, Hurdle MF, Locketz AJ, Wisniewski SJ. Ultrasound-guided piriformis injection: technique description and verification. Arch Phys Med Rehabil. 2006 Dec; 87(12):1664–67.

54. Stewart JD. The piriformis syndrome is overdiagnosed. Muscle & Nerve. 2003 Nov; 28(5):644–46.

55. Monnier G, Tatu L, Michel F. New indications for botulinum toxin in rheumatology. Joint Bone Spine. 2006 Dec; 73(6):667–71.

56. Paluska SA. An overview of hip injuries in running. Sports Med. 2005; 35(11):991–1014.

57. Walker P, Kannangara S, Bruce WJ, Michel D, Van der Wall H. Lateral hip pain: does imaging predict response to localized injection? Clin Orthop Relat Res. 2007 Apr; 457:144–49.

58. Brignall CG, Brown RM, Stainsby GD. Fibrosis of the gluteus maximus as a cause of snapping hip. A case report. J Bone Joint Surg Am. 1993 Jun; 75(6):909–10.

59. Malanga G, Nadler S. *Physical examination of the hip. Muscloskeletal physical examination: An evidence-based approach.* Philadelphia, PA: Elsevier Mosby; 2006. p. 251–79.

60. Ganz R, Parvizi J, Beck M, Leunig M, Notzli H, Siebenrock KA. Femoroacetabular impingement: a cause for osteoarthritis of the hip. Clinical Orthopedics and Related Research. 2003 Dec; (417):112–20.

61. Leunig M, Podeszwa D, Beck M, Werlen S, Ganz R. Magnetic resonance arthrography of labral disorders in hips with dysplasia and impingement. Clinical Orthopedics and Related Research. 2004 Jan; (418):74–80.

62. Birrell F, Croft P, Cooper C, Hosie G, Macfarlane G, Silman A. Predicting radiographic hip osteoarthritis from range of movement. Rheumatology (Oxford, England). 2001 May; 40(5):506–12.

63. Monteleone GP, Jr. Stress fractures in the athlete. The Orthopedic Clinics of North America. 1995 Jul; 26(3):423–32.

64. Johnson AW, Weiss CB, Jr., Wheeler DL. Stress fractures of the femoral shaft in athletes—more common than expected. A new clinical test. Am J Sports Med. 1994 Mar–Apr; 22(2):248–56.

65. Seror P, Seror R. Meralgia paresthetica: clinical and electrophysiological diagnosis in 120 cases. Muscle & Nerve. 2006 May; 33(5):650–54.

66. Rab M, Ebmer And J, Dellon AL. Anatomic variability of the ilioinguinal and genitofemoral nerve: implications for the treatment of groin pain. Plast Reconstr Surg. 2001 Nov; 108(6):1618–23.

67. Filler AG. Axonal transport and MR imaging: prospects for contrast agent development. J Magn Reson Imaging. 1994 May–Jun; 4(3):259–67.

68. Grant SR, Salvati EP, Rubin RJ. Levator syndrome: an analysis of 316 cases. Dis Colon Rectum. 1975 Mar; 18(2):161–63.

69. Rao SS, Paulson J, Mata M, Zimmerman B. Clinical trial: effects of botulinum toxin on Levator ani syndrome – a double-blind, placebo-controlled study. Aliment Pharmacol Ther. 2009 May 1; 29(9):985–91.

70. Papasterigou C, Koukoulias N, Tsitoridis I, Natsis C, Parisis C. Circumflex femoral vein thrombosis missed as acute hamstring strain. British Journal of Sports Medicine. 2007; 41:460–61.

71. McCrory P, Bell S. Nerve entrapment syndromes as a cause of pain in the hip, groin and buttock. Sports Med. 1999 Apr; 27(4):261–74.

72. Arnoldussen WJ, Korten JJ. Pressure neuropathy of the posterior femoral cutaneous nerve. Clin Neurol Neurosurg. 1980; 82(1):57–60.

73. Andersson G, Deyo R. History and examination in patients with herniated lumbar discs. Spine. 1996; 21(Suppl. 24): 10–8S.

74. Stankovic R, Johnell O, Maly P, Willner S. Use of lumbar extension, slump test, physical and neurological examination in the evaluation of patients with suspected herniated nucleus pulposus; a prospective clinical study. Man Ther. 1999; 4(1):25–32.

75. Manchikanti L, Cash KA, Pampati V, McManus CD, Damron KS. Evaluation of fluoroscopically guided caudal epidural injections. Pain Physician. 2004 Jan; 7(1):81–92.

76. Revel M, Poiraudeau S, Auleley GR, Payan C, Denke A, Nguyen M, et al. Capacity of the clinical picture to characterise low back pain relieved by facet joint anesthesia. Proposed criteria to identify patients with painful facet joints. Spine. 1998 Sep 15; 23(18):1972–76; discussion 77.

77. Beatty RA. The piriformis muscle syndrome: a simple diagnostic maneuver. Neurosurgery. 1994 Mar; 34(3): 512–14; discussion 14.

78. Solheim L, Siewars P, Paus B. The piriformis muscle syndrome; sciatic nerve entrapment treated with section of the piriformis muscle. Acta Orthp Scand. 1981; 52:73–75.

79. Hetrick DC, Ciol MA, Rothman I, Turner JA, Frest M, Berger RE. Musculoskeletal dysfunction in men with chronic pelvic pain syndrome type III: a case-control study. J Urol. 2003 Sep; 170(3):828–31.

80. Papastergiou S, Koukoulias N, Tsitoridis I, Natsis C, Parisis C. Circumflex femoral vein thrombosis misinterpreted as acute hamstring strain. BJSM. [case report]. 2007; 41:460–61.

81. Verrall GM, Slavotinek JP, Barnes PG, Fon GT. Diagnostic and prognostic value of clinical findings in 83 athletes with posterior thigh injury: comparison of clinical findings with magnetic resonance imaging documentation of hamstring muscle strain. The American Journal of Sports Medicine. 2003 Nov–Dec; 31(6):969–73.

82. Orchard J, Best TM, Verrall GM. Return to play following muscle strains. Clin J Sport Med. 2005 Nov; 15(6): 436–41.

83. Askling CM, Tengvar M, Saartok T, Thorstensson A. Acute first-time hamstring strains during high-speed running: a longitudinal study including clinical and magnetic resonance imaging findings. The American Journal of Sports Medicine. 2007 Feb; 35(2):197–206.

84. Schneider–Kolsky ME, Hoving JL, Warren P, Connell DA. A comparison between clinical assessment and magnetic resonance imaging of acute hamstring injuries. The American Journal of Sports Medicine. 2006 Jun; 34(6):1008–15.

85. Connell DA, Schneider–Kolsky ME, Hoving JL, Malara F, Buchbinder R, Kouloris G, et al. Longitudinal study comparing sonographic and MRI assessments of acute and healing hamstring injuries. AJR Am J Roentgenol. 2004 Oct; 183(4):975–84.

86. Gibbs NJ, Cross TM, Cameron M, Houang MT. The accuracy of MRI in predicting recovery and recurrence of acute grade one hamstring muscle strains within the same season in Australian Rules football players. J Sci Med Sport. 2004 Jun; 7(2):248–58.

87. Lempainen L, Sarimo J, Mattila K, Vaittinen S, Orava S. Proximal hamstring tendinopathy: results of surgical management and histopathologic findings. The American Journal of Sports Medicine. 2009 Apr; 37(4):727–34.

88. Schache AG, Kouloris G, Kofoed W, Morris HG, Pandy MG. Rupture of the conjoint tendon at the proximal musculotendinous junction of the biceps femoris long head: a case report. Knee Surg Sports Traumatol Arthrosc. 2008 Aug; 16(8):797–802.

89. Kujala UM, Orava S, Karpakka J, Leppavuori J, Mattila K. Ischial tuberosity apophysitis and avulsion among athletes. Int J Sports Med. 1997 Feb; 18(2):149–55.

90. Rossi F, Dragoni S. Acute avulsion fractures of the pelvis in adolescent competitive athletes: prevalence, location and sports distribution of 203 cases collected. Skeletal Radiol. 2001 Mar; 30(3):127–31.

91. Hill PF, Chatterji S, Chambers D, Keeling JD. Stress fracture of the pubic ramus in female recruits. J Bone Joint Surg Br. 1996 May; 78(3):383–86.

92. Isdale AH. Stress fractures of the pubic rami in rheumatoid arthritis. Ann Rheum Dis. 1993 Sep; 52(9):681–84.

93. Clanton TO, Coupe KJ. Hamstring strains in athletes: diagnosis and treatment. J Am Acad Orthop Surg. 1998 Jul–Aug; 6(4):237–48.

94. Lequesne M, Zaoui A. Misleading "hip" or buttock pain: proximal arteritis or lumbar spinal stenosis?]. Presse Med. 2006 Apr; 35(4 Pt 2):663–68.

95. Wong M, Chung CH, Ngai WK. Hip pain and childhood malignancy. Hong Kong Med J. 2002 Dec; 8(6): 461–63.

96. Rudwaleit M, Sieper J. [Diagnosis and early diagnosis of ankylosing spondylitis]. Z Rheumatol. 2004 Jun; 63(3):193–202.

97. Sieper J, Rudwaleit M. Early referral recommendations for ankylosing spondylitis (including pre-radiographic and radiographic forms) in primary care. Ann Rheum Dis. 2005 May; 64(5):659–63.

The knee triangle

Introduction

Large numbers of athletes present with knee pain on an annual basis; indeed, some studies report that up to 54% of all sports medicine consultations are related to the knee.[1] This may in part be due to the exposed nature of the joint, but also to its use in most sporting activity. Some specific sports, such as American football and skiing, report the knee as their most common site of injury. In the adolescent and younger athlete, it has been seen that injuries to the knee are the most common, either ligamentous injury,[2] or the anterior structures and extensor mechanisms.[3] The International Olympic Committee (IOC) developed a consensus statement on anterior cruciate ligament (ACL) injuries in the female athlete, due to a much higher incidence of ACL injuries in females in sports such as basketball and team handball. The study concluded that risk factors included: being in the pre-ovulatory phase of the menstrual cycle, compared with the post-ovulatory phase; a decreased intercondylar notch width on plain film radiography; and developing increased knee abduction moment during impact on landing.[4]

The high injury rate is not surprising, given the nature of the action of the knee. It must flex and extend, often with explosive force, all the while withstanding the torque, acceleratory, and de-acceleratory forces imposed on it by the quadriceps and hamstring complex, when changing direction and braking.

Rotation at the hip joint and ankle place valgus and varus strains through the knee, which must be absorbed by the soft tissue structures within and around the joint, which are its primary stabilizers. The knee therefore is a complex joint, and a thorough understanding of the anatomy is vital in understanding the discriminatory process of identifying possible injury, as you will see. It is not just the menisci and the cruciates!

Learning objectives

The landmarks of the knee triangle

The pain-generating structures of the region

Significant joints, ligaments, and muscle actions and properties

The presenting symptoms of pathology of each of these structures, to allow differentiation between them

Discriminative examinations and maneuvers to alter (reduce/increase) the presenting pain

Evidence-based examinations to confirm the clinical diagnosis

The joint

The knee is the largest joint in the human body, and is a synovial hinge joint, articulating the two femoral condyles and the tibial condyles (or plateaus), along with the patellofemoral joint—a synovial plane joint. There is some rotational movement of the knee; this occurs mainly at terminal extension, where a "screw home" mechanism of medial rotation of the femur ensures joint stability. Being a synovial joint, the knee is enclosed by a capsule, with intra- and extracapsular ligaments. Both the femoral and tibial condyles are covered in hyaline cartilage, and sitting on the tibial condyle are the meniscal cartilages (Fig. 7.1).

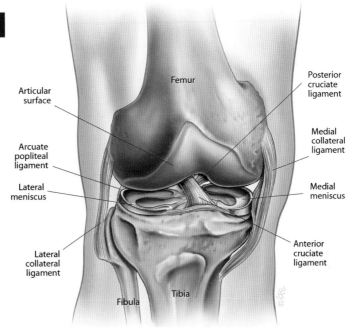

Figure 7.1 The knee joint

Articular surface

Arcuate popliteal ligament

Lateral meniscus

Lateral collateral ligament

Fibula

Tibia

Femur

Posterior cruciate ligament

Medial collateral ligament

Medial meniscus

Anterior cruciate ligament

Menisci

The menisci serve to improve the surface contact area of the femoral condyle with the tibia. The medial and lateral menisci are fibrocartilaginous discs. They sit between the femoral condyles and tibial condyles, and attach to the lateral aspect of the tibial condylar articular facets. The peripheral margin of the meniscus is attached to the tibia, and is much thicker than the free medial edge, which creates a triangular construction in cross-section.

Both lateral and medial menisci have an anterior horn and a posterior horn. The horns of the menisci are attached to the non-articular intercondylar area of the tibial plateau, and receive their blood supply from the medial and lateral geniculate arteries, branches of the popliteal artery. Only 10–30% of the peripheral medial meniscus border, and 10–25% of the lateral meniscus border receive a direct blood supply;[5] this has implications for healing in the event of injury.

The posterior articular branch of the posterior tibial nerve, and the terminal branches of the obturator and femoral nerves innervate the knee joint. Nerve fibers penetrate the joint capsule, along with the vascular supply, and innervate the menisci.[6]

The medial differs from the lateral meniscus in a number of aspects. The medial meniscus is semicircular and wider posteriorly than anteriorly, whereas the lateral meniscus is almost a complete disc and is a similar thickness throughout. The anterior horns of the menisci attach to the intercondylar facet, anterior to the insertion of the anterior cruciate ligament. The posterior horns attach at the intercondylar ridge, posterior to the attachment of the posterior cruciate ligament.

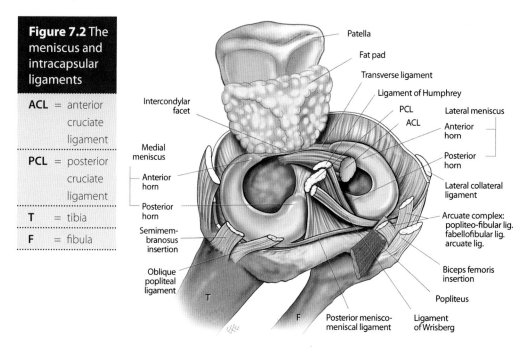

Figure 7.2 The meniscus and intracapsular ligaments

ACL = anterior cruciate ligament

PCL = posterior cruciate ligament

T = tibia

F = fibula

Patella
Fat pad
Transverse ligament
Ligament of Humphrey
PCL
ACL
Lateral meniscus
Anterior horn
Posterior horn
Lateral collateral ligament
Arcuate complex: popliteo-fibular lig. fabellofibular lig. arcuate lig.
Biceps femoris insertion
Popliteus
Ligament of Wrisberg
Posterior menisco-meniscal ligament

Intercondylar facet
Medial meniscus
Anterior horn
Posterior horn
Semimembranosus insertion
Oblique popliteal ligament
T
F

Synovial capsule

The synovial capsule is lined with synovial membrane, and is attached to the margins of the articular surfaces. Proximally, the capsule attaches superiorly to the borders of the articular surface of the femoral condyles. Posteriorly, it is attached above the intercondylar notch. Anteriorly, the capsular fibers do not attach to the bone, but to the patella and patellar ligament, via the medial and lateral patella retinaculum, with which they blend. Inferiorly, the capsule of the knee joint is attached medially and laterally to the borders of the articular surface of the tibial condyles, and to the fibular head. It invests with the medial and lateral coronary ligaments, to attach the medial and lateral menisci to the tibia. Posteriorly, the capsular fibers are attached to the posterior border of the tibial condyles. The popliteus exits through a passage in the synovial capsule which is strengthened by the arcuate popliteal ligament.

Bursae of the knee

There is much debate about bursae of the the knee, and their true purpose and indeed existence. Three clear spaces in the prepatellar region have been identified[7] (Fig. 7.5). The first lies between the layer of subcutaneous fat and the fascia late, the second is a prepatellar space between the superficial fascia and the intermediate oblique aponeurosis layer, and the third is a prepatellar sub-aponeurotic space between the oblique intermediate layer, and the rectus femoris tendon.

Laterally, much is made of the bursae deep to the iliotibial band (ITB) insertion, adjacent to Kaplan's fibers, attaching to the lateral condyle and the investing fibers into the tibial condyle. The authors' work, and that of others, does not demonstrate the existence of a bursa in this location, but merely a fat pad.[8, 9]

Intracapsular ligaments

Anterior cruciate ligament

The anterior cruciate ligament (ACL) is a band-like structure made up of dense collagen. It originates from the posterior part of the inner surface of the lateral femoral condyle. The ACL attachment is lateral to the midline, and the size of its bony attachment is significant, between 11 and 24 mm.[10] From its femoral origins, the ligament runs anteriorly, medially, and distally to the tibia, where it inserts into a fossa anterolateral to the medial tibial spine. The tibial attachment is wider and broader than the femoral. There are some investing fibers to the anterior and posterior horn of the lateral meniscus.

Functionally, the ACL is divided into two bundles – the anteromedial and posterolateral bundles. The posterior is the larger of the two. With the knee in extension, the fibers of the ACL run longitudinally. During flexion, there is slight lateral rotation of the ligament, and initially the anterior bundle spirals around the posterior, due to the bony attachment.

The ACL plays a critical role in joint stability. Its principal role is to prevent the anterior translocation of the tibia relative to the femur, but in addition, when the joint is in near-full extension, the ligament plays a part in resisting external rotation and tibial angulation.[11]

Posterior cruciate ligament

The posterior cruciate ligament (PCL) is stronger than the ACL. It runs from the femoral attachment at the roof and medial side of the interfemoral condylar notch (being up to 20 mm at its attachment[10, 12]), posteriorly to the small superior aspect of the tibial shelf.

Again there are two main bundles – the anterolateral and posteriomedial. The anterior attaches mainly to the roof of the notch, and the posterior to the medial wall. The posterior fibers are the longest, and the anterior fibers become slack when the knee is extended, but taut in flexion. Again critical for stability, the PCL prevents the posterior translocation of the tibia about the femur.

The meniscofemoral (MFL) ligaments[13] are comprised of the anterior MFL of Humphrey and the posterior MFL of Wrisberg. The aMFL of Humphrey is angled across the distal aspect of the PCL in the flexed knee, attaching to the femur distally to the PCL; its fibers merge with the PCL, to insert into fibers at the posterior horn of the lateral meniscus.

The pMFL of Wrisberg extends between the medial wall of the femoral intercondylar notch, and the posterior horn of the medial meniscus. These ligaments are not present in all knees, but when present, have a breaking strain equivalent to that of the PCL, so are significant structures. The aMFL is slack in the extended knee and tightens with flexion, whereas the pMFL is taut in the extended knee and relaxes with flexion.

Medial collateral ligament

The medial collateral ligament (MCL) is broad, and runs between the femoral condyle and the medial shaft of the tibia. It is integral to the joint capsule, and three distinct layers have been described.[14] The capsular layer is the deepest, and bound to the superficial MCL; beneath this, the fibers thicken to form the deep MCL, running from the femoral condyle to the meniscus, and from the meniscus to the tibial condyle.

The superficial layer is part of the fascia, merging with the pes anserinus and tibial periosteum distally. It covers the sartorius and quadriceps proximally, the retinaculum anteriorly, and forms the deep crural fascia posteriorly.[15]

Between these layers is a third layer, beginning within the posteromedial capsule as a posterior oblique ligament arising from the adductor tubercle, whereas the MCL arises from the medial condyle, 1 cm anterior and distal to the adductor tubercle. The posterior medial capsule is joined by the semimembranosus tendon, inserting into the posteromedial tibia just below the joint line, with extensions into the posterior capsule.[14]

Extracapsular ligaments

Lateral collateral ligament

In the normal gait cycle, the lower limb varus angulation is maximal during the stance phase in full knee extension. The lateral structures are under the most tension at this point. The lateral collateral ligament (LCL) is a pencil-like cord, which is extracapsular to the synovial capsule.[16] It is attached to the femur in a semicircular saddle, between the lateral condyle and the supracondylar process, anterior to the lateral head of the gastrocnemius.

The LCL is angulated posteriorly and laterally as it descends distally from its femoral attachment, inferiorly to its fibular attachment (Fig. 7.3). As it approaches its insertion, the medial fibers insert into a groove at the lateral edge of the fibular head, whereas the lateral fibers pass medially to the long head of the biceps femoris muscle, and end as an investment into the fascia late, over the peroneal compartment.

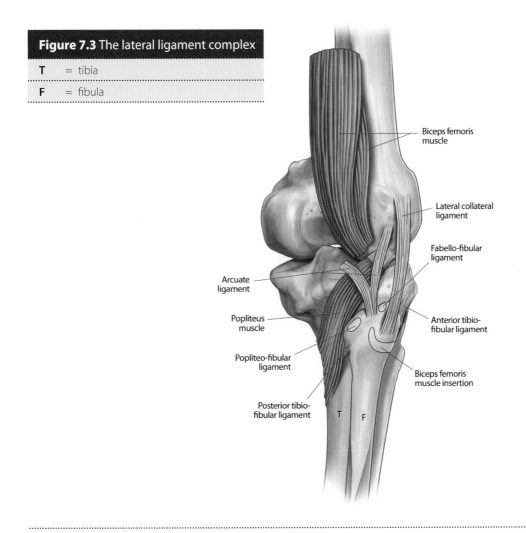

Figure 7.3 The lateral ligament complex

| T | = tibia |
| F | = fibula |

Biceps femoris muscle

Lateral collateral ligament

Fabello-fibular ligament

Arcuate ligament

Popliteus muscle

Popliteo-fibular ligament

Anterior tibio-fibular ligament

Biceps femoris muscle insertion

Posterior tibio-fibular ligament

Arcuate complex: popliteal and oblique popliteal ligaments

The arcuate popliteal complex is made up of the arcuate ligament, the popliteofibular ligament, and the fabellofibular ligament (Fig. 7.3). These ligaments run from the styloid process of the fibula, superomedially over the tendon of popliteus, into which they emit connecting fibers, and then divide to attach to the lateral femoral condyle, and to the posterolateral capsule. Posterolateral corner instability is one of the consequences when this complex is ruptured; the severity of the injury depends on the survival of the PCL. The lateral collateral ligament and biceps femoris tendon are closely opposed, and they may both be injured concomitantly.

The **oblique popliteal ligament** runs from the insertion of the semimembranosus, at the posterior part of the medial tibial condyle, superiorly and laterally. It invests into the posterior surface of the capsule of the knee joint, and inserts into the intercondylar line, and the lateral femoral condyle.

The **popliteofibular ligament** is one of the most important stabilizers in the posterolateral corner, and inserts on the posterior medial fibular styloid, and attaches to the popliteus tendon, just proximal to the myotendinous junction.

The **fabellofibular ligament** attaches to the posterolateral aspect of the fabella (a small sesamoid bone located in the lateral head of the gastrocnemius), and inserts on the fibular styloid. This ligament can be present even in the absence of a fabella, which is present in 30% of individuals.

The **arcuate popliteal ligament** is extracapsular and Y-shaped. Originating, as seen in Figure 7.3, from the fibular head, it arches over the popliteus, and attaches to the intercondylar area of the tibia. A second slip passes over to the lateral epicondyle of the femur, and diverges into the lateral head of the gastrocnemius.

Landmarks of the knee triangle

The specific anatomical landmarks and boundaries of the knee triangle are set out in Figure 7.4.

The anatomical apex points are:

> medial femoral condyle (superior aspect)

> lateral femoral condyle (superior aspect)

> tibial tuberosity

Figure 7.4 The knee triangle

VL	= vastus lateralis
RF	= rectus femoris
VM	= vastus medialis
Sar	= sartorius
Gr	= gracilis
QT	= quadriceps tendon
GC	= gastrocnemius
Sol	= soleus

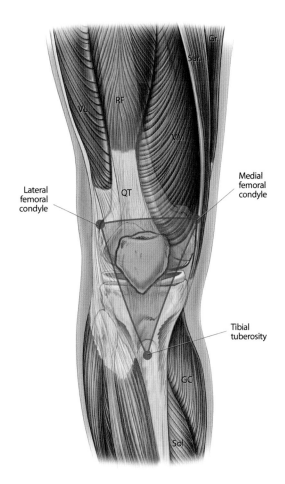

Anatomical relationships of the borders of the anterior knee triangle

Lateral border

The structures encountered moving from proximal to distal are:

> femoral condyle

> origin of lateral collateral ligament

> anterior joint line

> tibial tuberosity

> patellar tendon

The lateral border of the triangle runs from the lateral femoral condyle, anteriorly to the tibial tuberosity. As one moves down this border of the triangle at the femoral condyle, it marks the origin of the lateral collateral ligament, and its fibers may be felt as one runs anteriorly over the synovial capsule, and onto the lateral meniscus, moving antero-inferiorly to cross the lower fibers of the lateral retinaculum. This fascial expansion attaches along the border from the lateral quadriceps tendon, lateral patellar border, and lateral edge of the patellar tendon. It invests with the lateral part of the capsule of the knee joint, before attaching to the inferior margin of the lateral tibial condyle. Continuing along the border takes us onto the tibial tuberosity, and the fibers of the patella tendon.

Medial border

The structures encountered moving proximally to distal are:

> medial femoral condyle

> origin of medial collateral ligament

> medial joint line

> patellar tendon

> tibial tuberosity

The medial border runs from the tibial tuberosity in a superomedial direction; it again crosses the retinaculum and the coronary ligament, before crossing obliquely the medial meniscus and the medial collateral ligament, ending where it originates, at the medial femoral condyle. At the apex of the triangle is the patellar tendon insertion into the tibial tuberosity, a site commonly referred to in sports medicine, due to insertional tendinopathy and Osgood-Schlatter disease (traction apophysitis).

More medial to this sits the pes anserinus. This is a "goose-foot" shaped bursa separating the structures which insert here, and is well described by Mochizuki and colleagues,[17] who first observed the aponeurotic membranes originating from the semitendinosus, gracilis, and sartorius tendons fusing with the fascia cruris in the medial calf region.

Moving superior from this, the clinician crosses the medial retinaculum. This fascial expansion attaches along the border from the medial quadriceps tendon, medial patellar border, and medial edge of the patellar tendon. It invests with the medial part of the capsule of the knee joint, before attaching to the inferior margin of the medial tibial condyle (Fig. 7.5).

Deep to this is the joint line, and the directly palpable medial meniscus. The tendons of the semitendinosus and gracilis invest, as previously described, into the medial collateral ligament, along with the semimembranosus, which inserts lateral to the joint line, and follows the border of the triangle to its margin at the medial femoral condyle. The medial collateral ligament has a superficial layer divided into posterior fibers, forming the posterior oblique ligament, and anterior fibers, which tension in knee flexion. The deep layer can be described as meniscofemoral and meniscotibial.

The muscles encountered medial to the triangle are listed as follows:

Gracilis originates from the anteroinferior border of the symphysis pubis and the pubic rami. The muscle runs inferiorly, develops into a rounded tendon passing around the medial femoral condyle, and flattens into the aponeurotic insertion of the pes anserinus into the medial

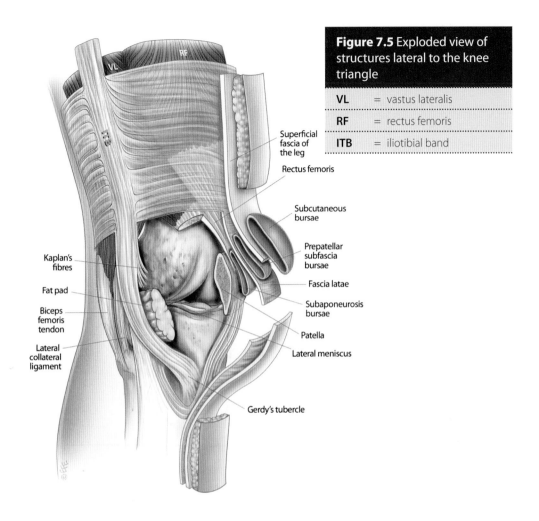

Figure 7.5 Exploded view of structures lateral to the knee triangle

VL	= vastus lateralis
RF	= rectus femoris
ITB	= iliotibial band

Superficial fascia of the leg

Rectus femoris

Subcutaneous bursae

Prepatellar subfascia bursae

Kaplan's fibres

Fascia latae

Fat pad

Subaponeurosis bursae

Biceps femoris tendon

Patella

Lateral collateral ligament

Lateral meniscus

Gerdy's tubercle

tibia. Supplied by the obturator nerve (L2, L3, L4), it adducts and flexes the hip, additionally causing some medial rotation of the knee.

Sartorius is superficial, and originates at the anterior superior iliac spine. It runs inferiorly and obliquely across the rectus femoris and vastus intermedius, passing deep to the tendinous insertion of the gracilis, to insert into the medial tibia as part of the pes anserine complex. It acts to flex, abduct, and laterally rotate the hip joint, but also rotates the tibia medially when the knee is flexed. It is supplied by the femoral nerve (L2, L3).

Semitendinosus originates from the inferomedial ischial tuberosity, by a tendon common to it and to the long head of the biceps femoris. The muscle is unique for its long tendinous insertion, which begins with the musculo-tendinous junction just inferior to the 3G point of the triangle. The tendon then lies medial to the popliteal fossa running medially around the femoral condyle, and overlies the medial collateral ligament, to insert as part of the three-part insertion at the pes anserinus. Supplied by the tibial nerve (L5, S1, S2), it acts to flex the knee, and extend the hip.

The origin of the **semimembranosus** is broad, and sweeps from the upper outer part of the ischial tuberosity. The muscle then winds around the insertion of the biceps femoris and semitendinosus, before running down the medial posterior part of the leg. The tendon is short, and inserts into the medial condyle of the tibia, at the posterior surface. Interestingly, the fibers diverge before the insertion, to invest in the popliteus, and also in the oblique popliteal ligament, contributing to knee joint stability. The muscle is supplied by the tibial nerve (L5, S1, S2), and acts to flex the knee and effect hip extension, with some degree of tibial rotation when the knee is flexed.

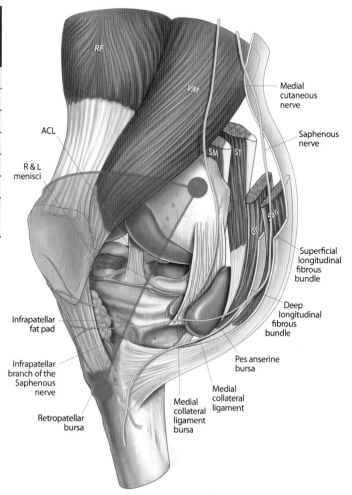

Figure 7.6 Exploded view of structures medial to the knee triangle

RF	= rectus femoris
VM	= vastus medialis
SM	= semimembranosus
ST	= semitendinosus
Gr	= gracilis
Sar	= sartorius
ACL	= anterior cruciate ligament

Superior border

The structures encountered, moving along the superior border, are as follows:

> medial femoral condyle

> vastus medialis

> quadriceps tendon

> vastus lateralis

> lateral femoral condyle

The superior border of the triangle runs horizontally between the condyles. Moving medially to laterally, the first structure encountered is the muscle bulk of the vastus medialis, palpable before the aponeurotic insertions of the rectus femoris and vastus lateralis, as they merge to form the quadriceps tendon. This runs superior to the patella, before one palpates the lateral femoral condyle.

Vastus medialis arises as an aponeurosis formed from a line running from the lower part of the neck of the femur, through to the linea aspera and the intermuscular septum. It also arises from the anterior, medial, and lateral shaft of the femur. The fibers converge to a broad common aponeurosis, which covers the anterior surface of the middle portion of the quadriceps tendon. It inserts into the patella, blending with the other portions of the quadriceps extensor. Acting to extend the knee, it is supplied by the femoral nerve (L2, L3, L4).

The largest of the quadriceps group, the **vastus lateralis** arises from a broad aponeurosis running between the intertrochanteric line, the greater trochanter, and the linea aspera. Slips from the gluteus maximus and the short head of the biceps femoris commonly invest in the lateral part of the muscle, which then runs inferiorly to insert obliquely into the quadriceps tendon, and via the patella into the tibial tuberosity. Supplied by the femoral nerve (L2, L3, L4), its sole action is to extend the knee.

Vastus intermedius is deep to the rectus femoris, and originates from the anterolateral surface of the femur. The muscle runs inferiorly, and inserts into the tibial tuberosity. The distal fibers cover the *articularis genu*, which inserts into the anterior synovial capsule from the anterior femur, and acts to elevate the capsule in knee extension, so as not to entrap the synovium. Supplied by the femoral nerve (L2, L3, L4), the muscle action of the vastus intermedius is knee extension.

Rectus femoris is a bipennate muscle originating from the anterior inferior iliac spine, and the reflected part from the acetabular rim. The muscle runs obliquely from this acetabular origin to form an aponeurosis, which travels inferiorly, inserting into the quadriceps tendon, and via the patella into the patellar tendon and tibial tuberosity. Supplied by the femoral nerve (L2, L3, L4), its action effects knee extension.

The posterior knee triangle

Superior border

Moving medially to laterally, the structures encountered are:

> semimembranous

> semitendinosus

> medial head of gastrocnemius

> popliteal artery

> tibial nerve

> popliteal vein

> common peroneal nerve

> lateral head of gastrocnemius

> insertion of biceps femoris

Again the landmarks are the same: the superior border of the triangle runs from the medial to lateral femoral condyles. Here the structures encountered are, in order, the aponeurotic insertions of the semimembranosus and semitendinosus, as they course toward their insertion, then the medial head of the gastrocnemius, before the popliteal fossa.

The fossa lies within the triangle, and is bounded by the biceps femoris muscle and lateral head of the gastrocnemius laterally, medially by the semitendinosus and semimembranosus muscles, and the medial head of the gastrocnemius. The first structure encountered is the deep popliteal artery, entering through a hiatus in the adductor magnus, as a continuation of the femoral artery. It divides at the lower border of the fossa, by dividing into anterior and posterior tibial arteries. The next structure is the popliteal vein, which ascends through the fossa medially, to the artery initially, but then passing deep to exit the fossa laterally.

The **tibial nerve**, a terminal branch of the sciatic nerve, runs through the fossa, initially lateral to the popliteal artery, then passing deep to it and lying medial. The nerve passes deep to the soleus to exit. A branch of the tibial nerve, the sural nerve, descends between the heads of the gastrocnemius. Moving laterally, the superior border passes over the common peroneal nerve, following the medial border of the biceps femoris, which is next encountered prior to the femoral condyle.

The apex of this triangle is an extrapolated point posteriorly from the tibial tuberosity, which defines the medial and lateral borders of the triangle, transecting the muscle bellies of the gastrocnemius, both medially and laterally.

The medial border of the triangle transects the muscle bulk of the medial head of the gastrocnemius, to a point extrapolated through from the anterior surface at the level of the tibial tuberosity.

The lateral border transects the muscle belly of the lateral head of the gastrocnemius to the same common apex.

Biceps femoris originates from two heads. The long head arises from the inferomedial aspect of the ischial tuberosity, along with the semitendinosus. The short head originates from a broad aponeurotic origin, along the linea aspera on the shaft of the femur; the two heads form a fusiform muscle, which extends down the posterior leg, to insert into the lateral fibula. Importantly, there is a slip, which invests the lateral collateral ligament of the knee. Both heads are supplied by the sciatic nerve, with the long head also supplied by the tibial nerve (L5, S1, S2), and the short head by the common peroneal nerve (S1, S2). The muscle effects knee flexion, and the long head effects extension of the hip.

The **popliteus** originates from the lateral aspect of the lateral femoral condyle; its fibers pass inferomedially, and attach to the posterior surface of the tibia. The muscle arises within the capsule, and its tendon divides the lateral meniscus from the lateral collateral ligament (Fig. 7.1). The muscle is supplied by the tibial nerve (S1, S2), and acts to effect medial rotation of the tibia on the femur. As the knee extends in weight-bearing exercise, the muscle acts inversely to effect lateral rotation of the femur on the tibia; this rotation reduces tension on the internal ligaments of the knee.

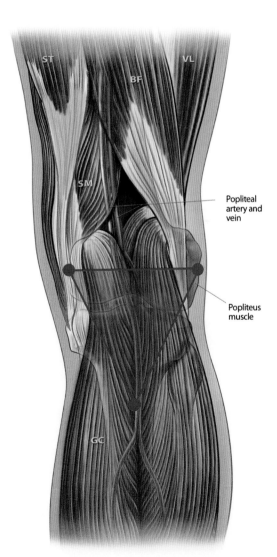

Popliteal artery and vein

Popliteus muscle

Figure 7.7 The posterior knee triangle

ST	=	semitendinosus
GC	=	gastrocnemius
SM	=	semimembranosus
BF	=	biceps femoris
VL	=	vastus lateralis

Gastrocnemius originates from two heads, the lateral from the lateral condyle and posterior surface of the femur, and the medial from the medial condyle and the femur. The two heads form a common insertion, via the achilles tendon, into the calcaneus. Supplied by the tibial nerve (S1, S2), the muscle acts to plantar flex the ankle, and has a lesser effect on knee flexion.

Soleus originates from the posterior surface of the proximal and middle thirds of the tibia, along with the posterior surface of the proximal third of the fibula. The muscle forms a conjoint tendon with the gastrocnemius, and inserts into the calcaneus via the achilles tendon. Supplied by the tibial nerve (S1, S2), the muscle acts to plantar flex the foot about the ankle.

The nerve supply

The **sciatic nerve** (L4, L5, S1, S2) divides just proximal to the upper margin of the popliteal fossa, to form the tibial and common peroneal nerves.

The **common peroneal nerve** (L5, S1) descends anterolaterally, to wind around the neck of the fibula. The nerve courses superficially, covered only by skin and subcutaneous tissue, and as such is exposed to potential injury. It then descends deep into the peroneus longus, where tethering can occur, before it branches to form the superficial and deep peroneal branches.

The superficial branch supplies the foot evertors (peroneus brevis, longus, and extensor digitorum brevis), along with sensation to the skin of the lateral calf and dorsum of the foot. The deep branch supplies the foot and toe dorsiflexors (tibialis anterior, peroneus tertius, extensor digitorum longus, and extensor hallucis longus), and has a small sensory component, which innervates only the skin of the web space between the first and second toes.

The **tibial nerve** (L4, L5, S1, S2, S3) branches in the popliteal fossa, to supply the popliteus, gastrocnemius, soleus, and plantaris. The nerve then passes into the deep posterior compartment of the leg, to supply the tibialis posterior, flexor hallucis longus (FHL), and flexor digitorum brevis (FDB), before passing behind the medial malleolus, to divide into medial and lateral plantar nerves. The sural nerve originates from the tibial nerve in the popliteal fossa. It descends between the two heads of the gastrocnemius, and continues inferiorly, lateral to the lateral margin of the talocalcaneal joint. It supplies the sensation to the skin of the posterolateral part of the lower third of the leg, and lateral border of the foot. The common peroneal nerve gives rise to the sural communicating nerve, and lateral sural cutaneous nerve in the popliteal fossa.

The **saphenous nerve** is the continuation of the femoral nerve (L3, L4), which pierces the fascia between the sartorius and gracillis, to emerge and descend on the medial leg, deep to the sartorius. At the lower end of the adductor canal, it forms an infrapatellar branch, which supplies skin over the medial side and front of the knee and patellar ligament. Below the knee, it is entirely sensory, and descends following the medial tibial border to the ankle, where cutaneous crural branches supply skin on the medial and dorsal aspects of the foot.

Muscle	Origin	Insertion	Nerve	Root
Rectus femoris	Straight head: anterior inferior iliac spine Reflected head: ilium above acetabulum	Quadriceps tendon into tibia tuberosity	Posterior division of femoral nerve	L2, L3, L4
Vastus lateralis	Upper intertrochanteric line, base of greater trochanter, lateral linea aspera, lateral supracondylar ridge, and intermuscular fascia	Lateral quadriceps tendon to patella and tendon to tibial tuberosity	Posterior division of femoral nerve	L2, L3, L4
Vastus intermedius	Anterior and lateral shaft of femur	Quadriceps tendon to tibial tuberosity	Posterior division of femoral nerve	L2, L3, L4
Vastus medialis oblique	Lower intertrochanteric line, medial linea aspera, and medial intermuscular fascia	Medial quadriceps tendon into medial patella and tibial tuberosity	Posterior division of femoral nerve	L2, L3, L4
Biceps femoris	Long head: upper inner quadrant of posterior ischial tuberosity Short head: middle third of line aspera, and lateral supracondylar ridge of femur	Styloid process of head of fibula, lateral collateral ligament, and lateral tibial condyle	Long head: tibial branch of sciatic nerve Short head: common peroneal branch of sciatic nerve	L5, S1, S2
Semimembranosus	Upper outer quadrant of posterior surface of ischial tuberosity	Medial condyle of tibia, fascia investing over popliteus, and oblique popliteal ligament	Tibial branch of sciatic nerve	L5, S1, S2
Semitendinosus	Upper inner quadrant of posterior surface of ischial tuberosity	Upper medial shaft of tibia behind gracilis	Tibial branch of sciatic nerve	L5, S1, S2
Gracilis	Outer margins of ishiopubic ramus	Upper shaft of tibia (pes anserinus) deep to sartorius	Anterior division of obturator nerve	L2, L3

Table 7.1 Origins, insertions and nerve supply to important muscles surrounding the knee joint

Table 7.1 Origins, insertions and nerve supply to important muscles surrounding the knee joint (continued)				
Muscle	**Origin**	**Insertion**	**Nerve**	**Root**
Sartorius	Below anterior superior iliac spine	Upper medial shaft of tibia (pes anserinus)	Anterior division of femoral nerve	L2, L3
Popliteus	Posterior shaft of tibia above soleal line, and below tibial condyles	Facet on lateral surface of lateral condyle of femur posterior and inferior to femoral condyle	Tibial nerve	L4, L5, S1
Gastrocnemius	Lateral head: posterior surface of lateral tibial condyle Medial head: posterior surface of femur above medial condyle	Achilles tendon into calcaneus	Tibial nerve	S1, L2
Soleus	Soleal line, middle ⅓ of posterior border of tibia, and upper quarter of posterior shaft of fibula	Achilles tendon into calcaneus	Tibial nerve	S1, L2

Medial to the knee triangle

Medial meniscal tears are commonly traumatic, and often result in vertical longitudinal tears, and can be coexistent with ligamentous injuries. They are associated with twisting injuries, and recent studies into clinical diagnosis have found the Thessaly test most sensitive.[18, 19] Although at times these settle spontaneously, they always have the potential to cause local inflammation, and potentially locking the knee.

Table 7.2 Prime movers of the key movements of the knee	
Flexion	**Extension**
Biceps femoris	Vastus intermedius
Semitendinosis	Vastus lateralis
Semimembranosus	Vastus medialis oblique
Sartorius	Rectus femoris
Gracilis	
Popliteus	
Gastrocnemius	

The **medial collateral ligament** is both intra and extracapsular, and functions to maintain medial knee stability under valgus load. Trauma can occur when the knee is placed into forced valgus, where the ligament tears more commonly at the proximal end. This can develop with time into Pellegrini-Stieda syndrome, where secondary ossification can occur, causing a palpable defect.[20] Given its predominant extracapsular nature, joint effusion is not always a sign, unless there is concomitant ligament injury, with ACL and medial meniscus involvement.[21]

The **pes anserine bursa** is particularly prone to inflammation, due to its anatomical position,[22] which is exacerbated by a valgus knee stance in gait. No independent risk factors have been identified; however, change in training load, volume, and running surface affect the valgus load, and exacerbate any predisposition to inflammation. Commonly palpable when inflamed, the bursa responds well to corticosteroid and local anesthetic treatment, to both confirm the diagnosis, and treat the condition.

Insertional tendinopathy of the semimembranosus and semitendinosus has been reported as a cause of medial knee pain, usually as a result of overuse,[35] and can be diagnosed by examination and ultrasound imaging. This can progress to a "snapping pes" due to the flicking of the tendons over the posteromedial border of the tibia.[36] Eccentric loading of the tendons appears effective as conservative management!

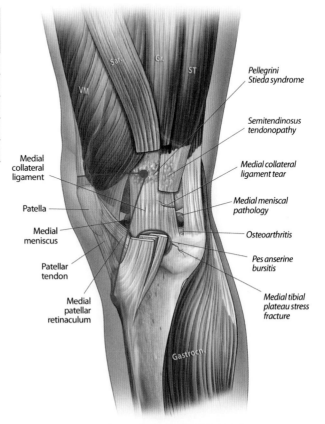

Figure 7.8 Medial to the knee triangle

VM	= vastus medialis
Sar	= sartorius
Gr	= gracilis
ST	= semitendinosus
Gastrocn	= gastrocnemius

Labels in figure: Sar, Gr, ST, VM, Pellegrini Stieda syndrome, Semitendinosus tendonopathy, Medial collateral ligament tear, Medial meniscal pathology, Osteoarthritis, Pes anserine bursitis, Medial tibial plateau stress fracture, Medial collateral ligament, Patella, Medial meniscus, Patellar tendon, Medial patellar retinaculum, Gastrocn

		Table 7.3 Medial to the knee triangle		
Define and align	Pathology	Listen and localize	Palpate and recreate	Alleviate and investigate
Medial to triangle	Medial meniscal pathology	Complains of immediate pain and swelling after twisting injury. Can leave a persistent clicking, and reduced joint range. History can be of a slow twisting injury with foot in contact with ground	McMurray test,[23] sensitivity 29%, specificity 95%, but Thessaly test[18] in conjunction with joint line tenderness improves to 93% sensitivity and 99% specificity[24]	MRI is most sensitive[25]
	Medial collateral ligament injury	Clear valgus stress to knee. Symptoms correlate with severity	Tenderness on palpation, valgus stress test 86% sensitivity[26]	Plain film will demonstrate gapping on a valgus stress view. MRI indicated as possible O'Donoghue's triad of ACL, MCL and medial meniscal injury[27]
	Pes anserinus bursitis assoc with semimembranosus and semitendinosus tendinopathy	Overuse injury common in runners on a change of camber or surface. Associated with rearfoot valgus, causing stress of MCL and associated attachments	Pain along medial joint line, bogginess to palpation at insertion of gracilis, sartorius, and semi-membranosus. Pain on resisted flexion	MRI with axial images to differentiate from Baker's cyst fluid with pes anserine bursa,[28] ultrasound examination of individual tendon
	Osteoarthritis, medial compartment	Usually >55years, previous injury, family history of OA	Joint line tenderness, bony exostosis, crepitus, effusion	PA weight-bearing plain film,[29] gadolinium contrast MRI,[30] high sensitivity for chondral disease
	Medial tibial condyle stress fracture	Associated with forefoot pronation and change in intensity of uphill running[31]	Difficult to differentiate from pes anserine issues, history different	Plain film not sensitive enough. Tc-bone scan but MRI as good[32, 33]
	Pellegrini-Stieda syndrome	Disruption of femoral origin of MCL. Complains of difficulty extending knee and when turning with foot on ground	Palpable lump in medial collateral ligament and decreased rotation at knee[20]	Plain film can demonstrate the ossification which characterizes the condition
	Snapping pes anserinus	Snapping and pain on active extension and flexion initiation[34]	Reproduction of symptoms	Ultrasound real-time demonstration of movement at gracilis and semitendinosus[24]

MRI	= magnetic resonance imaging		**OA**	= osteoarthritis
MCL	= medial collateral ligament		**PA**	= posteroanterior
ACL	= anterior cruciate ligament		**Tc**	= techniciam

Osteoarthritis is common, and the presenting symptoms are the gradual onset of pain, worsening over time and throughout each day. There is frequently an associated joint effusion, and it is a progressive disease with much morbidity. Although it can affect only a single joint, it is more common to have bilateral symptoms, unless preceded by unilateral joint injury.

Stress fractures of the tibial plateau are rare,[37] but care should be taken to exclude **Ewing's sarcoma**; Ewing's is responsible for 7% of all bone malignancy and, with a five-year survival rate of 25%, is particularly aggressive.

Lateral to the knee triangle

Laterally, the lateral retinaculum and fascial insertions into the patella are often attributed to "excessive lateral pressure syndrome"; in fact, this is only important due to the secondary changes on the cartilaginous undersurface of the joint. The fascial and capsular attachments have been discussed earlier, and, as discussed previously, the patella is strongly attached laterally and medially. The biomechanics of altered pull rest primarily with the balance of the quadriceps muscles, and as such are often amenable to treatment by reconditioning the quadriceps with neuromuscular firing-pattern synchronicity..

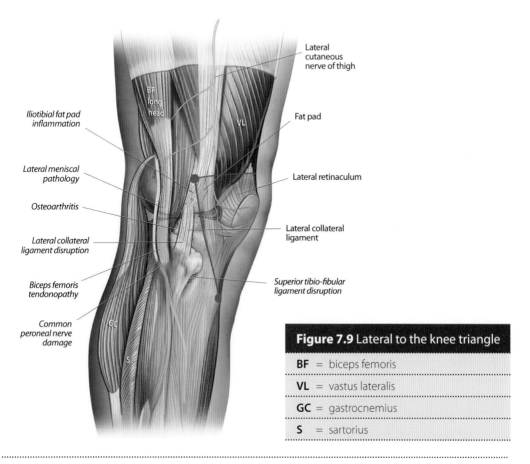

Figure 7.9 Lateral to the knee triangle

BF	= biceps femoris
VL	= vastus lateralis
GC	= gastrocnemius
S	= sartorius

The insertion point of the "iliotibial band" is easily confused. Traditionally, it has been thought of as a distinct entity, but it is actually merely a thickening of the fascia late that is attached laterally at the femoral condyle via Kaplan's fibers (Fig. 7.5) and the tibial condyle. Between these lies a fat pad, which is richly innervated, and as such is the likely source of the pain in iliotibial band friction syndrome. Here the tension in the fascial attachment is altered, usually due to tense fascia late or gluteus medius involvement, which result in the rubbing of the fat pad between the fascia and bone. It often responds well to a local anesthetic injection.

The lateral collateral ligament is rarely damaged in isolation, in part due to its extracapsular nature, but it can be damaged in significant trauma to the knee with other ligamentous rupture.

Osteoarthritic changes in the knee, characterized by osteophyte/bony exostosis, joint space narrowing, effusion, and crepitus, are common with advancing age and previous injury; indeed, it is the commonest cause of non-acute knee pathology. Lateral compartment disease, less common than medial compartment disease, presents with tenderness in the lateral area to the triangle overlying the joint line.

Biceps femoris tendinopathy is more commonly associated with proximal disease. Here in the insertional portion, it is more common to see acute tendinitis as an inflammatory response to load.

The proximal tibiofibular joint is intracapsular and, as Figure 7.2 on page 265 shows, is closely related to the arcuate ligament complex, popliteus, lateral collateral ligament, and biceps femoris tendon. The ligament resists the torsional load applied to the lower limb, and this injury mimics an LCL tear. Falkenberg describes a knee flexion injury, with ankle extension and foot inversion as the propagating injury.[38]

Common peroneal nerve damage can occur with local trauma, and in conjunction with superior tibiofibular joint disruption and fibula fracture, due to the close approximation of the common peroneal and the fibula neck, as the deep branch and superficial branch divide and descend through the shank of the leg.

The **ACL** is injured at different rates in different sports, and by gender. A meta-analysis of available data demonstrated that the female to male ratio was 3:1 and, significantly, year-round female soccer and basketball players have a 5% annual chance of rupture.[44] This difference is clearly related to multiple factors, including ligament laxity and varus angle. It is reported as being more common in non-contact injury and, due to significant morbidity, many studies are looking at possible prevention.[45, 46]

Chondral surfaces can be damaged by direct impact forces, or more torsional force commonly associated with ligamentous injury. Prevalence is high in symptomatic knees, some studies suggesting between 22 and 50%.[47] Due to its poor vascularity, there is a poor response to injury, with little chondrocyte migration and sparsity of mitotic action, along with continuous use of the joint.[48]

Tibial plateau fractures are rare, and usually associated with high-velocity trauma in motor or racing sports, but result in significant morbidity, with chondral damage along with bony

Table 7.4 Lateral to the knee triangle				
Define and align	**Pathology**	**Listen and localize**	**Palpate and recreate**	**Alleviate and investigate**
Lateral to triangle	Lateral meniscal pathology	Can present acutely with effusion and joint line tenderness, but also more chronically with vague, poorly located pain	Joint line tenderness, McMurray test,[26] sensitivity 29%, specificity 95%, but Thessaly test[18] in conjunction with joint line tenderness improves to 78% sensitivity and 99% specificity[27]	MRI is most sensitive[28]
	Lateral collateral ligament disruption	Unusual in isolation. Feeling of instability and pain on movement	Varus stress test much less sensitive, 25%[29]	MRI high sensitivity but poor correlation with clinical exam[39]
	Iliotibial band insertion/fat pad inflammation	History of increased change of load, or surface, worsens with exercise	Tenderness over Kaplan's fat pad and Gerdy's tubercle on tibia, Ober's test irritates	Plain film to exclude Gerdy's avulsion fracture vs Segond fracture
	Biceps femoris tendinopathy	Pain on commencing exercise, settles with warm up and worsens post exercise, started when accelerating or decelerating	Pain on palpation, weakness on hamstring bridging/resisted flexion	Ultrasound imaging will help demonstrate
	OA lateral compartment	Age > 55, family history, previous injury	Joint line tenderness, bony exostosis, crepitus, effusion	PA weight-bearing plain film,[32] gadolinium contrast MRI,[33] high sensitivity for chondral disease
	Superior tibiofibular joint disruption	Pain distal to the joint, worse on change of direction and twisting, fall with hyperextended knee with inverted foot[38]	Axial twisting on weight-bearing foot reproduces pain[40]	Plain film, distraction view, but CT if subtle can help delineate
	Lateral retinaculum/patello-femoral dysfuction (excessive lateral pressure syndrome)	Pain in patella and lateral knee, worse on flexion	Pain on patellar glide	Kinematic MRI[41] clinical examination
	Common peroneal nerve entrapment	Describe difficulties in dorsiflexion, sensory changes on dorsum of foot and peroneal compartment	Weakness in extensor digitorum brevis[42]	Plain film to exclude fibular fracture and nerve conduction studies or needle electromyography[43]

MRI = magnetic resonance imaging

PA = posterior anterior, in respect of beam direction for x-ray

CT = computerized tomography

reconstruction. Stress fractures have been covered earlier, but are less common in the tibial plateau than in the distal third of the tibial shaft.

Synovial plicae are somewhat controversial; they are folds of the synovium, and inflammation may cause pain, and chronic inflammation may lead to thickening and fibrosis. They occur usually in both supra- and infrapatellar, and medial and lateral locations. Hardaker[49] described plica syndrome as being painful impingement in the presence of an abnormal hypertrophic plica, but it is an arthroscopic diagnosis, and controversial, as the presence of plicae is not universal.

Table 7.5 Within the knee triangle – intracapsular				
Define and align	**Pathology**	**Listen and localize**	**Palpate and recreate**	**Alleviate and investigate**
Within the triangle – intracapsular	ACL injury	Common. Female predominance. Often non-contact, landing from jump, or decelerating, audible pop then knee giving way in valgus and extension. Immediate pain	Anterior drawer test poor sensitivity 40%,[29] improves to 90%[50] when under anesthesia and Lachman's up to 99% sensitive[50]	Abnormal alignment and lateral tibial avulsion by stress plain film.[51] MRI gold standard[52] and will assess posterolateral corner meniscus[53]
	PCL injury	More common contact injury, hyperextension injury with dorsiflexed foot and tackled. Poorly localized pain, little swelling due to extracapsular. Commonly with co-existent injury	Quadriceps active test 98% sensitivity and 100% specificity by Daniel et al.,[54] also posterior sag test	Plain film lateral across table to look for posterior sag. MRI[55] can identify associated injury to MCL and bone[56]
	Osteochondral lesion (osteochondritis dissecans)	Often concurrent with ligament injury and detected on imaging. Male predominance, commoner in <20s[57]	Not distinguishable from other injury	Tc-bone scan,[58] or MRI T2-weighted[59]
	Tibial plateau fracture	High-speed contact injuries. Non-weightbearing in severe pain. Varus or valgus force	Pain on overlying joint line and posterior to knee. Unable to extend knee fully	Plain film then CT with axial, coronal, and sagittal planes[60]
	Synovial plicae	Folds of synovium inside capsule, normally asymptomatic. Can be associated with knee swelling and pain	No specific test, occasionally palpated as thickened ridge under medial patella	MRI,[61] arthroscopy

Within the triangle – extracapsular

Within the triangle, but outside of the joint-stability ligaments, lie many of the pain-generating structures in anterior knee pain. The layered construction of the fascia and capsule has been described earlier, but the convergence of the quadriceps tendon into the patella is not often thought of as a structure prone to damage. A number of authors have drawn attention to tendinitis of the insertion primarily of the vastus medialis. Pfirrmann et al.[62] found, unlike with the patellar tendon, unusually high degrees of calcification, perhaps related to the force of generation.

Bursitis is common, and normally resolves without intervention from the clinician, but occasionally can be aided by USS-guided local anesthetic and corticosteroid injection.

The etiology of **patellar tendinopathy** is much debated in current literature,[63, 64] along with treatment,[65] but in making the diagnosis, the clinician is aided by good examination, usually with Ultrasound imagery looking specifically for hypo-echoic tendon degeneration and new blood vessel formation, and exclusion of other diagnoses.

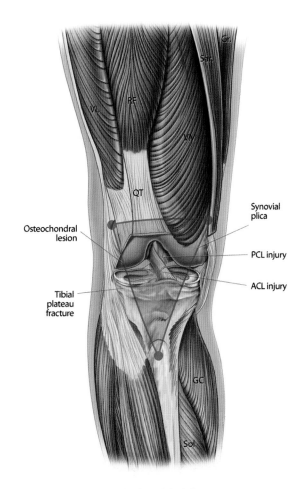

Figure 7.10 Within the knee triangle

VL	=	vastus lateralis
RF	=	rectus femoris
VM	=	vastus medialis
QT	=	quadriceps tendon
Sar	=	sartorius
Gr	=	gracilis
GC	=	gastrocnemius
Sol	=	soleus
PCL	=	posterior cruciate ligament
ACL	=	anterior cruciate ligament

The fat pad is intracapsular but extrasynovial, and anteriorly it is sandwiched between the patellar tendon and the synovium of the capsule. Posteriorly, it projects into the intercondylar notch via two synovial folds, which fuse, forming the infrapatellar plicae. Superiorly, the fat pad attaches to the inferior surface of the patella, and extends to the cartilage overlying the anterior aspect of the distal femur. Inferiorly, it is attached to the periosteum of the tibia, and the anterior horns of the menisci, and it abuts the deep infrapatellar bursa.

Hoffa described **Hoffa's disease**, or fat pad impingement, in 1904, as trauma resulting in hemorrhage and inflammation. The trauma may be a result of repetitive hyperextension, or rotational strain. The fat pad hypertrophies, and becomes impinged between the femoral and tibial condyles anteriorly, causing the characteristic Hoffa's sign or pain.

Patellar instability can commonly follow a patellar dislocation, resulting in recurrence, anterior knee pain, or frequent subluxation. It can also be a result of patella alta, a bony abnormality, making tracking of the patellofemoral joint more difficult. Even in recent times, some clinicians have recommended a lateral release and a surgical approach to this, but there is no evidence to support this.[75]

Osgood-Schlatter disease and **Sinding-Larsen–Johansson syndrome** are common in adolescence, when they are overuse injuries affecting opposing insertions of the patellar tendon into the tibial tuberosity and patella, respectively. They cause significant pain and discomfort, and often result in reduction or even withdrawal from sport, but they are self-limiting and soon settle.

Chondromalacia patella has significant overlap with patellofemoral disease and, although it technically refers to a softening of the articular cartilage, it presents in the same way. It may

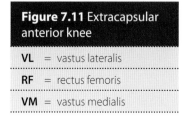

Figure 7.11 Extracapsular anterior knee

VL	= vastus lateralis
RF	= rectus femoris
VM	= vastus medialis

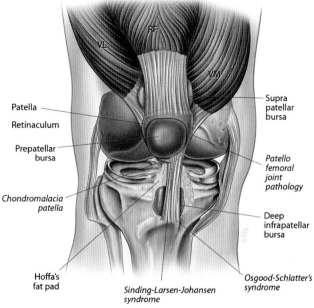

Table 7.6 Within the knee triangle – extracapsular				
Define and align	**Pathology**	**Listen and localize**	**Palpate and recreate**	**Alleviate and investigate**
Within the triangle – extra-capsular	Bursitis – prepatellar, suprapatellar, infrapatellar	Swelling, pain on movement	Tenderness and pain on palpation	Local anesthetic injection +/– ultrasound guidence
	Quadriceps tendinopathy	Focal swelling at insertion into patella, overuse injury, commonly VMO, predominance in beach volleyball[62]	Pain on resisted knee extension, delayed vastus medialis (VMO) firing	USS demonstrates tendon thickening and hypoechogenicity[62]
	Patellar tendinopathy	Repetitive jumping loading, worsens on starting exercises, then manageable, worse the day after	More common tenderness at inf pole patella, thickening of tendon, decline squat aggravates pain	Plain film can exclude Sinding-Larsen, USS correlates with surgical findings[66] and highlights neovascularization[67]
	Hoffa's fat pad inflammation	Kicking or uncontrolled hyperextension, or direct blow, pole around inferior pole of patella	Puffy inferior pole of patella with patella displacement, active extension painful	Plain film may demonstrate posterior tilt of inferior pole of patella, MRI differentiates well[68]
	Patellofemoral joint disease	Retropatellar pain, prolonged sitting, gradually worsens with exercise	Medial or lateral facet joint pain, patella glide test +ve, occasional crepitus, PFJ taping may reduce pain, poor correlation of test with surgical findings[69]	Plain film can exclude patellofemoral CT if surgical consideration,[70] MRI to image osteochondral surface[71]
	Patellar instability	Feeling of apprehension or that patella dislocates and sideways movement	Patella hyper mobility and lateral apprehension +ve	Kinematic MRI[41]
	Osgood-Schlatter disease	F 10–12, M 13–15 years, anterior knee pain on exercise, higher incidence in jumping, squatting, and kicking sports, stops participation	Tenderness over tibial tuberosity and clinical history	Plain film not normally indicated but may show fragmentation of apophysis of tibial tuberosity
	Chondromalacia patella	Retropatellar pain, crepitus and swelling	Patellar tap and grind test,[72] knee effusion	MRI subchondral bone changes, may progress to OA

Define and align	Pathology	Listen and localize	Palpate and recreate	Alleviate and investigate
	Sinding-Larsen–Johansson syndrome	Difficult to differentiate from patellar tendinopathy at first, presents in a younger age range with anterior knee pain[73]	Tenderness at inferior pole, no neovascularisation	Plain film again would show traction, apophyseal changes at inferior pole of patella and soft tissue swelling
	Patellar dislocation	Underlying dysplastic patella, recurrent dislocation or post surgical intervention	Apprehension test[74]	Plain film – skyline view to detect fracture, axial CT with quadriceps contraction[70] to diagnose, and MRI to demonstrate osteochondral damage

Table 7.6 Within the knee triangle – extracapsular (continued)

VMO	=	vastus medialis oblique
USS	=	ultrasound scan
OA	=	osteoarthritis
MRI	=	magnetic resonance imaging
CT	=	computerized tomography

progress to an osteochondral defect following a traumatic knee injury, where it is detectable on MRI.

Conventionally in this book, we have utilized the relationships around one triangle to delineate both the anatomy and pathology. In the knee, the pathology lends itself to the use of two triangles, one anteriorly and a second posteriorly.

Posterior to the triangle

The accompanying figure (Fig. 7.12) helps to delineate this area, but it is bordered by the medial and lateral heads of the gastrocnemius, and the posterior margin of the knee joint line. Deep to the triangle lie the posterior capsule, popliteus, and oblique and arcuate popliteal ligaments, and running through it are the tibial artery and vein, the tibial nerve, and the space for a Baker's cyst.

The joint line here is difficult to palpate due to the overlying structures, yet in the posterolateral corner of the meniscus lies a common site of missed injury, and this lies within the triangle, so the reader should identify this in patients presenting with posterior pain.

Gastrocnemius tears are more common at the medial head, as a result of the muscle action on active ankle plantar flexion, under eccentric load, and are occasionally referred to as "tennis leg". The medial head also contributes to the posterior stability of the knee, and as such may be prone to increased load. The clinical signs are commonly confused with the clinical signs of DVT, due to the fluid collection between the gastrocnemius and soleus,[81] and care should be taken to differentiate these in the history.

Hamstring injuries are common,[82] with significant morbidity. There are several predisposing factors, including fatigue, hamstring weakness, decreased flexibility, and fascial loading across the pelvis, alongside previous hamstring injury.[83] At the musculo-tendinous junction, both the biceps femoris and semimembranosus can present with posterior knee swelling, due to the collection of edema.

Baker's cysts are common, with two age-incidence peaks of 4 to 7 years, and 35 to 70 years.[84] While usually asymptomatic and non-detectable, they are commonly associated with other pathology in the older patient. There is often a connection between the joint and bursa,

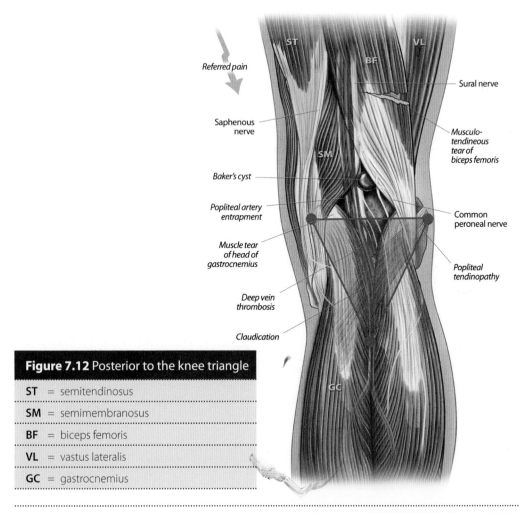

Figure 7.12 Posterior to the knee triangle

ST	=	semitendinosus
SM	=	semimembranosus
BF	=	biceps femoris
VL	=	vastus lateralis
GC	=	gastrocnemius

Table 7.7 Posterior to the knee triangle				
Define and align	**Pathology**	**Listen and localize**	**Palpate and recreate**	**Alleviate and investigate**
Posterior to triangle	Medial/ lateral head of gastrocnemius	More common in medial head, sudden burst with a sprint or lunge, sharp tearing pain on eccentric load	Tenderness in muscle belly, stretching of gastrocnemius reproduces pain, Thompson's squeeze test to exclude achilles rupture	Ultrasound examination will allow accurate assessment of muscle and musculo-tendinous junction
	Biceps femoris/ semimembranosus muscle tear	Deceleratory injury, in sport, associated with muscle tightness and poor flexibility, and with muscle tear – patient described the tear or pull of muscle	Pain on resisted flexion and eccentric loading	Ultrasound examination of tendon and musculo-tendinous junction useful, may need MRI to examine full muscle to exclude tears
	Popliteus tendinopathy	Feeling of instability when knee extended, insidious onset	Tenderness on palpation of muscle, Garrick test[76] of external rotation of flexed knee	Ultrasound examination of tendon
	Deep vein thrombosis (DVT)	Risk factors of immobility, smoking, increased BMI	Homans' sign[77]	D-dimer, doppler ultrasound imaging
	Baker's cyst (semimembrano-susgastrocnemius bursa)	Stiffness of knee with chronic joint effusion, insidious onset	Swelling in popliteal fossa, on occasion ruptures and mimics calf swelling	Ultrasound-guided aspiration, doppler to exclude DVT
	Popliteal artery entrapment	Hypertrophy of gastrocnemius,[78] claudicant pain brought on by exercise settles on cessation, worse on walking	Possible popliteal bruit (rare), nil to find on examination	Post-exercise ankle brachial pressure and doppler ultrasound[79]
	Referred pain	Co-existent back pain, sensation of numbness or tingling in foot	Braggard's[80] or slump tests reproduce symptoms	MRI imaging for level and degree of involvement, +/– epidural relieving injection
	Claudication (atherosclerotic)	Exercise-related pain in calf, night pain relieved by hanging leg over side of bed, occasional breakdown of skin and discoloration of skin of toes and foot	Decreased pedal pulses, bruit over site of atherosclerotic lesion (groin, mid thigh, or popliteal triangle)	Angiography

allowing synovial fluid from the joint into the bursa, with subsequent distension, producing these cysts. Some, however, have no connection, and the cysts arise primarily as bursitis of the bursa between the gastrocnemius and semimembranosus.

Popliteus tendinopathy may be caused by a variety of causes, including calcification[85], snapping of the tendon,[86] or an extension injury.[87] It is difficult to exclude on examination alone, but the reader should be aware of its existence.

Deep vein thrombosis (DVT) mainly affects the saphenous and popliteal veins. Risk factors include bed rest, cigarette smoking, leg fractures, recent pregnancy, obesity, recent pelvic surgery, estrogen-containing medicine, and periods of immobility, especially associated with long plane flights. The end result of venous congestion is leg swelling, which also leads to pain. At its most obvious, a difference in leg diameter can be seen, and low molecular-weight heparin should be given at an appropriate dose, until doppler ultrasound confirmation can be performed.

The **popliteal artery** can become entrapped between the heads of the gastrocnemius, resulting in symptoms of claudication and exercise-related pain. It is felt that anatomical variations in the artery,[88, 89] or in the medial head of the gastrocnemius,[90] are the predisposing factors, and athletic development of the muscle can exacerbate this.

Intermittent claudication is the result of arterial insufficiency to the gastrocnemius and soleus, and the distal foot muscles. It classically has a gradual onset of pain, which resolves quickly with rest. Predisposing factors include existing peripheral vascular disease, which is associated with hypertension, hypercholesterolemia, smoking, and diabetes mellitus.

Sciatic-type pain radiating from the lumbar spine should be considered in the absence of local features, and the hip and ankle should also be considered as sources of knee symptoms.

Ottawa knee rules

To aid the less experienced physician as to when to request plain radiography of the knee, in a similar fashion to the Ottawa ankle rules,[91] a set of validated knee rules has been produced:[92]
1. age 55 years or older
2. tenderness of head of fibula
3. isolated patella tenderness
4. inability to flex the knee to 90°
5. inability to walk four weight-bearing steps immediately after the injury

Plain film imaging is, however, often very useful when reported by an expert musculoskeletal radiologist who has been supplied with accurate information on the request referral. The reader is referred to the excellent and comprehensive text *Atlas of imaging in sports medicine,*[93] where the full use of the plain film is revealed.

Referred pain and malignancy

The lower limb is commonly the site of radiculopathy from the lumbar spine. The knee, and musculature surrounding it, has five nerve roots within its supply, and is particularly prone to nerve root irritation. The examination of the knee should therefore routinely include a lumbar spine examination, and a combination of a slump test and Braggard's test, to exclude nerve root irritation.[94]

It is vital to include direct questioning about red flags such as systemic signs of illness (night sweats, weight loss), and night pain. This is common to all the triangles, and beyond the scope of each table. Malignancy in the lower limb is thankfully uncommon, and most bone tumors are benign, and discovered incidentally on plain film, but there are malignant tumors affecting bone. While multiple myeloma is the most common malignancy in bone, Ewing's sarcoma presents between the ages of 5 and 20, and most frequently in the lower limb, and can be particularly aggressive. Care should be taken to have a high index of suspicion where appropriate.

Inflammatory arthritis

In any joint which is swollen, one should consider the possibility of inflammatory or reactive arthritis. Reiter's syndrome is common in the younger population, and the knee is commonly affected. Associated with a gastrointestinal or urological infection, it is a cause of monoarthritis. Other seronegative spondyloarthropathies can affect the knee, and a single swollen joint should raise suspicions to look for other joint involvement. Serological blood tests, and plain film imaging can often be of assistance.

Septic arthritis

One must always consider the possibility of septic arthritis. It is common, with over 20,000 reported cases per year in the US.[95] Indeed, the most common infective organism is neisseria gonorrhoea,[94] a sexually transmitted infection more prevalent in the younger population. The organisms can infect the joint either directly, or through surrounding tissue infection; the most common route is, however, via the blood.[96]

In the history, it is important to take a detailed history of both sexually transmitted infections and also tick exposure, as this is a common presentation of Lyme disease.[97]

Presenting signs can be the mono- or polyarticular manifestation of systemic illness. Investigation must include a joint aspiration to culture, and also blood ESR and CRP, along with possible leucocytosis.

Summary

It has been seen that the knee is the source of much local and referred pathology, and also systemic illness. These latter conditions do not fit our anatomically structured approach as well as the former. This is due to the more systemic presentation, but they should be considered when addressing a presentation on any of the triangles or tables. The triangles aim to direct the reader to the most appropriate differential diagnosis based on our anatomical groundings. The wider differential can be considered, should no localizing signs be identified.

As always in musculoskeletal medicine, the joints above and below the symptomatic one should be examined to exclude their involvement, and compared with the asymptomatic side. We have presented the most evidence-based examinations and diagnostic tests for each condition and, although some are in less common use, they are supported by evidence.

Case histories

Case 1

A 55-year-old schoolteacher presents with a two-week history of knee pain. He has been playing squash for the first time for a number of years, since challenged by his students. He was determined to keep up and lunged for every ball; he felt very sore on the inside of his knee that evening, and the next morning it also felt quite sore, and hurt when he tried to get out of bed.

Step 1: Define and align
Expose the patient properly; a pair of sports shorts will allow physical access and aid visibility.

Define the triangle: locate the medial and lateral femoral condyles, and the tibial tuberosity.

Align the patient's pain on the triangles. Here the pain is located to the medial side of the triangle.

The patient has localized the pain to the area "medial to the triangle". From this point we recommend that the reader attempt to exclude the potential pathologies. From Table 7.3, the potential causal structures are:

differential diagnosis
> medial meniscal pathology
> medial collateral ligament injury
> pes anserinus bursitis
> osteoarthritis medial compartment
> Pellegrini-Stieda syndrome

We proceed to differentiate between these structures, step 2.

Step 2: Listen and localize
Addressing medial meniscal injury we ask:

Q *Was there a moment you felt your knee twisted?*

A No, not really, it didn't give way or twist.

Q *Was there any swelling?*
A Yes, a little on the inside of my knee, the morning after the match.

Addressing medial collateral ligament injury we ask:
Q *Have you injured this knee before?*
A Not really, but I stopped squash because of recurrent hamstring strains, I felt I was just getting too old.

Addressing pes anserine bursitis we ask:
Q *Have you been increasing your activity lately?*
A Yes, I've been doing a bit of running, and going to the gym.
Q *Is there any associated clicking or snapping?*
A Yes, on occasion, when straightening my knee.

Addressing osteoarthritis we ask:
Q *Does your knee swell up from time to time?*
A No, I've had no problems with the knee at all.
Q *Does the knee feel stiff when you wake up, or at the end of the day?*
A No. (The patient describes no knee pain previously at all.)

Addressing Pellegrini-Stieda syndrome we ask:
Q *Do you have problems pushing off that knee, or twisting?*
A Yes, the main pain is when I push off, not so much with turning.

This will narrow our differential diagnosis somewhat, and we proceed to examination to narrow it further.

Differential diagnosis

More likely
> pes anserinus bursitis
> medial meniscal injury

Less likely
> medial collateral ligament injury
> osteoarthritis medial compartment
> Pellegrini-Stieda syndrome

By palpating painful structures, and recreating the pain through diagnostic maneuvers, we move toward a diagnosis, step 3.

Step 3: Palpate and re-create

We palpate the medial joint line, and we find tenderness at the posterior part of the line; this is worse in extension, but we cannot palpate any clicking or movement.

McMurray test: the knee is passively flexed and extended while internally and externally rotated, feeling for a click and watching for re-creation of pain. The test was negative, but the Thessaly test was positive (the patient stands barefoot on the affected leg, flexing to 5°, and rotates the knee and body in and out three times; the test is repeated with the knee flexed 20°, then the test is done on the involved or injured leg). Given step 2 and the results of our palpation, it is likely that this is an posteromedial meniscal tear. Given the age of the patient, it may be chronic and degenerative, rather than acute, explaining why the swelling was minimal. It is difficult to advise the patient further without further investigation.

We may now proceed to step 4 to confirm our clinical suspicion via imaging. The most evidence-based test is MRI.

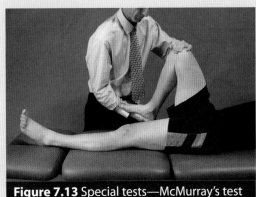

Figure 7.13 Special tests—McMurray's test

Case 2

A 19-year-old road cyclist comes to you complaining of left knee pain. The knee pain has started gradually, following a 180 km ride two weeks ago. It has been sore mainly on riding uphill since then, but occasionally on flat, faster paced rides. He is now struggling. He has a new bike, but it was set up for him by a professional race biomechanist, and is the same riding position and crank length as previously.

Step 1: Define and align

Expose the patient properly; a pair of sports shorts will allow physical access and aid visibility.

Define the triangle: locate the medial and lateral femoral condyles, and the tibial tuberosity.

Align the patient's pain on the triangles. Here the pain is located to the lateral side of the triangle.

The patient has localized the pain to the area "lateral to the triangle". From this point we recommend that the reader attempt to exclude the potential pathologies. From Table 7.4, the potential causal structures are:

Differential diagnosis

> lateral meniscal pathology

> lateral collateral ligament disruption

> iliotibial band insertion/fat pad inflammation

> biceps femoris tendinopathy

> OA lateral compartment

> superior tibiofibular joint disruption

> lateral retinaculum/patellofemoral dysfuction (excessive lateral pressure syndrome)

> common peroneal nerve entrapment

We proceed to differentiate between these structures, step 2.

Step 2: Listen and localize

Addressing lateral meniscal injury we ask:

Q *Was there a moment when you had a fall, or felt your knee twisted?*

A No, I have not fallen for some time, and the pain started after a long ride.

Addressing lateral collateral ligament disruption we ask:

Q *Have you recently changed your bike set up?*

A I have a new bike, but have trained in the same position and set up. My new pedals were a problem to start with, as they were a bit on the stiff side to clip in and out, but they are fine now.

Q *Have you had any crashes recently?*

A No.

Addressing iliotibial band insertion inflammation we ask:

Q *Do you do any running/triathlon training?*

A No, I'm a dedicated road cyclist – I have a massage after every ride, and a swim recovery session twice a week, but no running.

Q *Has your training load/intensity changed?*

A I'm building up distance, but have been doing so gradually.

Q *Does the pain stay with you in a ride, and go away overnight?*

A No, it's worse at the start of a ride, and in the morning rides. It seems to get a bit better when on the bike, unless riding uphill for more than 30 minutes, and then the following morning it starts again.

Addressing biceps femoris tendinopathy we ask:

Q *Do you notice a change in the pain when you accelerate?*

A Yes, the pain is sharp, and worse for a few minutes.

CLINICAL SPORTS ANATOMY

Addressing osteoarthritis, the patient is outside the normal age range for this condition, so to be thorough we check for previous trauma, and we ask:

Q *Do you have any previous history of knee trauma?*

A No.

This excludes superior tibiofibular joint dysfunction, but for completeness we ask:

Q *Is the pain on riding associated with any clicking in the knee?*

A No, I get some hip clicking on occasion, but nothing where I get the pain.

Addressing peroneal nerve entrapment we ask:

Q *Do you get any numbness, pins or needles in your leg or foot?*

A No, only the normal in both feet after long rides.

Differential diagnosis

Most likely
> biceps femoris tendinopathy
> iliotibial band insertion/fat pad inflammation

Least likely
> lateral meniscal pathology
> lateral collateral ligament disruption
> OA lateral compartment
> superior tibiofibular joint disruption
> lateral retinaculum/patellofemoral dysfuction (excessive lateral pressure syndrome)
> common peroneal nerve entrapment

This narrows our differential diagnosis somewhat, and we can isolate the condition to either biceps femoris tendinopathy, or perhaps some signs of iliotibial band irritation. We can proceed to examination to narrow it further. By palpating painful structures, and recreating the pain through diagnostic maneuvers, we move toward a diagnosis, step 3.

Step 3: Palpate and re-create

We palpate the lateral joint line, and find it pain-free. We test the superior tibiofibular joint, and find it non-painful, but the patient does have some tenderness over the biceps tendon. He is able to bridge when loading his hamstring, with the knee flexed to 90°, but when the knee is extended, he is unable to tolerate the bridge. His Ober's test is then performed.

In this test, the patient lies on the unaffected side, with hip and knee flexed. The clinician then stabilizes the pelvis, flexing the knee and extending the hip, while abducting the limb. When the limb is brought posterior to the neutral plane, the test is said to be positive if TFL/ITB contracture prevents adduction of the hip. The patient's Ober's test is negative, although he does have some gluteus medius trigger points bilaterally.

Given step 2 and the results of our examination, it is likely that this is biceps femoris tendinitis/opathy. It is difficult to advise the patient further without further investigation.

We may now proceed to step 4 to confirm our clinical suspicion via imaging. The most convincing examination here is ultrasound examination of the biceps tendon, as it is close to the skin, and a good view can be obtained

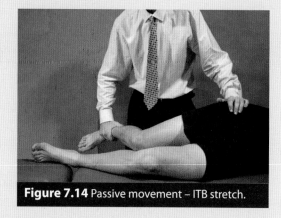

Figure 7.14 Passive movement – ITB stretch.

with ultrasound. If this confirms the diagnosis, then consideration for local anesthetic injection with corticosteroid can be given, to alleviate the pain and confirm the diagnosis.

Case 3

A 58-year-old recreational jogger presents with knee pain. He describes the injury as developing over a year or so. He cannot be more precise. He never runs more than three kilometers at an easy pace, but does so daily. Over the last year, he has noticed it becoming increasingly difficult. He feels pain in his knee, more so when he stretches out before running, and then just as his heel makes contact with the ground. He has tried replacing his running shoes, running on tan bark, sand, and even a treadmill, but none of those changes made a difference. His family doctor organized a plain x-ray of his knee while standing, and said he had no signs of osteoarthritis.

Step 1: Define and align

Expose the patient properly; a pair of sports shorts will allow physical access and aid visibility.

Define the triangle: locate the medial and lateral femoral condyles, and the tibial tuberosity.

Align the patient's pain on the triangles. Here the pain is located to the posterior of the triangle.

The patient has localized the pain to the area "posterior to the triangle". From this point we recommend that the reader attempt to exclude the potential pathologies. From Table 7.7, the potential causal structures are:

Differential diagnosis
> medial/lateral head of gastrocnemius
> hamstring tendon insertional tendinitis/opathy
> popliteus tendinopathy

> > deep vein thrombosis
> > Baker's cyst (semimembranosus–gastrocnemius bursa)
> > popliteal artery entrapment
> > referred pain
> > claudication (atherosclerotic)

We proceed to differentiate between these structures, step 2.

Step 2: Listen and localize

Addressing gastrocnemius injury we ask:

Q *When the injury started, do you remember a tearing pain, or a sudden injury?*

A No, it has been really rather gradual, but definitely worse now.

Q *Is the pain located to one side or the other?*

A No, it feels deep behind the knee.

Addressing hamstring tendinopathy we ask:

Q *Do you get pain on starting exercise, which eases off during the run?*

A No, it is really constant stiffness, rather than pain, but not worse before or after the run. In fact running aggravates it, but it doesn't seem to change much.

Q *Do you gain pain when accelerating or decelerating?*

A No, not really; occasionally the pain is worse when stepping off the kerbside, but really only with a straight leg.

Addressing popliteus tendinopathy we ask:

Q *Is the pain worse when your leg is straight?*

A Yes, it seems to be worse with a straight leg, it hurts if I lie down on the sofa and lift up my leg. Not a sharp pain but pressure.

Addressing deep vein thrombosis we ask:

Q *Do you smoke? Have you had any foreign travel? Have you broken a leg or had any other injury, which might have kept you immobile?*

A No, I have not been immobile, I do travel a lot with work, and spend over 10 hours a week on flights, but am aware of DVT and do exercise. I smoke the occasional cigar.

Addressing gastrocnemius/semimembranosus bursa we ask:

Q *Have you noticed the knee swelling?*

A It seems to swell after I've been on my feet all day, or after running. It's not so puffy at the front, but mainly at the back.

Addressing popliteal artery entrapment and claudication we ask:

Q *When you stop exercising, does the pain go away?*

A No, it is there really all the time, and certainly doesn't go away after a run. It might get a bit worse.

Q *Do you get rest pain, or night pain?*

A Occasional rest pain, but no night pain, or sleep problems, and in fact it seems a bit better after I've had my feet up for a while.

Addressing referred pain we ask:

Q *Do you get any pins and needles, or numbness in your toes or knee?*

A No, not numbness. My feet feel normal to me.

Q *Do you get any back pain?*

A Not really, unless after a long flight, when we all do, don't we?

As the reader can see, this has narrowed the diagnosis to a smaller group. We can now consider:

Differential diagnosis

Most likely

> deep vein thrombosis

> gastrocnemius/semimembranosus bursa

Least likely

> hamstring tendon insertional tendinitis/opathy

> popliteus tendinopathy

> Baker's cyst (semimembranosus–gastrocnemius bursa)

> popliteal artery entrapment

> referred pain

> claudication (atherosclerotic)

When we examine the patient, we find a swelling in the popliteal fossa, which is difficult to differentiate, and subjectively warmer than the other knee. There is some swelling of the calf, which is 1.5 cm larger than the non-affected side, but muscle definition seems normal. There are no sensation changes, and all other knee examination is normal. We can see here that the examination findings have not helped to narrow the diagnosis further; in fact, they have added one of the common diagnoses, that of inflammatory arthritis.

We would need to go back and address the screening questions more closely, asking for signs of systemic disease affecting the eyes, mucous membranes, bladder, and bowels, and consider excluding these with hematological tests.

Investigations which are appropriate here need to differentiate the differential diagnoses. A D-dimer may help with the DVT risk, but a USS doppler would help to delineate a Baker's cyst and a

DVT resulting in oedema. It may be helpful to aspirate the joint, which is warm and tender, although the duration of the history makes septic arthritis less likely. Hematological investigations would include a C-reactive protein to look for signs of infection; should this be raised, then a more targeted investigation would be appropriate, to elicit the sources of potential infection, if the history did not reveal more on further questioning.

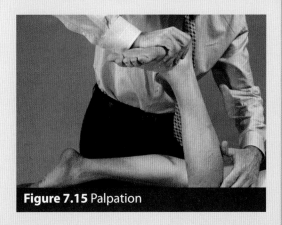

Figure 7.15 Palpation

Case 4

A 30-year-old tennis player presents to you with a month-long history of knee pain. She has started to take things more seriously this season, and is playing doubles as well as her singles ladder. In order to improve her fitness for this, she has enrolled in a "bootcamp" outdoor fitness class, three times a week before work.

Step 1: Define and align
Expose the patient properly; a pair of sports shorts will allow physical access and aid visibility.

Define the triangle: locate the medial and lateral femoral condyles, and the tibial tuberosity.

Align the patient's pain on the triangles. Here the pain is located to within the triangle.

The patient has localized the pain to the area "within the triangle". From this point we recommend the the reader attempt to exclude the potential pathologies. From Table 7.6, the potential causal structures are:

Differential diagnosis
> ACL injury
> PCL injury
> osteochondral lesion (osteochondritis dissecans)
> tibial plateau fracture
> synovial plicae
> bursitis – prepatellar, suprapatellar, infrapatellar
> quadriceps tendinopathy
> patellar tendinopathy

> Hoffa's fat pad inflammation

> patellar femoral joint disease

> patellar instability

> Osgood-Schlatter disease

> chondromalacia patella

> Sinding-Larsen–Johansson syndrome

> dislocating patella

We proceed to differentiate between these structures, step 2.

Step 2: Listen and localize

Addressing intra-articular pathology we ask:

Q *Have you ever had any traumatic injury to your knee?*

A No, my knees have always been ok. I had a bad ankle injury when playing netball at school, which took about a year to recover, but have not had any problems with it since.

Q *Does the knee ever lock or give way?*

A No, it has not locked, and only feels as if it might give way when I'm lunging at full length for a shot, but it hasn't as I can tolerate the pain it causes.

Q *Does your knee swell after exercise, or during it?*

A No, not really, I sometimes think my knee looks a little bit puffy, but this might be due to kneeling in my bootcamp class.

Q *Did the pain come on suddenly following an injury?*

A No, it has got worse over the last few weeks, but I can't remember when it actually started.

So an acute intra-articular injury is unlikely from the history. We cannot exclude it completely, but go on to address the extra-articular causes. Addressing bursitis we ask:

Q *Do you get the pain on movement?*

A Yes, the pain is there throughout the full range of motion, although I notice it most when I'm lunging for a shot on court, or running downhill in bootcamp training.

Q *Does your knee feel tight and restricted in its movement?*

A Not really, I can still get down for the low drop shots, but struggle to control my knee.

Addressing quadriceps tendinopathy we ask:

Q *Is there a specific area of soreness?*

A Yes, more in the tendon below my patella, not really above it in my thigh.

Addressing patellar tendinopathy we ask:

Q *Is the pain below the kneecap?*

A Yes, it feels on or just below the kneecap, but I couldn't feel anything when I had a look myself.

Q *Does the pain get a little better with exercise?*

A Not really, it is fine if I'm running on a flat surface, but changing direction and lunging make it worse, more so when I'm decelerating and stopping.

Q *Is the pain worse the day after tennis?*

A Yes, it is worse in the morning after tennis.

Addressing Hoffa's entrapment we ask:

Q *Have you started to do more kicking in the bootcamp, or have you had a sudden jerk or straightening of your leg?*

A No, not at all.

Addressing patellofemoral joint dysfunction we ask:

Q *Is the pain behind your kneecap?*

A No, it is more below or at the bottom of it. There is no grinding or clicking of my knee at all.

Q *Does it feel as if your patella is dislocating when you exercise?*

A No, my knee always feels stable until I lunge, when it feels as if it might give way.

The patient is of the wrong age to present with Osgood-Schlatter disease or Sinding-Larsen–Johansson syndrome – but she may have suffered as a child, so it is important to ask, as this may be secondary to an apophyseal fracture. Her history of netball certainly puts her at risk of this and Osgood-Schlatter. This can exacerbate patellar tendinopathy at the enthesis, and make it particularly refractory to treatment in later life.

As we proceed to palpate and re-create, we can see we have narrowed the diagnosis a little, but it is difficult to fully exclude on history alone here. The early-morning stiffness and enthesis pain should make the reader think outside the triangle, to the inflammatory arthropathy. There are enough indicators to need to more formally exclude these conditions here, and a full joint examination and more detailed systemic history are indicated to exclude rheumatoid and other inflammatory conditions, including Systemic Lupus Erythematosus (SLE), which may present in this age group.

Differential diagnosis

Most likely
> synovial plicae
> bursitis – prepatellar, suprapatellar, infrapatellar
> quadriceps tendinopathy
> patellar tendinopathy
> Hoffa's fat pad inflammation

Least likely
> ACL injury
> PCL injury

> osteochondral lesion (osteochondritis dissecans)

> tibial plateau fracture

> patellar femoral joint disease

> patellar instability

> Osgood-Schlatter disease

> chondromalacia patella

> Sinding-Larsen–Johansson syndrome

> dislocating patella

As you examine the knee, you confirm that there is some tenderness of the patellar tendon, at both its origins at the inferior pole of the patella, and also at its insertion into the tibial tuberosity. There is no bursitis or fat pad tenderness that you elicit, and ligament testing appears normal, with anterior draw and Lachman's, along with valgus and varus strain tests, all clinically normal. Meniscal testing revealed no tenderness.

To narrow down the diagnosis, an ultrasound examination of the patellar tendon may reveal signs of hypo-echogenicity or calcification. But to fully exclude intra-articular injury, it may be necessary to proceed to MRI imaging. The reader is encouraged to have confidence in the specificity and sensitivity of the knee ligament tests in negative findings. The modern increased reliance on imaging does the expert clinician no justice, and there is good evidence in combinations of investigations that they can have high diagnostic ability.

Conclusion

Clearly these cases are designed to lead the reader through the process of the triangle approach and the tables. The real-life situation is not always as clear, but the principles are the same. The localization of the pain always helps with narrowing the diagnosis, and the tables lead the reader to the most evidence-based discriminatory tests where available in the current literature.

References

1. Calmbach WL, Hutchens M. Evaluation of patients presenting with knee pain: Part I. History, physical examination, radiographs, and laboratory tests. Am Fam Physician. 2003 Sep 1; 68(5):907–12.
2. Louw QA, Manilall J, Grimmer KA. Epidemiology of knee injuries among adolescents: a systematic review. Br J Sports Med. 2008 Jan; 42(1):2–10.
3. Hughston JC. Subluxation of the patella. J Bone Joint Surg Am. 1968 Jul; 50(5):1003–26.
4. Renstrom P, Ljungqvist A, Arendt E, Beynnon B, Fukubayashi T, Garrett W, et al. Non-contact ACL injuries in female athletes: an International Olympic Committee current concepts statement. Br J Sports Med. 2008 Jun; 42(6):394–412.
5. Arnoczky SP, Warren RF. Microvasculature of the human meniscus. Am J Sports Med. 1982 Mar–Apr; 10(2):90–95.
6. Schutte MJ, Dabezies EJ, Zimny ML, Happel LT. Neural anatomy of the human anterior cruciate ligament. J Bone Joint Surg Am. 1987 Feb; 69(2):243–47.

7. Kaufmann P, Bose P, Prescher A. New insights into the soft-tissue anatomy anterior to the patella. Lancet. 2004 Feb 21; 363(9409):586.

8. Sanchez AR 2nd, Sugalski MT, LaPrade RF. Anatomy and biomechanics of the lateral side of the knee. Sports Med Arthrosc. 2006 Mar; 14(1):2–11.

9. Fairclough J, Hayashi K, Toumi H, Lyons K, Bydder G, Phillips N, et al. The functional anatomy of the iliotibial band during flexion and extension of the knee: implications for understanding iliotibial band syndrome. Journal of Anatomy. 2006 Mar; 208(3):309–16.

10. Duthon VB, Barea C, Abrassart S, Fasel JH, Fritschy D, Menetrey J. Anatomy of the anterior cruciate ligament. Knee Surg Sports Traumatol Arthrosc. 2006 Mar; 14(3):204–13.

11. Swenson TM, Harner CD. Knee ligament and meniscal injuries. Current concepts. Orthop Clin North Am. 1995 Jul; 26(3):529–46.

12. Amis AA, Gupte CM, Bull AM, Edwards A. Anatomy of the posterior cruciate ligament and the meniscofemoral ligaments. Knee Surg Sports Traumatol Arthrosc. 2006 Mar; 14(3):257–63.

13. Gupte CM, Smith A, McDermott ID, Bull AM, Thomas RD, Amis AA. Meniscofemoral ligaments revisited. Anatomical study, age correlation and clinical implications. J Bone Joint Surg Br. 2002 Aug; 84(6):846–51.

14. Warren LF, Marshall JL. The supporting structures and layers on the medial side of the knee: an anatomical analysis. J Bone Joint Surg Am. 1979 Jan; 61(1):56–62.

15. Wymenga AB, Kats JJ, Kooloos J, Hillen B. Surgical anatomy of the medial collateral ligament and the posteromedial capsule of the knee. Knee Surg Sports Traumatol Arthrosc. 2006 Mar; 14(3):229–34.

16. Espregueira M, da Silva MV. Anatomy of the lateral collateral ligament: a cadaver and histological study. Knee Surg Sports Traumatol Arthrosc. 2006 Mar; 14(3):221–28.

17. Mochizuki T, Akita K, Muneta T, Sato T. Pes anserinus: layered supportive structure on the medial side of the knee. Clin Anat. 2004 Jan; 17(1):50–54.

18. Karachalios T, Hantes M, Zibis AH, Zachos V, Karantanas AH, Malizos KN. Diagnostic accuracy of a new clinical test (the Thessaly test) for early detection of meniscal tears. J Bone Joint Surg Am. 2005 May; 87(5):955–62.

19. Grossman JW, De Smet AA, Shinki K. Comparison of the accuracy rates of 3-T and 1.5-T MRI of the knee in the diagnosis of meniscal tear. AJR Am J Roentgenol. 2009 Aug; 193(2):509–14.

20. Wang JC, Shapiro MS. Pellegrini–Stieda syndrome. Am J Orthop. 1995 Jun; 24(6):493–97.

21. Shelborne KD, Nitz PA. The O'Donoghue triad revisited. Combined knee injuries involving anterior cruciate and medial collateral ligament tears. Am J Sports Med. 1991 Sep–Oct; 19(5):474–77.

22. Alvarez-Nemegyei J. Risk factors for pes anserinus tendinitis/bursitis syndrome: a case control study. J Clin Rheumatol. 2007 Apr; 13(2):63–65.

23. Fowler PJ, Lubliner JA. The predictive value of five clinical signs in the evaluation of meniscal pathology. Arthroscopy. 1989; 5(3):184–86.

23. Ray JM, Clancy WG, Jr, Lemon RA. Semimembranosus tendinitis: an overlooked cause of medial knee pain. Am J Sports Med. 1988 Jul–Aug; 16(4):347–51.

24. Konan S, Rayan F, Haddad FS. Do physical diagnostic tests accurately detect meniscal tears? Knee Surg Sports Traumatol Arthrosc. 2009 Apr; 28.

24. Bollen SR, Arvinte D. Snapping pes syndrome: a report of four cases. J Bone Joint Surg Br. 2008 Mar; 90(3): 334–35.

25. Daffner RH, Martinez S, Gehweiler JA, Jr, Harrelson JM. Stress fractures of the proximal tibia in runners. Radiology. 1982 Jan; 142(1):63–65.

25. Muellner T, Weinstabl R, Schabus R, Vecsei V, Kainberger F. The diagnosis of meniscal tears in athletes. A comparison of clinical and magnetic resonance imaging investigations. Am J Sports Med. 1997 Jan–Feb; 25(1):7–12.

26. Harilainen A. Evaluation of knee instability in acute ligamentous injuries. Ann Chir Gynecol. 1987; 76(5): 269–73.

27. Norwood LA, Jr., Cross MJ. The intercondylar shelf and the anterior cruciate ligament. Am J Sports Med. 1977 Jul–Aug; 5(4):171–76.

28. Rennie WJ, Saifuddin A. Pes anserine bursitis: incidence in symptomatic knees and clinical presentation. Skeletal Radiol. 2005 Jul; 34(7):395–98.

29. Rosenberg TD, Paulos LE, Parker RD, Coward DB, Scott SM. The forty-five-degree posteroanterior flexion weight-bearing radiograph of the knee. J Bone Joint Surg Am. 1988 Dec; 70(10):1479–83.

30. Williams A, Gillis A, McKenzie C, Po B, Sharma L, Micheli L, et al. Glycosaminoglycan distribution in cartilage as determined by delayed gadolinium-enhanced MRI of cartilage (dGEMRIC): potential clinical applications. AJR Am J Roentgenol. 2004 Jan; 182(1):167–72.

31. Vossinakis IC, Tasker TP. Stress fracture of the medial tibial condyle. Knee. 2000 Jul 1; 7(3):187–90.

32. Fredericson M. Diagnosing tibial stress injuries in athletes. West J Med. 1995 Feb; 162(2):150.

33. Fredericson M, Bergman AG, Hoffman KL, Dillingham MS. Tibial stress reaction in runners. Correlation of clinical symptoms and scintigraphy with a new magnetic resonance imaging grading system. Am J Sports Med. 1995 Jul–Aug; 23(4):472–81.

34. Karataglis D, Papadopoulos P, Fotiadou A, Christodoulou AG. Snapping knee syndrome in an athlete caused by the semitendinosus and gracilis tendons. A case report. Knee. 2008 Mar; 15(2):151–54.

38. Falkenberg P, Nygaard H. Isolated anterior dislocation of the proximal tibiofibular joint. J Bone Joint Surg Br. 1983 May; 65(3):310–11.

39. Mirowitz SA, Shu HH. MR imaging evaluation of knee collateral ligaments and related injuries: comparison of T1-weighted, T2-weighted, and fat-saturated T2-weighted sequences—correlation with clinical findings. J Magn Reson Imaging. 1994 Sep–Oct; 4(5):725–32.

40. Thomason PA, Linson MA. Isolated dislocation of the proximal tibiofibular joint. J Trauma. 1986 Feb; 26(2): 192–95.

41. Shellock FG, Stone KR, Crues JV. Development and clinical application of kinematic MRI of the patellofemoral joint using an extremity MR system. Med Sci Sports Exerc. 1999 Jun; 31(6):788–91.

42. Piton C, Fabre T, Lasseur E, Andre D, Geneste M, Durandeau A. [Common fibular nerve lesions. Etiology and treatment. Apropos of 146 cases with surgical treatment]. Rev Chir Orthop Reparatrice Appar Mot. 1997; 83(6):515–21.

43. McCrory P, Bell S, Bradshaw C. Nerve entrapments of the lower leg, ankle and foot in sport. Sports Med. 2002; 32(6):371–91.

44. Prodromos CC, Han Y, Rogowski J, Joyce B, Shi K. A meta-analysis of the incidence of anterior cruciate ligament tears as a function of gender, sport, and a knee injury-reduction regimen. Arthroscopy. 2007 Dec; 23(12): 1320–25, e6.

45. Alentorn–Geli E, Myer GD, Silvers HJ, Samitier G, Romero D, Lazaro–Haro C, et al. Prevention of non-contact anterior cruciate ligament injuries in soccer players. Part 2: a review of prevention programs aimed to modify risk factors and to reduce injury rates. Knee Surg Sports Traumatol Arthrosc. 2009 Aug; 17(8):859–79.

46. Alentorn–Geli E, Myer GD, Silvers HJ, Samitier G, Romero D, Lazaro–Haro C, et al. Prevention of non-contact anterior cruciate ligament injuries in soccer players. Part 1: Mechanisms of injury and underlying risk factors. Knee Surg Sports Traumatol Arthrosc. 2009 Jul; 17(7):705–29.

47. Shelborne KD, Jari S, Gray T. Outcome of untreated traumatic articular cartilage defects of the knee: a natural history study. J Bone Joint Surg Am. 2003; 85-A Suppl 2:8–16.

48. Mankin HJ. The response of articular cartilage to mechanical injury. J Bone Joint Surg Am. 1982 Mar; 64(3): 460–66.

49. Hardaker WT, Jr, Garrett WE, Jr, Bassett FH, 3rd. Evaluation of acute traumatic hemarthrosis of the knee joint. South Med J. 1990 Jun; 83(6):640–44.

50. Donaldson WF, 3rd, Warren RF, Wickiewicz T. A comparison of acute anterior cruciate ligament examinations. Initial versus examination under anesthesia. Am J Sports Med. 1985 Jan–Feb; 13(1):5–10.

51. Rijke AM, Tegtmeyer CJ, Weiland DJ, McCue FC, 3rd. Stress examination of the cruciate ligaments: a radiologic Lachman test. Radiology. 1987 Dec; 165(3):867–69.

52. Yao L, Gentili A, Petrus L, Lee JK. Partial ACL rupture: an MR diagnosis? Skeletal Radiol. 1995 May; 24(4):247–51.

53. Miller TT, Gladden P, Staron RB, Henry JH, Feldman F. Posterolateral stabilizers of the knee: anatomy and injuries assessed with MR imaging. AJR Am J Roentgenol. 1997 Dec; 169(6):1641–47.

54. Daniel DM, Stone ML, Barnett P, Sachs R. Use of the quadriceps active test to diagnose posterior cruciate-ligament disruption and measure posterior laxity of the knee. J Bone Joint Surg Am. 1988 Mar; 70(3):386–91.

55. Gross ML, Grover JS, Bassett LW, Seeger LL, Finerman GA. Magnetic resonance imaging of the posterior cruciate ligament. Clinical use to improve diagnostic accuracy. Am J Sports Med. 1992 Nov–Dec; 20(6):732–37.

56. Patten RM, Richardson ML, Zink–Brody G, Rolfe BA. Complete vs partial-thickness tears of the posterior cruciate ligament: MR findings. J Comput Assist Tomogr. 1994 Sep–Oct; 18(5):793–99.

57. Linden B. The incidence of osteochondritis dissecans in the condyles of the femur. Acta Orthop Scand. 1976 Dec; 47(6):664–67.

58. Mesgarzadeh M, Sapega AA, Bonakdarpor A, Revesz G, Moyer RA, Maurer AH, et al. Osteochondritis dissecans: analysis of mechanical stability with radiography, scintigraphy, and MR imaging. Radiology. 1987 Dec; 165(3): 775–80.

59. De Smet AA, Ilahi OA, Graf BK. Untreated osteochondritis dissecans of the femoral condyles: prediction of patient outcome using radiographic and MR findings. Skeletal Radiol. 1997 Aug; 26(8):463–67.

60. Kode L, Lieberman JM, Motta AO, Wilber JH, Vasen A, Yagan R. Evaluation of tibial plateau fractures: efficacy of MR imaging compared with CT. AJR Am J Roentgenol. 1994 Jul; 163(1):141–47.

61. Ghelman B, Hodge JC. Imaging of the patellofemoral joint. Orthop Clin North Am. 1992 Oct; 23(4):523–43.

62. Pfirrmann CW, Jost B, Pirkl C, Aitzetmuller G, Lajtai G. Quadriceps tendinosis and patellar tendinosis in professional beach volleyball players: sonographic findings in correlation with clinical symptoms. Eur Radiol. 2008 Aug; 18(8):1703–99.

63. Cook JL, Purdam CR. Is tendon pathology a continuum? A pathology model to explain the clinical presentation of load-induced tendinopathy. Br J Sports Med. 2009 Jun; 43(6):409–16.

64. Franklyn-Miller A, Falvey E, McCrory P. Fasciitis first before tendinopathy; Does the anatomy hold the key? Br J Sports Med. 2009 Jan; 9.

65. Rees JD, Wolman RL, Wilson A. Eccentric exercises; why do they work, what are the problems and how can we improve them? Br J Sports Med. 2009 Apr; 43(4):242–46.

66. Kalebo P, Sward L, Karlsson J, Peterson L. Ultrasonography in the detection of partial patellar ligament ruptures (jumper's knee). Skeletal Radiol. 1991; 20(4):285–89.

67. Gisslen K, Gyulai C, Soderman K, Alfredson H. High prevalence of jumper's knee and sonographic changes in Swedish elite junior volleyball players compared to matched controls. Br J Sports Med. 2005 May; 39(5): 298–301.

68. Morini G, Chiodi E, Centanni F, Gattazzo D. [Hoffa's disease of the adipose pad: magnetic resonance versus surgical findings]. Radiol Med. 1998 Apr; 95(4):278–85.

69. O'Shea KJ, Murphy KP, Heekin RD, Herzwurm PJ. The diagnostic accuracy of history, physical examination, and radiographs in the evaluation of traumatic knee disorders. Am J Sports Med. 1996 Mar–Apr; 24(2):164–67.

70. Guzzanti V, Gigante A, Di Lazzaro A, Fabbriciani C. Patellofemoral malalignment in adolescents. Computerized tomographic assessment with or without quadriceps contraction. Am J Sports Med. 1994 Jan–Feb; 22(1):55–60.

71. Elias DA, White LM. Imaging of patellofemoral disorders. Clin Radiol. 2004 Jul; 59(7):543–57.

72. Solomon DH, Simel DL, Bates DW, Katz JN, Schaffer JL. The rational clinical examination. Does this patient have a torn meniscus or ligament of the knee? Value of the physical examination. JAMA. 2001 Oct 3; 286(13):1610–20.

73. Medlar RC, Lyne ED. Sinding–Larsen–Johansson disease. Its etiology and natural history. J Bone Joint Surg Am. 1978 Dec; 60(8):1113–16.

74. Sallay PI, Poggi J, Speer KP, Garrett WE. Acute dislocation of the patella. A correlative pathoanatomic study. Am J Sports Med. 1996 Jan–Feb; 24(1):52–60.

75. Colvin AC, West RV. Patellar instability. J Bone Joint Surg Am. 2008 Dec; 90(12):2751–62.

76. Brukner P, Khan K. *Clinical sports medicine.* 3rd ed. McGraw–Hill Australia; 2007.

77. Ng KC. Deep vein thrombosis: a study in clinical diagnosis. Singapore Med J. 1994 Jun; 35(3):286–89.

78. Stager A, Clement D. Popliteal artery entrapment syndrome. Sports Med. 1999 Jul; 28(1):61–70.

81. Yilmaz C, Orgenc Y, Ergenc R, Erkan N. Rupture of the medial gastrocnemius muscle during namaz praying: an unusual cause of tennis leg. Comput Med Imaging Graph. 2008 Dec; 32(8):728–31.

82. Brooks JH, Fuller CW, Kemp SP, Reddin DB. Incidence, risk, and prevention of hamstring muscle injuries in professional rugby union. Am J Sports Med. 2006 Aug; 34(8):1297–306.

83. Orchard JW. Intrinsic and extrinsic risk factors for muscle strains in Australian football. Am J Sports Med. 2001 May–Jun; 29(3):300–03.

84. Handy JR. Popliteal cysts in adults: a review. Semin Arthritis Rheum. 2001 Oct; 31(2):108–18.

85. Shenoy PM, Kim DH, Wang KH, Oh HK, Soo LC, Kim JH, et al. Calcific tendinitis of popliteus tendon: arthroscopic excision and biopsy. Orthopedics. 2009 Feb; 32(2):127.

86. Mariani PP, Mauro CS, Margheritini F. Arthroscopic diagnosis of the snapping popliteus tendon. Arthroscopy. 2005 Jul; 21(7):888–92.

87. Blake SM, Treble NJ. Popliteus tendon tenosynovitis. Br J Sports Med. 2005 Dec; 39(12):e42; discussion e.

88. Aktan Ikiz ZA, Ucerler H, Ozgur Z. Anatomic variations of popliteal artery that may be a reason for entrapment. Surg Radiol Anat. 2009 May; 6.

89. Lambert AW, Wilkins DC. Popliteal artery entrapment syndrome. Br J Surg. 1999 Nov; 86(11):1365–70.

90. Moore W, Krabak BJ. Chronic lateral knee pain in a cyclist: popliteal artery entrapment. Clin J Sport Med. 2007 Sep; 17(5):401–03.

91. Stiell IG, Greenberg GH, McKnight RD, Wells GA. Ottawa ankle rules for radiography of acute injuries. N Z Med J. 1995 Mar 22; 108(996):111.

92. Anderson J, Read J. *Atlas of imaging in sports medicine*. McGraw–Hill, Sydney, Australia; 2008.

93. Stiell IG, Wells GA, McDowell I, Greenberg GH, McKnight RD, Cwinn AA, et al. Use of radiography in acute knee injuries: need for clinical decision rules. Acad Emerg Med. 1995 Nov; 2(11):966–73.

94. Stankovic R, Johnell O, Maly P, Willner S. Use of lumbar extension, slump test, physical and neurological examination in the evaluation of patients with suspected herniated nucleus pulposus. A prospective clinical study. Man Ther. 1999 Feb; 4(1):25–32.

95. Goldenberg DL, Cohen AS. Acute infectious arthritis. A review of patients with nongonococcal joint infections (with emphasis on therapy and prognosis). Am J Med. 1976 Mar; 60(3):369–77.

96. Broy SB, Schmid FR. A comparison of medical drainage (needle aspiration) and surgical drainage (arthrotomy or arthroscopy) in the initial treatment of infected joints. Clin Rheum Dis. 1986 Aug; 12(2):501–22.

97. Rice PA. Gonococcal arthritis (disseminated gonococcal infection). Infect Dis Clin North Am. 2005 Dec; 19(4):853–61.

98. Aubert B, Barate R, Boutigny D, Couderc F, Karyotakis Y, Lees JP, et al. Search for the rare decay B0-->tau+tau- at BABAR. Phys Rev Lett. 2006 Jun 23; 96(24):241802.

The foot and ankle triangle

Introduction

A cute ankle injuries, such as lateral ligament sprains, have the highest incidence at 16–21% of all athletic injury,[1-3] and lateral ligament injuries account for 60% of all ankle sprains.[4] Overuse injuries, such as peroneal tendinopathy or stress fractures of the navicular bone, are also seen in the athletic population, and the differentiation of such injuries is difficult, but, unlike other joints such as the shoulder, much of the anatomy of the ankle is palpable. An accurate understanding of the anatomy of the area facilitates diagnosis.

Where an ankle injury is poorly rehabilitated, the athlete is more likely to suffer repeat injury, and develop joint damage. The morbidity may be considerable. It is estimated that 40% of athletes who suffer a forced inversion will develop chronic ankle instability.[5] Proper rehabilitation may prevent this, but requires a correct diagnosis.

The midfoot and forefoot are equally frustrating in terms of both making the diagnosis and understanding the palpable anatomy. The foot transmits significant forces and torsional loads, and accounts for some 15% of sports injuries.[6] Its relatively complex arrangement of bone, ligament, and overlying tendons makes an anatomical approach daunting. We guide the reader through the relevant anatomy and, by appreciating relationships to the key landmarks, make an anatomical approach digestible.

There are two triangles utilized in this chapter to enable the reader to fully appreciate the relationships between structures. These, as always, utilize bony landmarks to construct relationships between various key tissues. The relationships anteriorly, inferiorly, posteriorly, and distally are common to both triangles, but within the triangle there are discrete relationships.

The joints

The ankle is composed of four joints. The **tibiotalar** or talocrural joint is formed between the tibia, fibula, and talus. This is a cartilaginous synovial hinge joint, allowing plantar and dorsiflexion in the sagittal plane. The normal range of movement is between 20° of dorsiflexion and 50° of plantar flexion. In the dorsiflexed position, the tibiotalar joint is at its most stable. In the neutral mid-stance position, it is heavily dependent on the ligament structure for its stability.

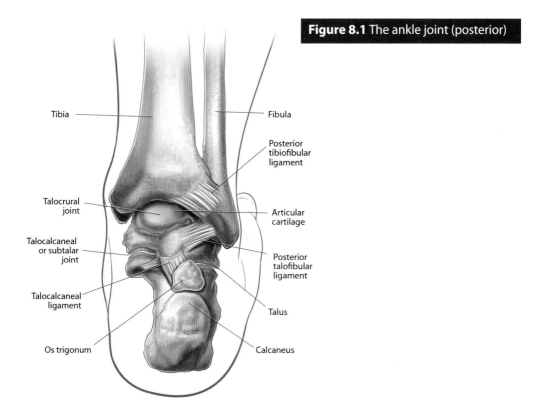

Figure 8.1 The ankle joint (posterior)

Tibia

Fibula

Posterior tibiofibular ligament

Talocrural joint

Articular cartilage

Talocalcaneal or subtalar joint

Posterior talofibular ligament

Talocalcaneal ligament

Talus

Os trigonum

Calcaneus

The **talocalcaneal** or subtalar joint is a synovial joint which forms a plane articulating the talus with the calcaneus. The subtalar joint allows hindfoot eversion and inversion. The range of motion is variable from subject to subject, but as a rule there is usually double the inversion compared to eversion at this joint, making up 40° of the range.

The **talocalcaneonavicular** joint is in effect two parts, made of the talocalcaneal, and the talonavicular, and again is synovial, and completes the base of integrity between the talus and the navicular. This is known variously as the transverse tarsal or "Chopart's joint". It allows for forefoot supination and pronation.

Finally, there is the **inferior tibiofibular** joint, a fibrous joint forming the closing part of the hinge joint, between the talus and the lower leg. The tibia forms the medial malleolus, and the fibula the lateral malleolus. The inferior tibiofibular joint is bound together by the strong tibiofibular ligaments, and is often called the "syndesmosis".

The structure of the ankle is maintained at an anatomical level by the integrity of the ligamentous attachments. In the acute setting, injury to ligaments causes pain, swelling, and dysfunction; if ligamentous laxity remains, the structural integrity of the joint may be affected, causing dysfunction and joint damage. As described above, these are the most common sites of athletic injury, and a comprehensive understanding is crucial.

Figure 8.2 The ankle joint (anterior)

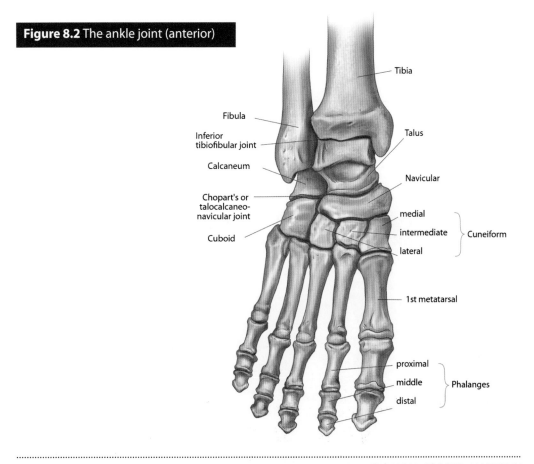

Lateral ankle ligaments

The **anterior talofibular ligament** (ATFL) is formed of two separate bundles, limits the anterior translocation of the talus. It is the weakest of all the lateral ligaments, and is incorporated in the joint capsule, passing from the anteroinferior margin of the lateral malleolus to the body of the talus, inserting just anterior to its cartilaginous margin. Importantly, it encroaches slightly into the tarsal tunnel, and so can "hang onto" the talus, preventing its anterior translocation. In plantar flexion, the lower part of the ligament remains relaxed, while the upper part becomes taut, and it is the converse in dorsiflexion. The ATFL is the primary restraint to inversion in the ankle. Strain patterns in the ligament increase movement from neutral to plantar flexion and inversion. This means that it is damaged in the motion of a forced inversion: inversion, plantar flexion, and internal rotation.[7]

The **calcaneofibular ligament** (CFL) is a strong, oval ligament arising from the distal part of the anterolateral margin of the lateral malleolus, below the inferior part of the ATFL. It runs obliquely inferiorly and posteriorly, to attach to the lateral surface of the calcaneum. It inserts onto a small tubercle postero-superiorly to the peronei muscle. This ligament is separate from the fibrous capsule, unlike the ATFL which is adherent to it, and its association with the peroneal tendon sheath may associate peroneal irritation with its disruption. The ligament bridges the subtalar and talocrural joints, both of which it stabilizes. The greatest strain patterns are noted when the ankle is inverted and dorsiflexed; the mechanism of injury therefore is most often inversion and ankle dorsiflexion.[7]

The **posterior talofibular ligament** (PTFL) is the strongest of all ligaments[8] in the lateral complex, running a line posteriorly from the articular surface of the lateral malleolus, horizontally to the posterior talus. Again the ligament is part of the fibrous capsule of the ankle. In plantar flexion and mid-stance, the ligament is relaxed, but in dorsiflexion and

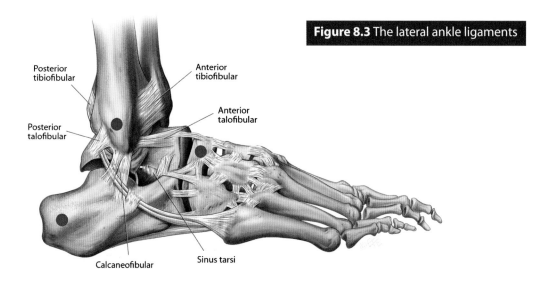

Figure 8.3 The lateral ankle ligaments

Posterior tibiofibular

Anterior tibiofibular

Anterior talofibular

Posterior talofibular

Calcaneofibular

Sinus tarsi

toe-off, the ligament is taut. The PTFL is rarely injured in isolation; this usually happens secondary to inversion.

The **anterior and posterior tibiofibular ligaments** are broad ligaments which cross the inferior tibiofibular joint, forming the distal part of the syndesmosis. This completes the structural integrity of the proximal talocrural joint, and forms the hinge of the joint. The syndesmosis is completed by the interosseous ligament between the medial edges of the bones.

The **calcaneocuboid ligament** is formed of two parts; the short part lies deep to the long plantar ligament, to connect the inferior surface of the calcaneus to the cuboid in a short but wide strong triangular ligament.[9] The long slip is attached posteriorly to the plantar surface of the calcaneal tuberosity, and in front to the tuberosity on the plantar surface of the cuboid, the more superficial fibers running forward to the bases of the second, third, and fourth metatarsals.

The **bifurcate ligament** runs anteriorly from the superior surface of the calcaneus into two slips, a calcaneocuboid slip inserting into the medial cuboid, and a calcaneonavicular slip inserting onto the lateral border of the navicular bone.

The medial ankle ligaments

The **deltoid ligament** is formed of the superficial tibiotalar, anterior deep tibiotalar, tibial calcaneonavicular or tibiospring ligament, tibiocalcaneal, and posterior deep tibiotalar ligaments.

The **tibionavicular** and **tibiocalcaneal** ligaments are in the more superficial layer of the ligament; these are important as they cross two joints – the talocrural and subtalar joints. The tibionavicular arises from the tip of the medial malleolus, and attaches to the navicular tuberosity, abutting the medial part of the spring or calcaneonavicular ligament. The tibiocalcaneal arises from the same common point (the apex of the deltoid), and runs inferiorly to the sustentaculum talus on the calcaneus. The posterior tibiotalar ligament arises from the same common origin, running posteriorly to the medial talar tubercle.

The deep layer is the deep tibiotalar ligament, which may have anterior and posterior divisions. It is intracapsular, running in the synovium of the joint capsule.

Cadaveric studies[10] of the ligament have shown that the function of the superficial and deep components is to act as the main restraint against valgus tilting of the talus, with the superficial and deep components being equally effective in this regard. The deep deltoid ligament appears to be the secondary restraint against both lateral and anterior talar excursion, with the lateral malleolus and supporting ligaments being the primary restraint.

The **spring ligament** runs from the sustentaculum tali, forward to the inferior edge of the navicular. It is supported by the tendons of the tibialis posterior and flexor hallucis, and helps to maintain the talar position.

The **tarsometatarsal ligaments** run between the superior surfaces of the cuneiforms and cuboid bones, and the respective bases of the metatarsals. The transverse ligaments run between the second and third, third and fourth, and fourth and fifth metatarsals respectively, but the second metatarsal has a transverse ligament running to the medial cuneiform, often termed "Lisfranc's ligament". This is the strongest and largest of the interosseus ligaments.

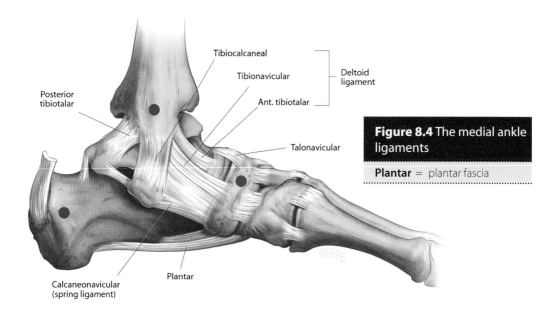

Figure 8.4 The medial ankle ligaments

Plantar = plantar fascia

The **cuneonavicular ligament** is a kite-shaped ligament running from the superior surface of the navicular bone, to insert into each of the three cuneiform bones.

The **cuneocuboid ligament** runs from the lateral cuneiform bone to the cuboid, along and across the superior (dorsal) surface.

The Y-shaped **bifurcate ligament** originates proximally at the anterolateral part of the calcaneus, deep to the extensor digitorum brevis (EDB), and runs via two slips; the medial part or calcaneonavicular ligament inserts on the lateral margin of the navicular bone, and the lateral slip inserts on the cuboid. This ligament stabilizes the respective joints.

Landmarks of the medial ankle triangle

> medial prominence of calcaneus

> medial border of navicular

> tip of medial malleolus

Anatomical relationships of borders of medial ankle triangle

The posterior border of the triangle runs in line with the posterior part of the deltoid ligament, but also overlies the flexor retinaculum. The border crosses the tarsal tunnel, and as such it is important to know the order in which the structures are palpable:

> tibialis posterior

> flexor digitorum longus

> posterior tibial artery

Figure 8.5 Ligaments of the dorsal foot

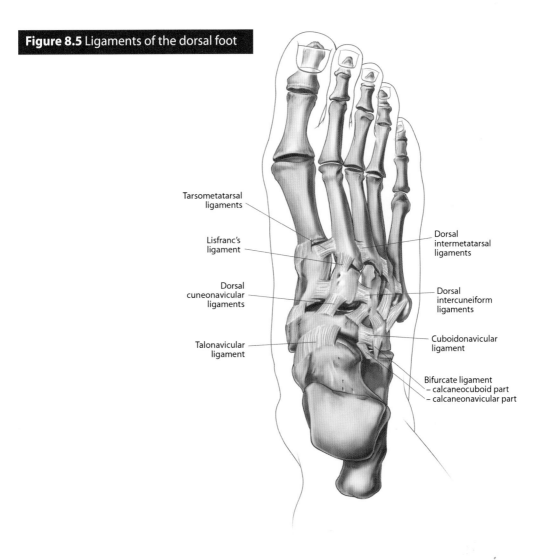

Tarsometatarsal ligaments

Lisfranc's ligament

Dorsal cuneonavicular ligaments

Talonavicular ligament

Dorsal intermetatarsal ligaments

Dorsal intercuneiform ligaments

Cuboidonavicular ligament

Bifurcate ligament
– calcaneocuboid part
– calcaneonavicular part

> tibial nerve:
- – medial plantar nerve
- – lateral plantar nerve
> flexor hallucis longus

The first structure is the tibialis posterior. A strong invertor of the foot, it originates from the posterior shafts of the tibia and fibula and the interosseus membrane, and runs under the flexor retinaculum, initially deep to the flexor digitorum, but superficially around the tip of the medial malleolus. It inserts into the navicular tuberosity, with further slips onto the bases of the second, third, and fourth metatarsals. Contraction of the tibialis posterior plantar flexes and inverts the foot, but it is primarily a stabilizer of the medial arch of the foot; dysfunction causes acquired flat foot.[11] It is supplied by the tibial nerve.

Figure 8.6 The medial ankle triangle

AbdHall	– abductor hallucis
FDB	= flexor digitorum brevis
EHL	= extensor hallucis longus
DL	= deltoid ligament
TA	= tibialis anterior
TP	= tibialis posterior
FDL	= flexor digitorum longus
FHL	= flexor hallucis longus
AT	= achilles tendon
MPN	= medial plantar nerve
LPN	= lateral plantar nerve

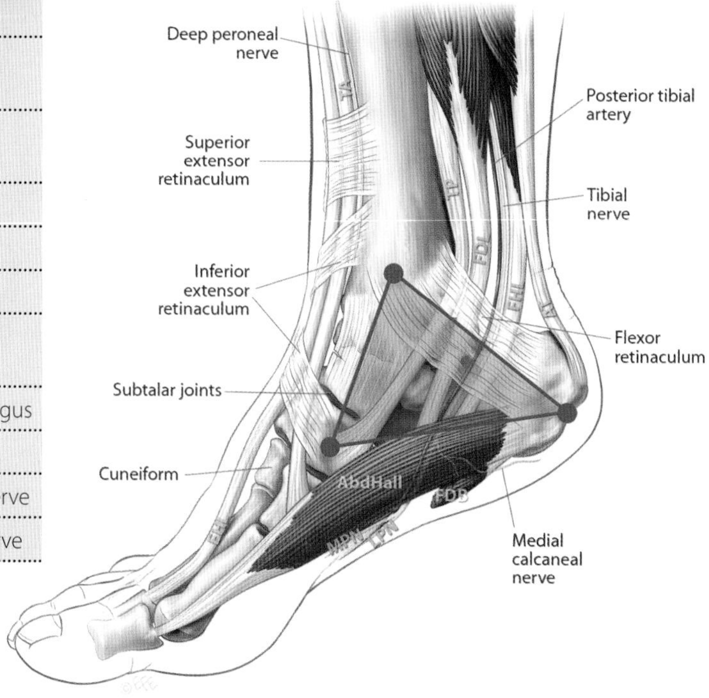

The next structure is the flexor digitorum longus, which arises from the posterior surface of the tibia, primarily in the mid-portion of the shaft. It is bipennate, however, with a further portion arising from the posterior fascia overlying the calf. The muscle tendon passes around the medial malleolus, deep to the flexor retinaculum, and then descends deep to the abductor hallucis, to divide into four tendons which insert into the base of the lateral four distal phalanges. Supplied by the posterior tibial nerve, it flexes the phalanges.

The posterior tibial artery is often palpable next, at the mid-point of the posterior border of the triangle. It arises from the tibial artery, and further divides under the inferior flexor retinaculum, to give the medial plantar artery, which follows the course of the medial plantar nerve, and the lateral plantar artery. It is accompanied by the tibial nerve, which divides to form the lateral and medial plantar nerves, and medial calcaneal nerve, just under the flexor retinaculum, where the posterior fibers of the deltoid ligament are palpable as they insert into the calcaneus.

The line here crosses the **tarsal tunnel**, which causes much anatomical confusion. It is composed of the medial part of the calcaneus, the lower part of the medial malleolus/tibia, the flexor retinaculum, and the talus. It contains the long flexor tendons, posterior tibial artery, tibial vein, and nerve.

The lateral plantar nerve (a branch of the tibial nerve) supplies the abductor hallucis longus, and may be subject to compression from various causes, such as scar tissue, varicose veins, or hypertrophy of the muscle itself (sometimes seen in athletes),[12] and this can reproduce paresthesia or pain in the muscle, should a hypertrophic muscle cause compression. The nerve gives off the medial calcaneal nerve, the most proximal and most posterior of all branches.

Tarsal tunnel syndrome itself is caused by compression proximally to the tarsal tunnel, at the level of the lower third of the gastrocnemius, within the tunnel beneath the flexor retinaculum, or at the division of the lateral plantar nerve as it enters the fascia within the abductor hallucis.

The last tendon which the posterior border line crosses is the flexor hallucis longus, before ending at the medial prominence of the calcaneum.

The anterior border of the triangle arises from the tip of the medial malleolus, following the line of the talonavicular ligament. There are no structures crossing this border, but at the landmark of the navicular bone is the insertion of the tibialis posterior to the navicular tubercle.

The inferior border of the triangle runs between the navicular and the calcaneus, in the line of the spring or calcaneonavicular ligament.

The spring ligament is not directly palpable, as it is covered by the abductor hallucis. Originating from the medial calcaneal tubercle and the plantar fascia aponeurosis, it runs along the line of the posterior border, and inserts into the base of the first phalanx. The flexor digitorum brevis also arises from the plantar aponeurosis, with an often-palpable slip to the calcaneal tubercle, before dividing into four tendons inserting into the base of each of the lateral distal phalanges. The tendons of the FHL, FDL, and TP are palpable as they exit the base of the triangle.

Within the triangle lie the tendons of the flexor digitorum longus, tibialis posterior, and flexor hallucis longus, as well as the deltoid ligament and the spring ligament.

The **tibialis posterior** (TP) arises from the proximal two-thirds of the lateral margin of the posterior tibia, the interosseus membrane, and the upper half of the posterior fibula. It runs inferiorly with the tendon beneath the flexor retinaculum behind the medial malleolus, and then courses anterior to the sustentaculum, and inserts into the navicular tuberosity. Slips then extend to the cuboid, three cuneiforms, and the bases of the second, third, and fourth metatarsals. It acts to plantar flex the foot at the talocrural joint, and acts to significantly support the medial longitudinal arch of the foot, and is therefore crucial in controlling pronation speed. It is supplied by the tibial nerve (L4, L5, S1).

The **flexor hallucis longus** (FHL) arises from the inferior posterior two-thirds of the fibula and the interosseus membrane. Running inferiorly and below the flexor retinaculum, behind the medial malleolus, it passes inferior to the sustentaculum tali, and inserts into the distal phalanx of the great toe, with attachments to the tendon of the flexor digitorum longus. It acts to flex the great toe, but also contributes to plantar flexing the foot at the talocrural joint, and contributes to maintaining the medial longitudinal arch. It is supplied by the tibial nerve.

The **flexor digitorum longus** (FDL) arises from the posterior surface of the tibia, mainly from the central third. The tendon passes along with the tibialis posterior and FHL, deep to the flexor retinaculum; indeed it receives an extension from the FHL. The tendon divides into four slips which insert in the bases of the distal phalanges two to five. In order to reach their insertions, they pass via an opening within the tendon of the flexor digitorum brevis. The muscle acts to flex the second to fifth toes, and also has a role in ankle plantar flexion and inversion. Due to its nature, it is also part of the integrity of the medial and lateral longitudinal arches. It is supplied by the tibial nerve.

Landmarks of the lateral ankle triangle

> lateral prominence of calcaneus

> lateral border of cuboid

> tip of lateral malleolus

Figure 8.7 The lateral ankle triangle

ADM	=	abductor digiti minimi
EDB	=	extensor digitorum brevis
PL	=	peroneus longus
PB	=	peroneus brevis
EDL	=	extensor digitorum longus
ATFL	=	anterior talofibular ligament

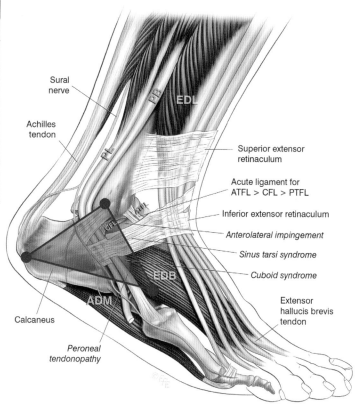

Sural nerve

Achilles tendon

Superior extensor retinaculum

Acute ligament for ATFL > CFL > PTFL

Inferior extensor retinaculum

Anterolateral impingement

Sinus tarsi syndrome

Cuboid syndrome

Extensor hallucis brevis tendon

Calcaneus

Peroneal tendonopathy

Anatomical relationships of borders of the lateral triangle

The anterior border of the lateral triangle runs from the tip of the fibula to the cuboid bone. There are few structures along this border, but the border transects the sinus tarsi at its mid-point. Structures palpable:

> sinus tarsi

> flexor retinaculum

> muscle belly of extensor digitorum brevis

The sinus tarsi is formed by the space between the talus and calcaneus. The talocalcaneona-vicular joint forms the anterior border or facet, and the posterior facet of the subtalar joint completes the facet. It runs posterior medially into the tarsal canal, in which run the interosseous talocalcaneal ligament and the roots of the inferior extensor retinaculum.

A retinaculum is defined as "keeping something in place", and contains collagen fibers similar to those found in the fascia of the lower limb. Retinacula serve as stirrups and blocks by which to secure tendons in the tunnels and grooves made with the tarsal bones, without which the muscle actions in the foot would be very different.

The extensor digitorum brevis lies anterior to the sinus tarsi and the distal point of the border.

The inferior border of the triangle runs from the calcaneus anteriorly to the cuboid bone. Running parallel but below the inferior line is the muscle belly of the abductor digiti minimi. Originating from the medial and lateral tubercles of the calcaneus, it runs anteriorly to insert at the base of the fifth proximal phalanx.

The posterior border of the lateral triangle runs from the tip of the fibula posteriorly to the calcaneum. Traversing this border from the superior margin are the tendons of the peroneus brevis, and deep to it the peroneus longus.

The peroneus brevis originates from the inferior half of the lateral shaft of the fibula, and the intramuscular septum between the tibia and fibula. It passes deep to the superior and inferior extensor retinaculum, running in a groove past the lateral malleolus, and then passes anteriorly along the calcaneus, before inserting onto the styloid process of the base of the fifth metatarsal. Acting to evert and plantar flex the foot, it is supplied by the superficial peroneal nerve (L5, S1).

The peroneus longus originates from the head of the fibula and the interosseous membrane, along with the upper third of the fibula. Following the same course as the brevis, it passes behind the lateral malleolus, before stirruping under the cuboid and traversing the longitudinal arch of the foot, inserting into the lateral border of the medial cuneiform and the base of the first metatarsal plantar surface. It has a notable sesamoid bone, the os peroneum, often originating just proximal to its insertion. It acts to evert and plantar flex the foot, at the subtalar and talocrural joints. It also provides significant support to the transverse arch, and is supplied by the superficial peroneal nerve (L5, S1).

The sural nerve passes down the posterolateral shank, superficially over the extensor retinaculum, and anteriorly down its course onto the dorsum of the lateral foot. The lateral calcaneal nerve and dorsal cutaneous nerve are branches. The nerve supplies sensation to the lateral and posterior third of the leg, as well as to the lateral ankle and foot.

Within the triangle lies the course of the peroneal tendons, under the extensor retinaculum, accompanied by the branches of the sural nerve.

Anterior to both triangles

The triangles both have common anterior structures on the dorsum of the ankle. The landmark following on from the apical triangle points is a horizontal line between the malleoli. This runs directly through structures superficial to the talus, and is in line with the anterior inferior

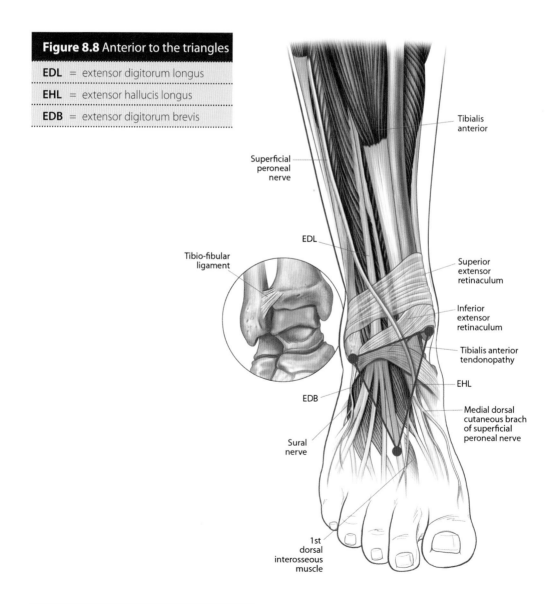

Figure 8.8 Anterior to the triangles

EDL	= extensor digitorum longus
EHL	= extensor hallucis longus
EDB	= extensor digitorum brevis

Tibialis anterior

Superficial peroneal nerve

EDL

Tibio-fibular ligament

Superior extensor retinaculum

Inferior extensor retinaculum

Tibialis anterior tendonopathy

EHL

EDB

Medial dorsal cutaneous brach of superficial peroneal nerve

Sural nerve

1st dorsal interosseous muscle

tibiofibular ligament, as shown in Figure 8.2 on page 308. These structures are largely retained by the flexor retinaculum. Structures encountered:

> tibialis anterior

> extensor hallucis longus

> common tendon of extensor digitorum longus, passing under inferior extensor retinaculum before separating into its four slips to the distal phalanges

> extensor digitorum brevis

The superficial peroneal nerve is a branch of the common peroneal nerve. As the deep peroneal nerve branch winds around the head of the fibula, the superficial branch runs inferiorly, and divides just distal to the inferior extensor retinaculum, into the medial dorsal cutaneous nerve, and the smaller, more lateral, dorsal cutaneous nerve.

Tibialis anterior (TA) arises from the lateral border of the tibia, from the lateral tibial condyle down to the proximal two-thirds of the tibia. It is bipennate, as it also arises from the anterior compartment fascia and the interosseus membrane. The muscle runs inferiorly, deep to the flexor retinaculum, to insert into the base of the first metatarsal, plantar surfaces, and the medial cuneiform. It acts to dorsiflex and invert the ankle, and is supplied by the deep peroneal nerve (L4, L5, S1).

Extensor digitorum longus (EDL) arises from the proximal two-thirds of the fibula, as well as the interosseous membrane and lateral condyle of the tibia. It runs inferiorly under the retinaculum, to insert into the dorsal surface of the middle and distal phalanges, via the medial expansion to the second to fifth. It acts to extend the second to fifth digits at the metatarsal phalangeal (MTP) and interphalangeal (IP) joints, and also dorsiflexes the foot and contributes to eversion. It is supplied by the deep peroneal nerve (L4, L5, S1).

Extensor hallucis longus (EHL) arises from the middle third of the anterior tibia and interosseous membrane, and descends in the anterior compartment of the leg, to insert into the dorsal surface of the great toe at the MTP joint. It acts to extend the great toe at the MTP joint, and to a lesser extent also to dorsiflex and invert the ankle. The muscle is innervated by the deep peroneal nerve (L4, L5, S1).

Extensor digitorum brevis (EDB) arises from the anterior superior surface of the calcaneus, and inserts into the proximal phalanx of the great toe, and into the extensor tendons of the EDL of the next three phalanges. It acts to dorsiflex the foot and extends the toes, and is innervated by the deep peroneal nerve (L4, L5, S1).

Posterior to both triangles

Posterior to both triangles lies the achilles tendon, as the common insertion of the gastrocnemius and soleus into the calcaneum. There are two bursae, one retrocalcaneal, sitting between the achilles tendon and the posterior calcaneus, and one superficial to the tendon but deep to the skin, although histologically this may actually be a fat pad.

Gastrocnemius arises from two heads, the lateral from the lateral condyle and posterior surface of the femur, and the medial from the medial condyle of the femur. The two heads form

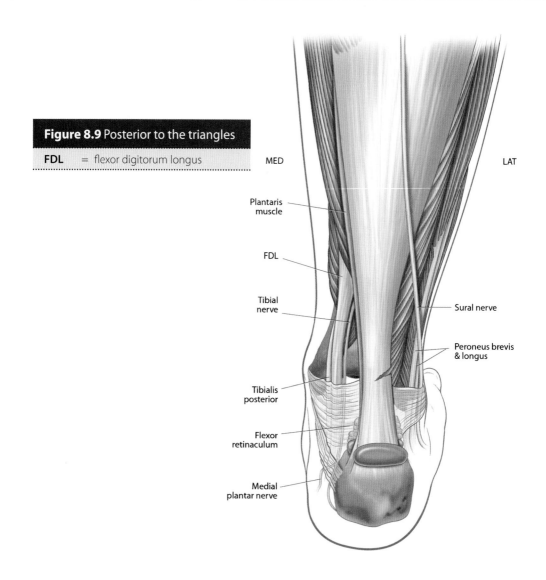

Figure 8.9 Posterior to the triangles

FDL = flexor digitorum longus

MED

LAT

Plantaris muscle

FDL

Tibial nerve

Sural nerve

Peroneus brevis & longus

Tibialis posterior

Flexor retinaculum

Medial plantar nerve

a common insertion, via the achilles tendon, into the calcaneus. Supplied by the tibial nerve (S1, S2), the muscle acts to plantar flex the ankle, and has a lesser effect on knee flexion.

Soleus arises from the posterior surface of the proximal and middle thirds of the tibia, along with the posterior surface of the proximal third of the fibula. The muscle forms a conjoint tendon with the gastrocnemius, and inserts into the calcaneus via the achilles tendon. Supplied by the tibial nerve (S1, S2), the muscle acts to plantar flex the foot about the ankle.

Plantaris arises from the distal posterolateral femur, superior to the lateral head of the gastrocnemius. It runs via a very long tendon inferiorly, to insert into the calcaneus via the achilles tendon. It acts to aid plantar flexion of the foot at the ankle, and is supplied by the tibial nerve (S1, S2).

Inferior to the triangles

Inferior to the triangles lies the sole of the foot and the intrinsic muscles. While we have previously endeavored to use the relationship of the triangle to describe the anatomy, here an original view is employed in order to best understand the anatomy.

Moving from superficial layers to deep, the intrinsic muscles and structures can be grouped into four layers. Most superficially is the skin and subcutaneous fat, and then the plantar fascia. As seen in Figure 8.11, the plantar fascia is made up of a central aponeurosis originating at the medial and lateral tubercles of the calcaneus, alongside the inferior surface, and runs distally to insert, by way of five slips, into the distal phalanges. The central slip is thick and stronger than the medial and lateral slips. The plantar fascia helps to maintain the longitudinal arch of the foot in a bowstring manner.

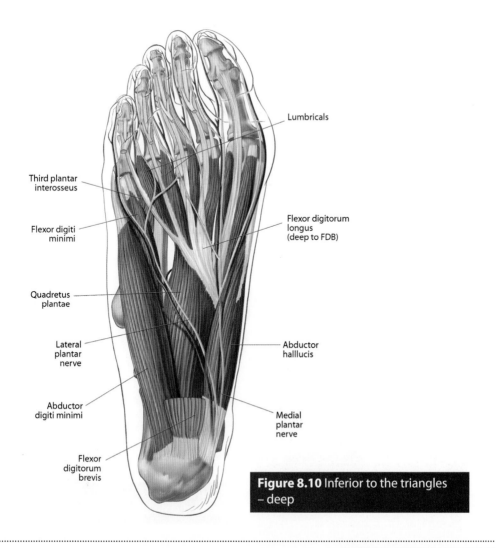

Lumbricals

Third plantar interosseus

Flexor digiti minimi

Flexor digitorum longus (deep to FDB)

Quadretus plantae

Lateral plantar nerve

Abductor halllucis

Abductor digiti minimi

Medial plantar nerve

Flexor digitorum brevis

Figure 8.10 Inferior to the triangles – deep

Deep to the plantar fascia lies a layer where, moving from lateral to medial, the abductor digiti minimi, flexor digitorum brevis, and abductor hallucis are present. These medial and lateral structures make up the immediate inferior borders of their respective triangles.

The **abductor digiti minimi** (ADM) originates from the medial and lateral tubercles of the calcaneus, along with slips from the flexor retinaculum and plantar aponeurosis. It runs anteriorly, to insert into the base of the proximal phalanx of the fifth toe, and forms a common insertion with that of the flexor digiti minimi brevis. It acts to abduct the little toe, and is supplied by the lateral plantar nerve (S1, S2), a terminal branch of the tibial nerve.

A small muscle, the **flexor digitorum brevis** arises from the medial tubercle of the calcaneus and the plantar aponeurosis, and divides into four tendons passing to phalanges two to five. Each of the individual tendons divides, to allow the transection of the FDL, and then inserts into the lateral and medial border of each of the middle phalanges. The muscle flexes the four toes (two to five) when not weight-bearing, and when loaded it acts to give form to the medial

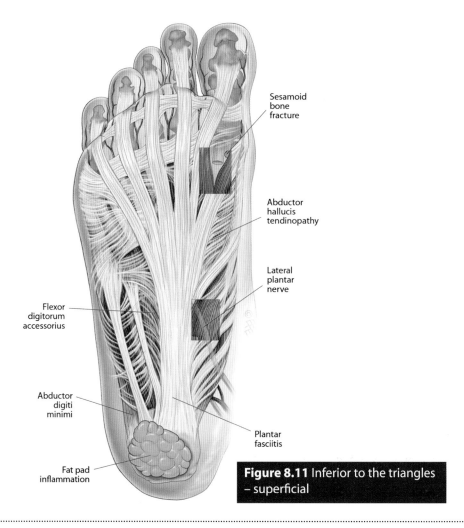

Sesamoid bone fracture

Abductor hallucis tendinopathy

Lateral plantar nerve

Flexor digitorum accessorius

Abductor digiti minimi

Plantar fasciitis

Fat pad inflammation

Figure 8.11 Inferior to the triangles – superficial

and lateral longitudinal arches. The muscle is supplied by the medial plantar nerve (S1, S2), which arises from the tibial nerve.

The **abductor hallucis** originates from the medial tubercle of the calcaneus, the lower border of the flexor retinaculum, and the plantar aponeurosis, to run anteriorly to the base of the proximal phalanx of the great toe, inserting at a common insertion with the flexor hallucis brevis. The muscle acts to flex and abduct the great toe when non-weight-bearing. It is supplied by the medial plantar nerve (S1, S2), again a terminal branch of the tibial nerve.

Moving deeper again, laterally is the flexor digiti minimi, centrally the quadratus plante and the tendons of the flexor digitorum longus, and medially the tendon of the flexor hallucis longus. The FDL and FHL are discussed earlier, where they pass the ankle joint.

The **flexor digiti minimi** (FDM) originates from the base of the fifth metatarsal and the distal tendon of the peroneus longus, to insert into the base of the proximal phalanx of the fifth toe. It acts to flex the toe at the metatarsophalangeal joint (MTPJ). The muscle is supplied by the lateral plantar nerve (S1, S2, S3).

Quadratus plante originates from two heads, arising from the medial and lateral calcaneus. They insert together into the lateral margin of the flexor digitorum longus tendon, and act as a "guy rope" to tension the action of the FDL to prevent it acting medially, but in turn it augments the flexion action of the FDL. It is supplied by the lateral plantar nerve (S1, S2).

The deepest layer starts laterally with the flexor digiti minimi, then moving medially, the interossei muscles, lumbricals, adductor hallucis, and medially the two heads of the flexor hallucis brevis.

The **lumbricals** in the foot vary in their presence and attachments. The first lumbrical arises from the tendon of the flexor digitorum longus, enroute to the second toe, and inserts into the base of the proximal phalanx of the toe. The second, third, and fourth lumbricals originate between the respective tendons of the FDL, to insert into their respective distal phalanges. The first lumbrical is supplied by the medial plantar nerve (S1, S2, S3), and the second to fourth by the lateral plantar nerve (S1, S2, S3).

The **plantar interossei** are small muscles originating from the medial aspect of the third to fifth metatarsals, and insert on the medial base of the same-toe proximal phalanx. They act to adduct the toes at the MTPJ, and are supplied by the lateral plantar nerve (S1, S2).

Adductor hallucis has an oblique head, which runs from the base of the second to fourth metatarsals and the tendon of the peroneus longus, to insert into the base of the proximal phalanx of the great toe. The transverse head originates from the transverse metatarsal ligaments, and inserts at the common insertion. The muscle acts to adduct the great toe, and also helps to support the transverse arch of the foot. It is supplied by the lateral plantar nerve (S2, S3).

Flexor hallucis brevis (FHB) originates from the base of the cuboid and lateral cuneiform bones, and inserts into the base of the proximal phalanx of the great toe. It acts to flex the great toe at the MTPJ. The distal tendon of this muscle contains the sesamoid bones of the foot, and as such is an important source of pathology. It is supplied by the medial plantar nerve (S1, S2).

The sole of the foot is supplied by two terminal branches of the tibial nerve:

The **medial plantar nerve** is a terminal branch of the tibial nerve, originating from the sciatic nerve, and dividing at the popliteal fossa. It originates as the nerve passes behind the posterior malleoulus, deep to the flexor retinaculum. It then passes distally along the medial border of the foot, deep to the abductor hallucis, and then in the space between the abductor hallucis and flexor hallucis brevis.

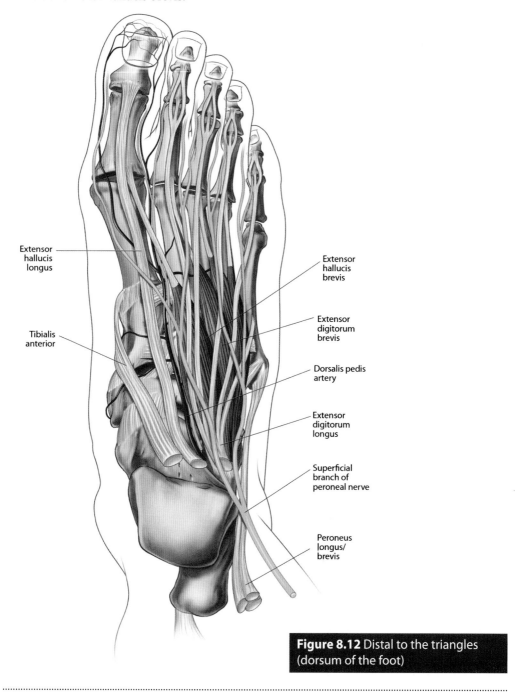

Extensor hallucis longus

Tibialis anterior

Extensor hallucis brevis

Extensor digitorum brevis

Dorsalis pedis artery

Extensor digitorum longus

Superficial branch of peroneal nerve

Peroneus longus/ brevis

Figure 8.12 Distal to the triangles (dorsum of the foot)

The **lateral plantar nerve** is the other terminal branch of the tibial nerve, and again originates deep to the flexor retinaculum, as it passes around the medial malleolus. It runs obliquely deep to the abductor hallucis, flexor digitorum brevis, and abductor digiti minimi. It does not pierce the quadratus plante, but divides to form a superficial branch which runs to become a fourth digital plantar nerve, and a deep branch which runs as a terminal arch across the metatarsal heads.

Distal to the triangles

Taking the structures distal to the line drawn between the two triangles anteriorly, this leaves the traditional midfoot and forefoot. Rather than divide the anatomy further, we encourage you to treat the foot as a whole, to look at the superficial tendon layers moving medial to laterally, the tibialis anterior, extensor hallucis longus, and extensor digitorum longus, and deep to this layer, the oblique muscle bellies of the extensor digitorum brevis.

Figure 8.5 highlights the palpable midfoot and forefoot bony landmarks and ligaments.

The dorsum of the foot carries the median branch of the superficial branch of the peroneal nerve. It divides in the mid-shank, to cross the anterior space of the triangles, superficial to the extensor retinaculum. It continues down the medial dorsum of the foot, with communicating branches to the saphenous and deep peroneal nerves, before dividing at the level of the metatarsal heads, to give two dorsal digital nerves as its terminal branches.

The lateral branch of the superficial peroneal nerve follows the same course; arising at a similar junction, it divides to form the dorsal digital nerves supplying the spaces between the third and fourth, and fourth and fifth toes respectively.

Table 8.1 Origins, insertions, and nerve supply to important muscles of the ankle				
Muscle	**Origin**	**Insertion**	**Nerve**	**Root**
Tibialis anterior	Upper half of lateral shaft of tibia and interosseous membrane	Inferomedial border of medial cuneiform and base of 1st metatarsal	Deep peroneal	L4, L5
Extensor hallucis longus	Mid-half of anterior shaft of fibula	Base of distal phalanx of great toe	Deep peroneal	L5, S1
Extensor digitorum longus	Upper ⅔ of shaft of anterior shaft of fibula, interosseus membrane, and superior talofibular joint	Extensor expansion of lateral 4 phalanges	Deep peroneal	L5, S1
Extensor digitorum brevis	Superior surface of calcaneus	4 tendon skips to base of proximal phalanx and long extensions to 2nd, 3rd, and 4th distal phalanges	Deep peroneal	L5, S1

Table 8.1 Origins, insertions, and nerve supply to important muscles of the ankle *(continued)*

Muscle	Origin	Insertion	Nerve	Root
Tibialis posterior	Upper ½ of posterior shaft of tibia and fibula, along with interosseus membrane	Navicular tuberosity	Tibial	L4, L5
Flexor hallucis longus	Lower ⅔ of posterior fibula, lower intramuscular septum and interosseus membrane	Base of distal phalanx of great toe	Tibial	S1, S2
Flexor digitorum longus	Posterior shaft of tibia and from fascial aponeurosis	Bases of distal phalanges of lateral 4 toes	Tibial	S2, S3
Gastrocnemius	Posterior surface of lateral femoral condyle and lateral condyle, posterior surface of femoral condyle	Calcaneum via common tendon	Tibial	S1, S2
Soleus	Soleal line and middle ⅓ of posterior border of tibia and upper ¼ of posterior shaft of fibula	Calcaneus via common tendon	Tibial	S1, S2
Plantaris	Lateral supracondylar ridge of femur above lateral head of gastrocnemius	Calcaneus (medial side deep to achilles)	Tibial	S1, S2
Peroneus longus	Upper ⅔ of lateral shaft of fibula, head of fibula and superior tibiofibular ligament	Plantar aspect of base of 5th metatarsal and medial cuneiform	Deep peroneal	L5, S1
Peroneus brevis	Lower ⅔ of shaft of fibula	Tuberosity to base of 5th metatarsal	Superficial peroneal	L5, S1
Flexor digitorum brevis	Medial process of calcaneus tuberosity	4 tendons to lateral 4 middle phalanx, separated by slips of FDL to distal phalanx	Medial plantar	S1, S2
Abductor digiti minimi	Medial and lateral processes of posterior calcaneal tuberosity	Base of proximal phalanx of 5th toe and metatarsal	Lateral plantar	S2, S3
Abductor hallucis	Posterior calcaneal tuberosity	Base of proximal phalanx of great toe incorporating sesamoid	Medial plantar	S1, S2

Table 8.2 Origins, insertions, and nerve supply to important muscles of the foot

Muscle	Origin	Insertion	Nerve	Root
Abductor digiti minimi	Calcaneal tuberosity	Base of proximal phalanx of 5th toe	Lateral plantar	S1, S2
Flexor digitorum brevis	Calcaneal tuberosity	Base of middle phalanges of 2nd to 5th toes	Medial plantar	S1, S2
Abductor hallucis	Calcaneal tuberosity	Base of proximal phalanx of great toe	Medial plantar	S1, S2
Flexor digiti minimi	Base of 5th metatarsal	Base of proximal phalanx of 5th toe	Lateral plantar	S1, S2
Quadratus plante	Medial and lateral calcaneus	Tendon of flexor digitorum longus	Lateral plantar	S1, S2
Lumbricals	1st medial tendon of FHL to 2nd toe, 2-5th arise between FHL tendons	Base of proximal phalanges 2-5th	1st medial plantar 2-5th lateral plantar	S1, S2
Plantar interossei	Medial aspect of 2nd to 5th metatarsals	Medial proximal phalanx	Lateral plantar	S1, S2
Adductor hallucis	Oblique: base of 2-4th metatarsals Transverse: deep transverse metatarsal ligaments	Base of proximal phalanx of great toe	Lateral plantar	S1, S2
Flexor hallucis brevis	Cuboid and lateral cuneiform	Base of proximal phalanx of great toe	Medial plantar	S1, S2

Table 8.3 Prime movers of ankle movements

Dorsi flexion	Plantar flexion	Eversion	Inversion
Tibialis anterior	Gastrocnemius	Peroneus longus	Tibialis anterior
Peroneus tertius	Flexor digitorum longus	Peroneus brevis	Tibialis posterior
Extensor digitorum longus	Flexor hallucis longus	Peroneus tertius	Flexor digitorum longus
Extensor hallucis longus	Peroneus longus	Extensor digitorum longus	Flexor hallucis longus
	Peroneus brevis		
	Plantaris		
	Soleus		
	Tibialis posterior		

Anterior to the triangles

Anterior to the triangles lies the talocrural joint, as seen in Figures 8.1 to 8.5. This is important, as it is the best place to palpate the accessible talus in the plantar flexed position.

Osteochondral damage is known to occur both chronically, as a consequence of previous injury, and acutely. The talar dome is particularly susceptible, due to its role as the wedge of the mortice (the subcrural joint). Histologically and radiologically, this may range from bone bruising to chondral fracture.

Most commonly, osteochondral damage occurs in the anterior third of the lateral talar dome and the posterior third of the medial dome.[13] Posterior medial fractures are commonly the result of forced plantar flexion, and inversion and external rotation of the ankle, and commonly result in more significant injuries than the lateral talar injury.

Grading of talar injuries[14, 15]

Grade 1: bone bruising; most heal due to increased vascularity, but some become avascular, and form a demarcation line
Grade 2: the presence of subchondral changes
Grade 3: the presence of an undisplaced, detached osteochondral fragment
Grade 4: a detached and displaced osteochondral fragment

Surgical intervention is limited in its ability to deal with chronicity, and these injuries are important to detect early.[16]

Anterior impingement syndrome is a consequence of the entrapment of the synovial capsule, tendons or fat pads, and bursae in the anterior joint space of the talocrural joint. There are a number of causes, including bony spurs, osteophytes,[17] and also ankle instability,[18] where anterior translocation of the joint ensues the entrapment. The tendons themselves can be responsible, along with the thickened synovium. It is common anterolaterally following inversion injury. The recovering ligament damage forms scar tissue, resulting in entrapment.[19]

Tibialis anterior is a critical muscle in the control of the normal gait cycle.[20] Over-activation and reliance on the extensor digitorum and hallucis longus in dorsiflexion causes weakness in this muscle, and exposes it to overuse and ultimately tendinopathy. This may be a factor in chronic exertional compartment syndrome, but the pathological cause of this is yet unknown. Gait re-education is vital in the rehabilitation process.

The bony construction, and the ligamentous control of the ankle, lend themselves to bony impingement both at the joint lines, but also in the areas where the tendons are secured with retinacula. Where nerve branches pass under these tunnels, the nerve is exposed to nerve entrapment, and this is seen anteriorly with the deep peroneal nerve under the extensor retinaculum of the ankle.[21] This entrapment is a less common cause of "deep peroneal nerve entrapment or anterior tarsal tunnel syndrome". More commonly seen is entrapment as the nerve passes around the fibula head,[22] and penetrates between the head of the peroneus longus, where a fibrous sheath is a common site of entrapment. In both cases, entrapment causes dysesthesia over the dorsum of the foot.

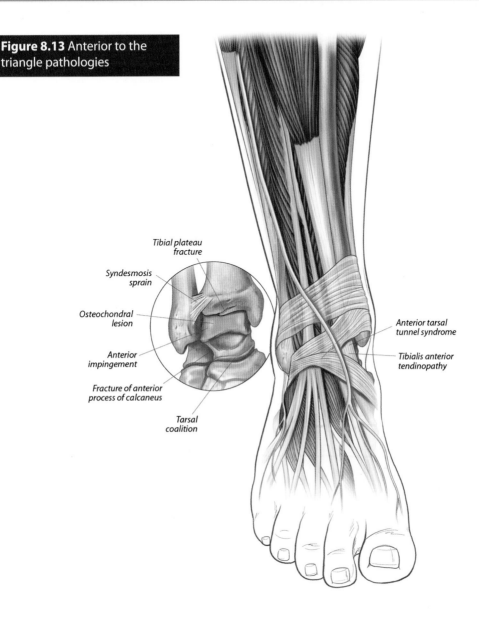

Figure 8.13 Anterior to the triangle pathologies

Tibial plateau fracture

Syndesmosis sprain

Osteochondral lesion

Anterior impingement

Fracture of anterior process of calcaneus

Tarsal coalition

Anterior tarsal tunnel syndrome

Tibialis anterior tendinopathy

Syndesmosis sprains have become increasingly diagnosed since Hopkinson suggested an incidence as low as 1% of all ankle sprains;[38] others report incidences as high as 20%.[39] As seen in Figure 8.1 and 8.2, the distal tibia and fibula are secured by the anterior inferior tibiofibular ligament and the posterior inferior tibiofibular ligament, alongside the interosseus ligaments. The mechanism of injury is commonly external rotation of a foot in fixed dorsiflexion,[40] and, although this is more common in contact sport, it can occur passively with a ski or toe catching and resulting in sudden unexpected movement. One should always consider a Maisonneuve fracture in syndesmotic sprains, due to the high forces, and examine the whole length of the fibula.

Define and align	Pathology	Listen and localize	Palpate and recreate	Alleviate and investigate
Table 8.4 Patho-anatomic approach; anterior to the triangle				
Anterior to triangle	Osteochondral lesion	Deep anterior ankle pain. Worse on impact, ankle pain persisting after 6 weeks	Ankle plantar flexed to 45°, palpate talus for tenderness[23]	MRI higher sensitivity than CT[24] and aids staging[25]
	Anterior impingement syndrome	Ankle pain worse on loaded/forced dorsiflexion	Tenderness along talocrural joint line along with palpation if osteophytes[26]	Plain x-ray dorsiflexion view, weight-bearing in lunge to demonstrate exostoses,[15] USS-guided LA injection[27]
	Tibialis anterior (TA) tendinopathy	Pain aggravated by running uphill. But precipitated by downhill running and tight lacing.[28] Nocturnal burning, midfoot burning, midfoot pain	Crepitis along TA tendon. Pain on resisted dorsiflexion and palpable swelling over tendon[29]	Ultrasound to compare with contralateral side. Thickening of tendon at insertion to medial cuneiform
	Anterior inferior tibio fibula ligament syndesmosis sprain "high ankle sprain"	Loss of toe-off power,[25] history of significant inversion injury, particularly with dorsiflexion	Tenderness over the AITFL. Rotation and dorsiflexion reproduce pain. Syndesmotic ligament test[30] or squeeze test[23]	Weight-bearing plain film,[31] USS[32] Exclude Maisonneuve fracture
	Deep peroneal nerve entrapment (and anterior tarsal tunnel syndrome)	Burning sensation over dorsum of foot extends to 1st webspace[33]	Tinel's test[34] to reproduce symptoms	Plain film to exclude exostosis, then EMG if non-resolving. Proximal lesions seen on MRI at proximal tib-fib joint, distal by USS under flexor retinaculum
	Fracture to anterior process of calcaneus	Persistent pain after ankle sprain associated with calcaneonavicular injury	Pain on palpation anterior to sinus tarsi, pain-free with ATFL injury[35]	Oblique plain film[15] images anterior calcaneus, if negative can proceed to CT
	Tibial plafond fracture	Fall from height onto feet	Pain on anterior talocrural joint line, palpation worse in dorsiflexion if posterior articular injury and plantar flexion if anterior articular injury[36]	MRI higher sensitivity than CT[24] as with ostechondral imaging

Table 8.4 Patho-anatomic approach; anterior to the triangle *(continued)*				
Define and align	Pathology	Listen and localize	Palpate and recreate	Alleviate and investigate
	Tarsal coalition	Lateral ankle pain locating to fibula, associated with slow response to lateral ankle healing in adolescent	Pes planus, with restriction on subtalar and mid-tarsal foot mobility. Pain on end of range of movement	Calcaneonavicular – oblique weight-bearing plain film Talocalcaneal – C sign and talar beaking on lateral plain film[37]
MRI	= magnetic resonance imaging			
CT	= computerized tomography			
EMG	= electromyography			
ATFL	= anterior talofibular ligament			
AITFL	= anterior inferior tibiofibular ligament			
USS	= ultrasound scan			
LA	= local anesthetic			

Tibial plafond fractures are high-energy injuries resulting in fracture from axial loading,[41] and commonly result in significant soft tissue damage and a "kissing lesion" with the talar dome. They are significant in terms of morbidity, and often require surgical intervention early on.

Tarsal coalition is an autosomal dominant inherited condition seen in children and adolescents, which results in abnormal fusion, either osseus or fibrous, between the bones of the midfoot. It can affect a number of joints, with the calcaneonavicular reported as more common, and it can occur bilaterally. It can present late or after concurrent injury with anterolateral ankle pain.

Posterior to the triangle

Posterior to the triangle, the most common pathology is that of the achilles tendon. This is somewhat of a perpetual hot topic in sports and exercise medicine, with the ongoing debate about the etiology and management behind tendinopathy.[42–44] What is clear is that there is a distinction to be made between two types of tendon injury. Mid-tendon disease, a more degenerative process, demonstrates an increase in fibroblast density and disordered neovascularisation,[45] which are features of degeneration.

Insertional tendon inflammation, seen in inflammatory arthropathy, is very different, commonly mistaken for sporting injury. This on occasion is the presentation of inflammatory arthritis, both in terms of tendon inflammation in juvenile inflammatory arthritis,[46] and the seronegative spondyloarthropathies.[47] The pathology is very different, and is part of systemic inflammation.

The presence of bony exostosis and posterior joint line impingement are common, either from the more traditional **Haglund's deformity**, where it is felt that the prominent posterosuperior spur causing pressure into the retrocalcaneal bursa is the cause, or others[48] such as previous injury to the synovial capsule, or osteophyte formation. Haglund's syndrome refers to the entrapment of both the retrocalcaneal bursa and then the superficial bursa to the achilles. A bony protuberence on the superior margin of the posterior sulcus may predispose a patient to this condition, which is sometimes termed Haglund's deformity. The superficial bursa is often inflamed by direct rubbing of the shoe-heel tab on the achilles tendon.

Posterior impingement is common in dancers, who frequently force their ankle into plantar flexion end range,[49] and is often a result of impingement of the posterior process of the talus, or an os trigonum between the bony surfaces of the tibia and calcaneum, as a result of repeated forced plantar flexion.

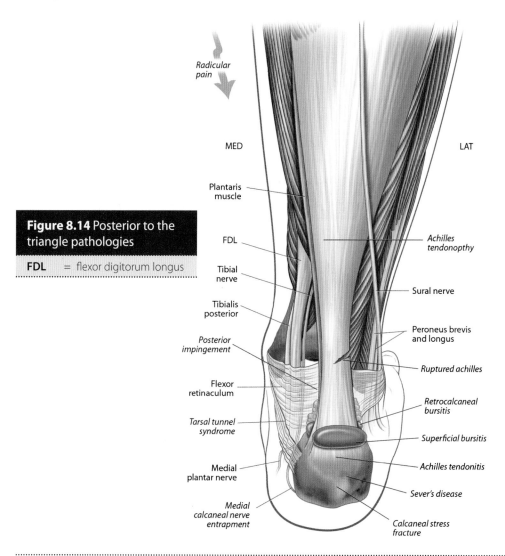

Figure 8.14 Posterior to the triangle pathologies

FDL = flexor digitorum longus

Radicular pain

MED

LAT

Plantaris muscle

FDL

Tibial nerve

Tibialis posterior

Posterior impingement

Flexor retinaculum

Tarsal tunnel syndrome

Medial plantar nerve

Medial calcaneal nerve entrapment

Achilles tendonopthy

Sural nerve

Peroneus brevis and longus

Ruptured achilles

Retrocalcaneal bursitis

Superficial bursitis

Achilles tendonitis

Sever's disease

Calcaneal stress fracture

Sever's disease is a common problem in children between the ages of 8 and 13 years. It has been more prevalent in males, but incidence in females is increasing with increases in exercise.[50] It is an apophysitis of the calcaneus, and is an overload injury, similar to Osgood-Schlatter disease, and is self-limiting.

Deep to the achilles tendon is the **retrocalcaneal or subtendinous bursa**, which is located between the achilles tendon and the calcaneus. A second subcutaneous calcaneal bursa, also called the achilles bursa, lies superficial to the tendon, between the skin and posterior aspect of the distal achilles tendon. Inflammation of either or both of these bursae can cause pain at the posterior heel and ankle region.[51]

Achilles tendon rupture can be either partial,[52] which is best identified on ultrasound examination, or complete tears. These are most common in the right foot of males aged 30–50 years old who are "weekend athletes", with a sudden eccentric force to a dorsiflexed foot.[53, 54] The classic presentation is so sudden that the athlete will often describe feeling as if they had been shot or struck by another player.

The mechanism of **tarsal tunnel entrapment** and the parasthesia encountered have been described earlier, but this is of multiple etiology, dependent on foot swelling, muscle hypertrophy, or concurrent injury. It may present with a similar clinical picture to that of referred pain from the sciatic nerve, and care should be taken to exclude this in the L4, L5, S1 distribution.

Medial calcaneal nerve entrapment involves the first branch of the medial plantar nerve, and is often referred to as Baxter's nerve entrapment.[55] Entrapment occurs at the point where the

Table 8.5 Patho-anatomic approach; posterior to the triangle				
Define and align	**Pathology**	**Listen and localize**	**Palpate and recreate**	**Alleviate and investigate**
Posterior to triangle	Achilles tendinopathy (mid-portion)	Gradual buildup of intensity of achilles pain, worsening with time and exercise. Usually not worse on waking	Thickened tender mid-achilles, painful focus which moves with passive dorsiflexion[57]	USS[58] with doppler to demonstrate neovasularisation
	Posterior impingement	Pain on forced plantar flexion or when running at toe-off	Positive posterior impingement test[59, 60]	USS-guided LA, or lateral plain film to exclude ostrigonum,[15] MRI[61]
	Insertional achilles tedinopathy	Often associated with Haglund's disorder or retrocalcaneal bursitis – pain on dorsiflexion[62] But also history of systemic disease in particular inflammatory spondyloarthropathy	Tenderness over insertion to calcaneus, no muscle weakness, worsened in plantar flexion. Can be associated with calcific nodularity[63]	USS,[58] ESR, CRP, and HLA-B27

Table 8.5 Patho-anatomic approach; posterior to the triangle *(continued)*

Define and align	Pathology	Listen and localize	Palpate and recreate	Alleviate and investigate
	Sever's disease	Presents between 7 and 10 yrs. Activity-related heel pain	Swelling and tenderness at insertion of achilles[64]	MRI demonstrates bone marrow edema metaphysis of calcaneus[65]
	Achilles bursitis	Posterior heel pain, worse when direct contact with shoe	Tenderness and swelling over calcaneus	USS-guided injection
	Ruptured achilles tendon	More likely male than female (10:1) and mid-40s. Describe a "shot in back of leg"	Simmonds'[66] and Mantle tests[67] if both positive have a sensitivity of 100%, O'Briens needle test[68]	Fat suppressed T2 STIR MRI
	Tarsal tunnel syndrome	Neuropraxia in plantar border of foot. Pain relieved by rest	Tinel's sign, altered sensation along L4 dermatome, tenderness over tarsal tunnel. Nerve compression test as plantar nerve enters abductor hallucis[21]	Nerve conduction studies[69] or provocation tests and clinical signs
	Medial calcaneal nerve entrapment	Burning pain over the medial aspect of calcaneus, radiates to longitudinal arch[70]	Tinel's tapping over nerve root reproduces pain, unlikely to reproduce heel pain if isolated medial calcaneal nerve[70]	LA injection, nerve conduction studies[71]
	Radicular pain	Pain following nerve distribution down posterior surface of calf and into foot	Braggard's[72] or slump tests reproduce symptoms	MRI for level and degree of involvement, ± epidural relieving injection
	Calcaneal stress fracture	Posterior calcaneal tuberosity pain in high-mileage runners,[73] persistant heel pain despite exclusion	Reactive effusion but requires careful history to discriminate from retrocalcaneal bursa	MRI and DEXA bone densitometry[74]

MRI = magnetic resonance imaging		**USS** = ultrasound scan	
CT = computerized tomography		**LA** = local anesthetic	
EMG = electromyography		**CRP** = C-reactive protein	

nerve turns laterally, between the thick lateral fascia of the abductor hallucis, symptomatically causing forefoot pain and nocturnal burning. If the symptoms extend back to include the heel, then often the entrapment is more proximal at the tarsal tunnel, rather than distally, but this makes it difficult to differentiate from plantar fasciitis.

Calcaneal stress fractures commonly present as a result of military training or distance running, but are occasionally due to insufficiency.[56] They are at low risk of progression, and present with tenderness along the medial and lateral calcaneus.

Radicular pain caused by nerve root irritation, either by degeneration or lumbar disc protrusion, can cause radiation of pain down the back of the calf into the ankle and foot. The distribution is usually dermatomal, and can be bilateral.

The medial triangle

The medial triangle encompasses the long flexor tendons, which may be partly responsible for tarsal tunnel pathology, or more likely tendinopathy, themselves, and are palpable as they run forward under the retinaculum.

The **tibialis posterior**, as earlier described, is responsible for maintaining the medial longitudinal arch, and controlling midfoot pronation during walking and running gaits.[75] It is particularly prone to inflammation in those with flattened arches and pes planus; indeed; spending a lot of time barefoot or in thongs on holiday is often the precipitant, or alternatively a change of running shoes.[11] An eccentric loading program is an effective management strategy, but gait re-education is vital to prevent recurrence.

Injuries to the **flexor hallucis longus** are typically overuse injuries due to repeated plantar flexion, although in dancers longitudinal tears are reported.[88] The more common tendinopathy and entrapment occur at the fibro-osseous tunnel along the posteromedial ankle, under the base of the first metatarsal, where the flexor digitorum longus (FDL) tendon crosses the FHL tendon, and where the FHL tendon passes between the great toe sesamoids, beneath the metatarsal head. With chronic disease, the tendon can become nodular, resulting in "triggering" of the great toe, and progression to hallux rigidus.[89]

The **deltoid ligament** is described earlier, and is injured by a force unstabilizing the pronated and abducted foot through external rotation,[90] placing a large abduction force onto the ankle and deltoid ligament. Because the forces required to injure the strong deltoid ligament are so great, the injury can be found to continue through the inferior syndesmosis, causing a much greater injury[91] with significant morbidity.

The **navicular bone** is crucial in maintaining the medial longitudinal arch, and its position close to the surface makes it palpable, as it is the anterior reference point in our medial triangle. It is commonly the site of avulsion fractures, but one in particular, of the tibialis posterior tendon from the navicular tuberosity, is a significant injury requiring surgical repair.

Coronal fractures have been classified by Sangeorzan,[92] with lateral displacement being of worse prognosis, but more frequently seen are stress fractures of the navicular bone. These are common in the military, and in athletes; Bennell[93] found an incidence of 15% of all stress fractures being navicular in track and field athletics. Torg[94] found a representative mean time

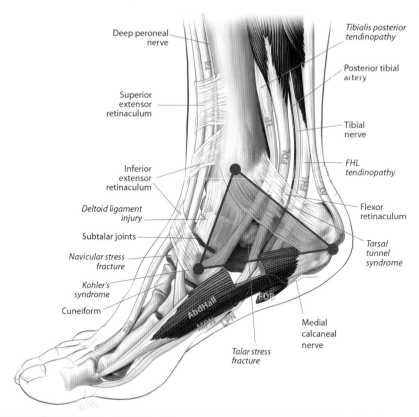

Figure 8.15 Medial to the triangle pathologies

AbdHall	= abductor hallucis	**FDL**	= flexor digitorum longus
FDB	= flexor digitorum brevis	**FHL**	= flexor hallucis longus
EHL	= extensor hallucis longus	**AT**	= achilles tendon
DL	= deltoid ligament	**MPN**	= medial plantar nerve
TA	= tibialis anterior	**LPN**	= lateral plantar nerve
TP	= tibialis posterior		

to diagnosis of seven months, as they are commonly misdiagnosed, and they are particularly slow to reunite.[95]

Talar stress fractures are rare, although they have been seen in gymnasts.[85, 86] They can be slow to demonstrate findings on plain film, and usually have a sagittal–oblique orientation.

Mid-tarsal sprains of the dorsal calcaneocuboid and bifurcate ligament can be associated with a fracture of the anterior process of the calcaneus, and are more common in footballers and gymnasts. These can be identified with a varus stress plain radiograph.

Kohler's disease, or osteochondritis of the navicular bone, is common in young children, in particular those between three and seven years old. It presents with a painful limp, and tenderness directly over the navicular bone.[87]

Table 8.6 Patho-anatomic approach; within the medial triangle				
Define and align	Pathology	Listen and localize	Palpate and recreate	Alleviate and investigate
Within the medial triangle	Tibialis posterior tendinopathy	Pain originating posterior to medial malleolus, radiating to longitudinal arch of foot	Resisted inversion causes pain and weakness, crepitus over tendon sheath[75]	USS examination[76] showed high sensitivity and specificity
	Flexor hallucis longus tendinopathy	Pain on plantar flexion, maximally around sustentaculum tali, associated with posterior impingement syndrome[77]	Resisted flexion of great toe or full dorsiflexion stretch. Associated snap or pop – in posteromedial ankle[75]	USS imaging preferable as fluid shut off in tendon sheath proximal to fibro-osseous canal makes MRI interpretation difficult[78, 79]
	Deltoid ligament injury	Pain on medial ankle and swelling with concomitant pain on dorsiflexion Injury commonly in external rotation and dorsiflexion	Resisted inversion of the foot, and palpable gap anteroinferior to medial malleolus [80]	Weight-bearing plain film to exclude syndesmosis injury[81] and full-length anteroposterior, lateral, and mortice views to exclude Maisonneuve fracture[15]
	Navicular stress fracture	Common in sports with explosive push off (rugby, track and field) Pain deep in foot	N spot tenderness[82] Percussion over navicular and hopping on plantar flexed foot[83]	Plain film with navicular view, CT[84]
	Talar stress fracture	Medial ankle pain with exercise.[85] High-distance runners most likely group	Single leg hop and heel tap when lying on couch with knee flexed reproduces pain[86]	MRI and CT[15]
	Mid-tarsal sprain (dorsal calcaneocuboid and/or bifurcate ligament)	Jumping sports, gymnasts and footballers. Pain in lateral midfoot worse on impact	Tenderness at calcaneocubid or overlying bifurcate ligaamnet. Pain with forefoot supination and plantar flexion	Plain film or MRI to examine for displacement
	Kohler's syndrome	Medial foot pain, painful limp, males 3–7 years	Navicular tenderness	Sclerosis and bony collapse on plain film[87]

MRI = magnetic resonance imaging   **USS** = ultrasound scan

CT = computerized tomography

The lateral triangle

The lateral triangle contains the most frequently injured structures of the lateral ligament complex. When the foot is in plantar flexion, the ATFL runs parallel to the axis of the leg,[96] therefore exposing the ligament, and is most frequently injured in inversion injury. Studies suggest that isolated, complete rupture of the ATFL is present in 65% of all ankle sprains.[4]

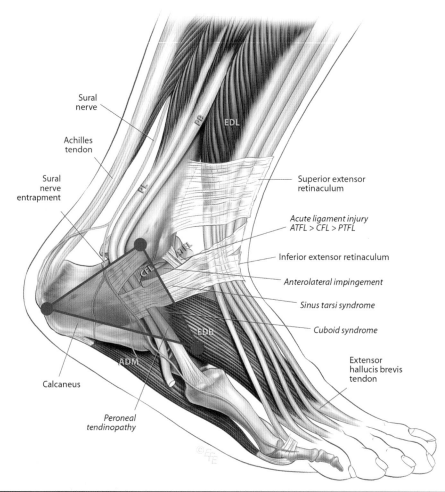

Figure 8.16 Lateral to the triangle pathologies

ADM	= abductor digiti minimi		**ATFL**	= anterior talofibular ligament
EDB	= extensor digitorum brevis		**CFL**	= calcaneofibular ligament
PL	= peroneus longus		**PiTFL**	= posterior talofibular ligament
PB	= peroneus brevis		**PTFL**	= posterotalofibular ligament
EDL	= extensor digitorum longus			

The CFL and PTFL are less commonly injured,[97] typically occurring in severe injuries, as the inversion dissipates force through the posterior structures after ATFL rupture. Isolated injuries of the CFL can occur when the ligament is under maximum strain with the foot in dorsiflexion, but injuries to the PTFL are extremely rare.

Tendinopathy of the peroneal muscles is often precipitated by an increase in training, and so has peak incidences in pre-season and in return from other injury.[98] This is more commonly an inflammatory reaction, and fluid is seen on ultrasound.[99] On occasion, tears, and degeneration of the tendon occur, but this is more frequently chronic in dancers with ankle instability.[100] Peroneus longus tendinopathy occurs most frequently at the cuboid, whereas peroneus brevis tendinopathy occurs at the lateral malleolus, and tears occur on the surface of the tendon.[15]

Sinus tarsi syndrome, or more accurately strain of the interosseus talocalcaneal ligament, presents as lateral foot pain with focal pain to palpation over the tarsal sinus, and commonly hindfoot instability. Commonly presenting following acute ankle inversion, there is still debate as to its pathology.[101] Increasingly it is felt that the damage is to the interosseus ligament or the joint, and as such it is misnamed.[102]

Anterolateral impingement occurs following relatively minor insult involving forced ankle plantar flexion and supination. Tearing of the anterolateral soft tissues and ligaments without substantial instability, and repetitive microtrauma, can result in synovial scarring, inflammation, and hypertrophy in the anterolateral recess of the tibiotalar joint, leading to impingement. Other contributing factors are thought to include hypertrophy of the inferior portion of the anterior tibiofibular ligament, and osseous spurs.[103] MRI is highly accurate in detecting soft tissue thickening, when compared to arthroscopic findings.[104]

Table 8.7 Patho-anatomic approach; within the lateral triangle				
Define and align	Pathology	Listen and localize	Palpate and recreate	Alleviate and investigate
Within the lateral triangle	Acute lateral ligament injury ATFL, CFL, PTFL, PiTFL	Acute injury of inversion, occasionally with audible pop and immediate swelling	Tenderness over ligament course but initially swelling++	Plain film to exclude fracture, MRI to delineate ligament injury
	Peroneal tendinopathy	Lateral ankle pain in sub-fascial tunnel posterior to lat malleolus, aggravated by activity, relieved by rest.[57] Associated with running on a camber, excessive pronation when running. Can be associated with tendon dislocation and snapping	Local tenderness and crepitus. Painful resisted eversion or passive inversion	MRI to include coronal and axial sections of metatarsals.[99] USS cannot differentiate peroneal tendon in cuboid tunnel

Table 8.7 Patho-anatomic approach; within the lateral triangle *(continued)*				
Define and align	**Pathology**	**Listen and localize**	**Palpate and recreate**	**Alleviate and investigate**
	Interosseous talocalcaneal ligament sprain, or sinus tarsi syndrome	Pain localized to anterolateral ankle. Follows acute ankle inversion or chronic instability	Pain reproduced on forced passive eversion.[106] Tenderness at opening of sinus tarsi	LA/CSI injection. MRI gives detailed imaging of ligament[107]
	Anterolateral impingement	Catching sensation of ankle with previous inversion injury	Pain can be reproduced in plantar flexion and eversion, but it is not reliable as difficult to compress the joint space[108]	Arthroscopy. MRI[61] specificity low
	Cuboid syndrome	Associated with plantar flexion and inversion injury. Common in dancers[109]	Pain on palpation of cuboid and sulcus sign,[110] along with pain on peroneal tendon on resisted inversion.[111] Weakness in push-off and inability to move from flat foot to demipointe	MRI not helpful. Oblique and plain lateral films can assist in confirming subluxation[112]
	Sural nerve entrapment	Associated with trauma over extensor retinaculum as nerve passes over it	Provocation test by placing the ankle as described by Styf:[113] pressure applied to anterior intramuscular septum with active dorsiflexion. Then, passive plantar flexion and inversion at ankle, maintaining passive stretch, gentle percussion is applied over course of the nerve	Imaging not helpful but nerve conduction studies if significant weakness in eversion[114]

ATFL	= anterior talofibular ligament		**CT**	= computerized tomography
CFL	= calcaneofibular ligament		**USS**	= ultrasound scan
PiTFL	= posterior talofibular ligament		**LA**	= local anesthetic
PTFL	= posterotalofibular ligament		**CSI**	= corticosteroid
MRI	= magnetic resonance imaging			

Cuboid syndrome refers to the pain due to a subluxing cuboid bone. Presenting as an inability to "work through" the foot and reproducible pain on manipulation, it is most commonly seen in dancers,[105] likely secondary to coexisting ligament injury of the calcaneocuboid ligament.

Sural nerve entrapment occurs at a number of sites in its course between the two heads of the gastrocnemius muscle. It descends along the lateral border of the achilles tendon with the short saphenous vein. The nerve divides just proximal to the ankle, into a lateral branch which supplies sensation to the lateral heel, and a branch which runs enclosed in the peroneal sheath. Entrapment causes primarily paresthesia over the fourth webspace and lateral heel.

Inferior to the triangles

Plantar fasciitis is one of the most common causes of heel pain.[115] It is relatively common in distance runners,[116] and in sedentary individuals who are overweight.[117] The plantar fascia acts as a mechanical bowstring which passively stabilizes the foot, maintaining the integrity of

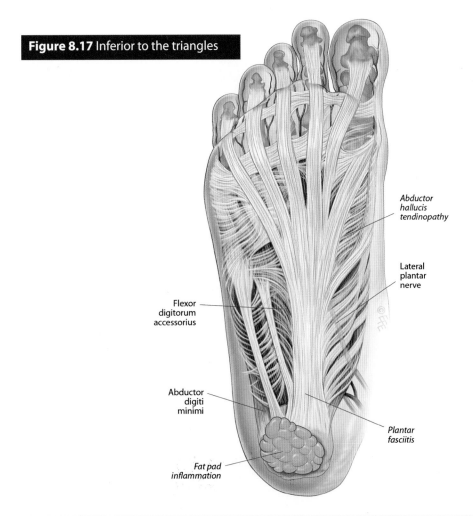

Figure 8.17 Inferior to the triangles

Abductor hallucis tendinopathy

Lateral plantar nerve

Flexor digitorum accessorius

Abductor digiti minimi

Plantar fasciitis

Fat pad inflammation

the medial longitudinal arch.[25] During the stance phase, the plantar fascia is stretched, and repetitive loading may cause microtears of the plantar fascia, contributing to the development and chronicity of plantar fasciitis.[118]

Fat pad inflammation can be a result of direct trauma to the heel, or biomechanical in its origins. Common in those overweight and in static standing jobs, it can be confused with plantar fascia pain, but is usually more laterally localizing. Known to be a sign of inflammatory arthropathy, care should be taken in the history to exclude such presentation.[119, 120]

Abductor hallucis tendinopathy or hypertrophy is often found as a causative factor in tarsal tunnel syndrome, but in isolation this tendon is rarely injured.[121] Ultrasound examination can clearly identify the muscle,[122] to show any tendinopathy or inflammation.

The sesamoids are two small, pea-like bones which form part of the metatarsophalangeal joint of the great toe. They act to absorb weight-bearing forces, decrease friction, and protect the flexor hallucis brevis tendons. In particular, they assist the leverage of the flexor hallucis brevis, and elevate the first metatarsal head to aid force dissipation.[123] Best imaged on plain film, the axial sesamoid view is a tangential view of the sesamoids and lesser metatarsal heads.[124] Injury ranges from acute trauma to repetitive injuries that cause stress fractures, or avascular necrosis.

Table 8.8 A patho-anatomic approach – inferior to the triangles				
Define and align	**Pathology**	**Listen and localize**	**Palpate and recreate**	**Alleviate and investigate**
Inferior to the triangles	Plantar fasciitis	Posterior medial heel pain, worse on first steps of the day, "walking on broken glass". Associated with increased weight	Tenderness over medial border of calcaneus, stretching fascia by dorsiflex, 1st MTPJ may reproduce[125]	Ultrasound demonstrates thickened fascia.[126] Plain film not indicated
	Heel fat pad inflammation	Pain on impact exercsize and standing, more lateral heel pain can be associated with inflammatory arthropathy[120]	Tenderness localized to calcaneus, not extending into fascia	No imaging required, can be seen on USS and MRI[119]
	Abductor hallucis tendinopathy	Pain along medial border of longitudinal arch	Tender to palpate muscle and insertion of AH into base of great-toe proximal phalanx	USS with doppler may highlight degeneration or inflammation
	Sesamoid bone fracture	Pain worse on forefoot, weight-bearing, walking on lateral border of foot. Hx of traumatic jump landing or increase in forefoot running	Tenderness overlying sesamoid bone. Flexion of 1st MTPJ associated with reproduction of pain[127]	Plain film,[124] MRI to exclude osteochondritis or necrosis[128]

Distal to the triangles

Here the main pathologies lie in the mid- and forefoot, and are discussed by frequency of occurrence. The anatomy again leads us to the diagnosis, as most are associated with a single joint or bony landmark.

The Lisfranc ligament (Fig. 8.5) is significant, and isolated injury is uncommon, but is more frequent in athletes following high-impact kicking or impact injury. It can equally be seen subtly following repetitive injury.[129] Lisfranc ligament injury ranges from sprain to complete rupture, and is often seen with concomitant metatarsal fracture, or injury to the midfoot bones forming the transverse arch (cuboid, three cuneiform bones, and base of the second metatarsal), or injury to the tarsometatarsal ligaments. Plain film imaging is useful

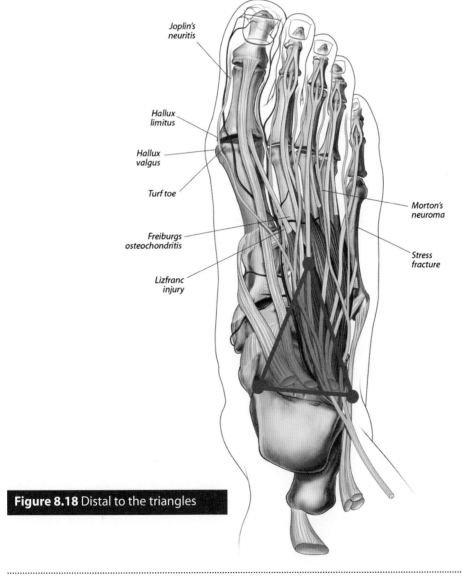

Joplin's neuritis

Hallux limitus

Hallux valgus

Turf toe

Freiburgs osteochondritis

Lizfranc injury

Morton's neuroma

Stress fracture

Figure 8.18 Distal to the triangles

to detect both congruence of the second metatarsal head and medial cuneiform, and also the longitudinal arch and transverse arch.

Hallux valgus is a common condition with a strong female-to-male ratio (9:1)[130] This is likely due to a combination of footwear choice and ligament laxity. The deformity is created by valgus deviation of the great toe, and varus (medial) deviation of the first metatarsal, creating

Table 8.9 A patho-anatomic approach – distal to the triangles				
Define and align	**Pathology**	**Listen and localize**	**Palpate and recreate**	**Alleviate and investigate**
Distal to the triangles	Hallux valgus	Initially asymptomatic with deformity noticed, pain on medial pressure from shoes[130]	Joint deformity and bony exostosis	Plain film
	Hallux limitus	Pain located to 1st MTPJ. Worsened by impact/exercise	Dorsal tenderness of 1st MTPJ, painful decreased range of motion[132]	Plain film to look for degenerative features
	Morton's neuroma	Forefoot pain radiating to toes, paresthesia in toes, pain on forefoot loading	Localized tenderness between metatarsals commonly 3rd and 4th. Palpable click of metatarsal heads[133]	Corticosteroid and local anesthetic injection relieve symptoms and confirm
	Freiberg's osteochondritis	Standing is painful, most frequent in adolescents, 2nd MT common location[134]	Tenderness of head of 2nd MT and swelling	Plain film can show flattened MT head, MRI more sensitive
	Joplin's neuritis	Pain along 1st MT into great toe, worse when wearing tight footwear & at end of the day	Tenderness over dorsal MTPJ and no joint deformity	Orthotic unloading of joint reduces symptoms
	Stress fracture Metatarsals	Forefoot pain worsened by impact activity, pain settles but worsens with activity, more common in F:M[135]	Focal tenderness over affected metatarsal	Plain film or MRI[136, 137]
	Lisfranc injury	Forefoot pain, worse on weight-bearing	Swelling at plantar border of forefoot, tenderness over tarsometatarsal joints. Pain on passive abduction and pronation[138]	Plain film – distance between MT bases not > 3 mm on weight-bearing[129]
	Turf toe	Pain over 1st MTPJ with history of bending of joint. Exclude gout if non-traumatic	Localized synovitis and tenderness. Plantar flexion and dorsiflexion worsen joint pain	Exlude osteoarthritis by plain film, consider aspiration if not settling for gout

a prominent joint line on the medial border of the foot. Due to the disruption of the joint, bony osteophytes develop, and an exostosis limits range in extension. Pain can occur due to irritation of the dorsal digital nerve, and it can also be associated with disruption of the cuneiform metatarsal joint. Many surgical options exist, each with their own proponents.[131]

Hallux limitus is characterized by a reduction in the ability to dorsiflex at the first MTPJ. The ability to dorsiflex the first MTPJ is essential for normal gait, requiring some 60° of flexion.[132] The condition can occur post-traumatically, or secondarily to exostosis due to inflammatory joint degeneration with inflammatory arthropathies, or alternatively, degeneration and loss of joint space with osteoarthritis.

Morton's neuroma is associated, commonly, with the irritation of the interdigital dorsal digital nerve (a terminal branch of the superficial peroneal), between the third and fourth metatarsals.[133] The pathology of the condition is not fully understood, but the metatarsal ligaments are thought to contribute to compression and scar tissue, in conjunction with trauma or altered gait biomechanics.

Freiberg's osteochondritis, first described by Freiberg in 1914, occurs primarily in adolescence and more commonly in females than males (5:1). It is characterized by the avascular changes of sclerois, fragmentation, and collapse of the second, third, and fourth metatarsal heads. It can lead to hallux limitus if left untreated.[134]

Joplin's neuritis,[139] or compression injury to the medial plantar digital nerve, is uncommon, and caused by entrapment along its course. It results in pain in the first webspace and great toe, which can be worsened by palpation of the webspace.[140]

Stress fractures are responsible for between 0.7 and 20% of all sports medicine presentations,[141] and metatarsal fractures are the second most frequently occurring stress fracture. They vary in location, with second-metatarsal fractures being common in dancers[142] due to potential biomechanical loading, and in military recruits and long-distance runners in the fifth metatarsal,[135, 136] leading to a Jones fracture if complete.

"Turf toe" occurs following an acute injury to the first metatarsophalangeal joint, usually in conjunction with a hyperextension or flexion injury; acute synovitis, swelling, and a painful range of motion characterize the condition, which must be carefully detailed to exclude a more inflammatory arthropathy.

Complex regional pain syndrome

Due to the frequency of injury of the ankle ligaments, and the exposed nature of the nerve supply, this is commonly a site of chronic pain post-traumatic injury,[143] but in the CRPS it can occur without precipitant injury, mimicking acute ankle ligament injuries, with spontaneous pain, hyperanalgesia, impairment of motor function, swelling, changes in sweating, and vascular abnormalities in the ankle.

Although the mechanism is not clear, this is not usually accompanied by nerve injury but allodynia, hyper- and hypo-analgesia, and changes to proprioception are common, along with anesthesia dolorosa (the absence of touch sensation, despite the pain sensation being intact, in the otherwise numb area).

Commonly a diagnosis is made by exclusion, but this condition is difficult to treat, with early mobilization and weight-bearing exercise essential[144] for improved outcome.

Ottawa ankle rules

To aid the less experienced physician or professional in deciding on the appropriateness of an x-ray,[145] the Ottowa ankle rules are reproduced here.

These rules assess physical findings in the ankle which correlate with risk of bony injury. A plain x-ray is required only if there is any pain in either malleolar region plus any of these findings:

1. bony tenderness from the tip of the lateral malleolus to include the lower 6 cm of the posterior border of the fibula
2. bony tenderness from the tip of the medial malleolus to the lower 6 cm of the posterior border of the tibia
3. the inability to walk four weight-bearing steps immediately after the injury and in the emergency department

Systemic illness and malignancy

These conditions are beyond the scope of the diagnostic triangles, and care should always be taken to exclude systemic illness. The cardinal features of malignancy include unexplained weight loss, night bone pain, and systemic illness, although of course commonly these are late-presenting signs. The clinician should always be aware of the potential for a musculoskeletal condition to mask an underlying systemic illness.

Osteoid osteoma is reported to occur in the cuneiform, cuboid, navicular, talus, and calcaneum bones. It is more common in 10–25 year olds, with a male-to-female ratio of 2:1. Located in the cancellous or subperiosteal bone, they are difficult to differentiate from other, more common pathologies. These benign tumors commonly present with night pain.[146] Plain imaging changes are often too subtle, but the lesion is readily seen on CT, while MRI is not as sensitive.[147]

Summary

As the reader has seen, there are many potential differential diagnoses in the foot and ankle, but all of these directly relate to the anatomy of the ankle, and the pathological structures. The triangles serve both to refresh and guide you to the appropriate structure, but also to help narrow the differential diagnosis from common to less common, in acute and chronic injury to the ankle. They are based on easily palpable landmarks, and as such the reader can familiarize the structures on him- or herself, and then apply the triangle construct to patients. While we categorize the conditions according to anatomical landmarks, the reader is reminded, particularly in the foot, of the potential for nerve entrapments higher in the ankle to reproduce distal symptoms. The foot and ankle should be considered together when addressing potential diagnoses, and for this reason we have not separated them.

Case histories

Case 1

A 55-year-old tennis player presents with a four-week history of ankle pain. He has been playing doubles for the last two years, due to occasional twinges in his ankle after a bad sprain on court. He has had some physiotherapy for the ankle, but due to work commitments has not completed the rehabilitation program. He had no imaging of his ankle on the last occasion, and was unable to play for six months. This is a presentation of ankle pain; as such proceed to step 1, define and align the ankle triangles.

Step 1: Define and align

Expose the patient properly; a pair of sports shorts will allow physical access and aid visibility.

Define the triangle: locate the calcaneus, the medial and lateral malleolus, and the navicular and cuboid bones.

Align the patient's pain on the triangles. Here the pain is quite specific to the talocrural joint line on the anterior side of the triangles.

The patient has localized the pain to the area "anterior to the triangle". From this point we recommend that the reader attempt to exclude the potential pathologies. From Table 8.4, the potential causal structures are:

differential diagnosis
> osteochondral lesion
> anterior impingement
> tibialis anterior tendinopathy
> anterior inferior tibiofibular ligament syndesmosis sprain
> deep peroneal nerve entrapment
> fracture to anterior process of calcaneus
> tibial plafond fracture

We proceed to differentiate between these structures, step 2.

Step 2: Listen and localize

Addressing osteochondral defect we ask:

Q *Is the pain worse on impact?*

A Yes, the ankle pain is sharp when I lunge for a low net shot. It feels like a burning pain, deep inside the ankle.

Q *Is there any associated ankle swelling?*

A Yes, after a match my foot and ankle become puffy. I always ice the ankle after playing, or else I struggle to walk the following day.

Addressing tibialis anterior tendinopathy we ask:

Q *Does the pain have an insidious onset, and is it worse if you are running uphill?*

A Not sure, I don't do much in the way of running outside tennis, but it is not really a gradual buildup of pain.

Addressing any nerve entrapments we ask:

Q *Do you experience any burning pain or numbness in your ankle or foot?*

A Not initially or during exercise, but I have noticed that I get some numbness if the ankle swells up after exercise.

Addressing fracture we ask:

Q *Did the pain ever go away after your previous injury?*

A Yes, it was fine for the last year, and I probably played more tennis than previously.

Q *Was it a twisting injury, or was it a fall?*

A No, it was a definite twisting injury, during the second set of a doubles match on court.

Addressing syndesmosis sprain we ask:

Q *Do you have problems pushing off that ankle to chase down a ball?*

A No, the main problem is stopping when I get the pain on lunging.

This narrows our differential diagnosis somewhat, and we proceed to examination to narrow it further. By palpating painful structures, and recreating the pain through diagnostic maneuvers, we move toward a diagnosis, step 3.

Step 3: Palpate and re-create

We palpate the anterior talocrural joint line, and find tenderness over the inferomedial joint line, worse on plantar flexion. The squeeze test and Tinel's test were negative.

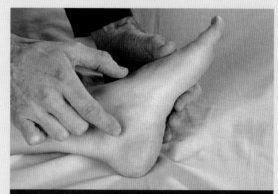

Figure 8.19 Tinels test: Tapping over the posterior tibial nerve may reproduce symptoms distal to tarsal tunnel

Differential diagnosis

More likely

> osteochondral lesion

> fracture to anterior process of calcaneus

Less likely

> anterior impingement

> tibialis anterior tendinopathy

> anterior inferior tibiofibular ligament syndesmosis sprain

> deep peroneal nerve entrapment

> tibial plafond fracture

We may now proceed to step 4 to confirm our clinical suspicion via imaging. The most evidence-based test is MRI.

The MRI confirms that there is bone edema of the talus, and this is an osteochondral lesion of the talus, secondary to the old injury.

Case 2

A 36-year-old masters triathlete presents with a two-month history of ankle pain. He has been training for an ironman distance triathlon, and increased his running load. He has also changed his training bike shoes, as he has picked up some sponsorship from a local bike shop. He put the pain down to the shoes to start with, and has managed to train through the pain, but after a 100 kilometer ride yesterday he is struggling to walk. This is a presentation of ankle pain; as such proceed to step 1, define and align the ankle triangles.

Step 1: Define and align

Expose the patient properly; a pair of sports shorts will allow physical access and aid visibility.

Define the triangle: locate the calcaneus, the medial and lateral malleolus, and the navicular and cuboid bones.

Align the patient's pain on the triangles. Here the pain is toward the back of the ankle.

The patient has localized the pain to the area "posterior to the triangle". From this point we recommend that the reader attempt to exclude the potential pathologies. From Table 8.5, the potential causal structures are:

Differential diagnosis

> achilles tendinopathy (mid-portion)

> posterior impingement

> insertional achilles tendinopathy

> Sever's disease

> achilles bursitis

> ruptured achilles

> tarsal tunnel syndrome

> medial calcaneal nerve entrapment

> radicular pain

> calcaneal stress fracture

We proceed to differentiate between these structures, step 2.

Step 2: Listen and localize

Addressing achilles tendinopathy we ask:

Q *Have you had the pain for some time?*

A Yes, the pain has been present when running and cycling for about two months. It seemed to start when changing cycling shoes.

Q *Does the pain get progressively worse?*

A Yes, after running and cycling, particularly hill work, the next day the ankle is stiff and painful, even getting out of bed.

Addressing posterior impingement we ask:

Q *Does the pain have sharpness on pushing off, or on jumping?*

A No, the pain is more stiffness then pain, not at all sharp.

Addressing old Sever's disease we ask:

Q *Did you experience ankle pain as a child or teenager?*

A No, I had no problems as a child, and did mini-athletics from seven years old.

Addressing tarsal tunnel syndrome we ask:

Q *Does the pain settle with rest?*

A No, in fact the pain seems to worsen with rest, for a couple of days after exercise.

Q *Do you experience any burning pain, or numbness in your ankle or foot?*

A No numbness in the foot or pain.

Addressing referred radicular pain we ask:

Q *Is the pain worse on one side?*

A Yes, it is mainly on the right ankle, but does affect my left side at times.

Q *Do you have any pain from your buttocks or the back of your leg?*

A No, just the back of the ankle and the achilles.

This narrows our differential diagnosis somewhat, and we proceed to examination to narrow it further. By palpating painful structures, and recreating the pain through diagnostic maneuvers, we move toward a diagnosis, step 3.

Differential diagnosis

Most likely

> achilles tendinopathy (mid-portion)

> insertional achilles tendinopathy

> achilles bursitis

> ruptured achilles

Least likely

> posterior impingement

> Sever's disease

> tarsal tunnel syndrome

> medial calcaneal nerve entrapment

> radicular pain

> calcaneal stress fracture

Step 3: Palpate and re-create

We palpate the posterior ankle, examining the structures in the triangle (Fig. 8.6). On palpation of the insertion of the achilles, there is no pain and Simmond's test is negative, but the mid-portion of the achilles is thickened and painful to touch.

Given step 2 and the results of our palpation, it is likely that this is mid-portion achilles tendinopathy. We may now proceed to step 4 to confirm our clinical suspicion via imaging. The most evidence-based test is ultrasound examination. This is easily imaged with a linear transducer with high-intensity

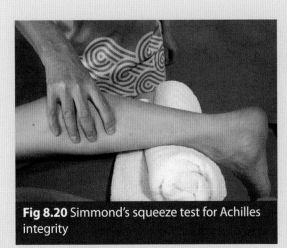

Fig 8.20 Simmond's squeeze test for Achilles integrity

imaging. The benefits include bedside interpretation and, significantly, the real-time monitoring of the rehabilitation process.

Case 3

A 22-year-old company dancer with the Royal Australian Ballet company presents with a four-month history of ankle pain. She has managed to rehearse, but has struggled with performances. She complains of impact pain on landing, and demipointe pain. Her whole foot is sore each day, and she is taking non-steroidal anti-inflammatory medication to get through the day.

Step 1: Define and align

Expose the patient properly; a pair of sports shorts will allow physical access and aid visibility.

Define the triangle: locate the calcaneus, the medial and lateral malleolus, and the navicular and cuboid bones.

Align the patient's pain on the triangles. Here the pain is located within the medial triangle.

The patient has localized the pain to the area "within the medial triangle". From this point we recommend that the reader attempt to exclude the potential pathologies. From Table 8.6, the potential causal structures are:

Differential diagnosis
> tibialis posterior tendinopathy
> flexor hallucis longus tendinopathy
> deltoid ligament injury
> navicular stress fracture
> talar stress fracture

We proceed to differentiate between these structures, step 2.

Step 2: Listen and localize

Addressing tibialis posterior tendinopathy we ask:

Q *Do you get pain when controlling your landing?*

A Yes, the pain is sharp, but when I run on the treadmill I do not get pain.

Q *Do you get pain down the inside of your leg, along with the ankle pain?*

A No, really the pain feels deep in the foot.

Addressing deltoid ligament injury we ask:

Q *Have you acutely injured or twisted the ankle?*

A No, not for at least three years, the ankle has been good.

Addressing navicular stress fracture we ask:

Q *Has the pain worsened over the four-month period?*

A Yes, it started off as a dull ache but with no sharp pains, and now it is sharper with the dull pain always being there.

Addressing talar stress fracture syndrome we ask:

Q *How long are you in rehearsal each day?*

A Normally 5 hours a day, and on performance days it could be 8 hours.

Q *Do you experience any burning pain, or numbness in your ankle or foot?*

A No numbness in the foot or pain.

Differential diagnosis

More likely

> navicular stress fracture

> talar stress fracture

Less likely

> tibialis posterior tendinopathy

> flexor hallucis longus tendinopathy

> deltoid ligament injury

This narrows our differential diagnosis somewhat, and we proceed to examination to narrow it further. By palpating painful structures, and recreating the pain through diagnostic maneuvers, we move toward a diagnosis, step 3.

Step 3: Palpate and re-create

We palpate the medial ankle, examining the structures in the triangle (Fig. 8.7). On palpation of the base of the triangle, there is navicular spot tenderness, and pain is reproduced on percussion and tuning-fork application to the navicular bone. It is important here to differentiate between insertional pain from the tibialis posterior insertion.

Given step 2 and the results of our palpation, it is likely that this is a navicular stress fracture. We may now proceed to step 4 to confirm our clinical suspicion via

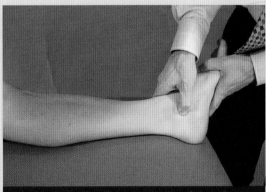

Figure 8.21 Tibialis posterior tendon palpation, posteromedial to medial malleolus to insertion at navicular bone

imaging. The most evidence-based test is MRI examination. There is some debate over this, as bone scan has been a traditional means of identifying stress fractures. The high radiation dose, and the high specificity of MRI, should begin to see it preferred. A plain film is of use with navicular views, and should be performed as a first line of investigation.

Case 4

A 24-year-old rugby league player presents with a 12-month history of ankle pain. He has just joined your club, and tells you he has struggled with his ankle throughout the last season, following a bad sprain in pre-season training. X-ray examination and MRI on the day of injury were "all fine" but he missed six games last season with it.

Step 1: Define and align

Expose the patient properly; a pair of sports shorts will allow physical access and aid visibility.

Define the triangle: locate the calcaneus, the medial and lateral malleolus, and the navicular and cuboid bones.

Align the patient's pain on the triangles. Here the pain is located within the medial triangle.

The patient has localized the pain to the area "within the medial triangle". From this point we recommend that the reader attempt to exclude the potential pathologies. From Table 8.6, the potential causal structures are:

Differential diagnosis
> acute lateral ligament injury: ATFL, CFL, PTFL, PTiFL, ATFL
> peroneal tendinopathy
> interosseous talocalcaneal ligament sprain or sinus tarsi syndrome
> anterolateral impingement
> cuboid syndrome
> peroneal nerve entrapment

We proceed to differentiate between these structures, step 2.

Step 2: Listen and localize

Addressing acute lateral ligament injury we ask:

Q *Have you reinjured your ankle recently?*

A No. It swells up a lot, but I have not sprained it again recently. The last injury was over 12 months ago.

Q *Do you get pain down the outside of your leg, along with the ankle pain?*

A No, the pain feels in the ankle; it does catch on occasions if I change directions, and there's a sharp pain down the outside of my ankle.

Addressing sinus tarsi syndrome we ask:

Q *Do you get pain on jumping?*

A Yes, the pain is mainly on landing, and again is lateral and anterior.

Addressing nerve entrapments we ask:

Q *Do you get any areas of numbness, or weakness?*

A No.

Differential diagnosis

More likely

> interosseous talocalcaneal ligament sprain or sinus tarsi syndrome

> anterolateral impingement

Less likely

> acute lateral ligament injury: ATFL, CFL, PTFL, PTiFL, ATFL

> peroneal tendinopathy

> cuboid syndrome

> peroneal nerve entrapment

This narrows our differential diagnosis somewhat, as both are common chronic injuries post-inversion injury, and we proceed to examination to narrow it further. By palpating painful structures, and recreating the pain through diagnostic maneuvers, we move toward a diagnosis, step 3.

Step 3: Palpate and re-create

We palpate the lateral ankle, examining the structures in the triangle (Fig. 8.7). There is swelling of the ankle, and tenderness over the sinus tarsi. On plantar flexion and eversion, there is also some pain, and it is difficult to differentiate. There is no pain over resisted eversion of the peroneal tendons.

Given step 2 and the results of our palpation, it is likely that this is sinus tarsi syndrome or anterolateral impingement. We may now proceed to step 4 to confirm our clinical suspicion. It may be beneficial

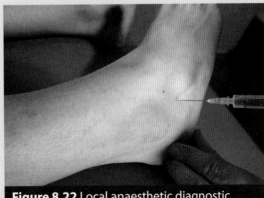

Figure 8.22 Local anaesthetic diagnostic injection to sinus tarsi 3

to consider a guided LA injection to the sinus tarsi before proceeding to MRI; this would have the advantage of excluding sinus tarsi syndrome, and may allow you to concentrate on ankle arthroscopy, suspecting anterior lateral impingement. A set of plain films is likely to be useful at this stage via imaging. The most evidence-based test is MRI examination.

Case 5

A 19-year-old track-and-field national athlete presents with right foot pain. She she has moved from long jump to triple jump this season, and is doing well but training heavily. The pain started three weeks ago, was quite sudden in onset, and is stopping her progress.

Step 1: Define and align

Expose the patient properly; a pair of sports shorts will allow physical access and aid visibility.

Define the triangles: locate the calcaneus, the medial and lateral malleolus, and the navicular and cuboid bones.

Align the patient's pain on the triangles. Here the pain is located inferior to the triangles.

The patient has localized the pain to the area "inferior to the triangles". From this point we recommend that the reader attempt to exclude the potential pathologies. From Table 8.8, the potential causal structures are:

Differential diagnosis
> plantar facsia disorders
> heel fat pad contusion
> abductor hallucis tendinopathy
> sesamoid bone pathology

We proceed to differentiate between these structures, step 2.

Step 2: Listen and localize

Addressing plantar fascia pain we ask:

Q *Is the pain worse when you get out of bed in the morning?*
A No. It worsens throughout the day and when training, there is no pain at all on waking.
Q *Do you get pain at your heel?*
A No, the pain feels more on the inside of the foot under the arch.

Addressing heel fat pad contusion we ask:

Q *Do you get pain on jumping and landing on your heels?*
A No, my heels are not sore at all.

Addressing abductor hallucis tendinopathy we ask:

Q *Is your foot painful when you push off?*

A Yes, it is painful when I push off the hop, and also when walking at the end of the day.

Addressing sesamoid bone involvement we ask:

Q *Have you changed shoes or orthotics?*

A No, I have not changed shoes, they're the same spikes as last year, and I've never had orthotics.

Q *Have you been jumping more than you were last season?*

A Yes, mainly for technique in the triple, with a lot of hopping and landing on the track.

Q *Are you menstruating, or have your periods stopped?*

A No, my periods are still regular, but lighter than when they first started at 14 years old.

Differential diagnosis

More likely

> adductor hallucis tendinopathy

> sesamoid bone involvement

Less likely

> plantar fascia pathology

> heel fat pad contusion

This narrows our differential diagnosis somewhat, and we proceed to examination to narrow it further. By palpating painful structures, and recreating the pain through diagnostic maneuvers, we move toward a diagnosis, step 3.

Step 3: Palpate and re-create

We palpate the muscle belly of the adductor hallucis, and find some tenderness at the insertion of the muscle, but there is significant pain on palpation of the FHL and the sesamoid bone. There is also some swelling under the first MTPJ and it feels boggy.

Given step 2 and the results of our palpation at step 3, it is likely that this is sesamoid bone pathology. Given the relatively short onset and the increase in training load and impact, it is likely that this is an acute fracture. We may now proceed to step 4 to confirm our clinical suspicion. It may be beneficial to consider a plain film. The sesamoid bone is usually ossified by the age of 8 in girls and 12 in boys, so one would expect it to be fused; in some people it is bipartite, so it may be beneficial to image

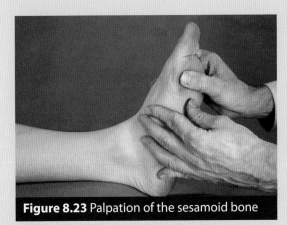

Figure 8.23 Palpation of the sesamoid bone

both feet. Ultrasound examination would assist in this, but is not sensitive for recent fractures. The plain film shows an acute fracture of the sesamoid, and confirms the diagnosis.

Case 6

A 16-year-old dancer presents with pain in her foot. It started slowly, and she was aware of it at the end of last year, but this year it seems to have been aggravated by more aerial work. She feels a sharp pain in her foot, which is worse on landing, and the movements feel stiff at the end of a session. She has had to reduce her sessions from eight per week to three.

Step 1: Define and align

Expose the patient properly; a pair of sports shorts will allow physical access and aid visibility.

Define the triangles: locate the calcaneus, the medial and lateral malleolus, and the navicular and cuboid bones.

Align the patient's pain on the triangles. Here the pain is located dorsally, distal to the triangles.

The patient has localized the pain to the area "distal to the triangles". From this point we recommend that the reader attempt to exclude the potential pathologies. From Table 8.9, the potential causal structures are:

Differential diagnosis
> hallux valgus
> hallux limitus
> Morton's neuroma
> Freiberg's osteochondritis
> Joplin's neuritis
> stress fracture metatarsals
> Lisfranc injury
> turf toe

We proceed to differentiate between these structures, step 2.

Step 2: Listen and localize

Addressing hallux valgus we ask:

Q *Have you noticed any misshapen toes, or pain when wearing shoes?*

A No. My feet feel and look the same, but I have noticed they swell up after a reherasal. Shoes seem to make things better than barefoot.

Q *Do the movements of your foot feel normal?*

A No, it is difficult to get up "en pointe", and when pushing off for a jump the pain is worse.

Q *Is the swelling in your toes?*
A No, it is much more in the middle of my foot.

Addressing nerve entrapment we ask:

Q *Do you get pain in or between the toes?*
A The pain does seem to move down between the second and third toes.
Q *Do you get any tingling or numbness in the toes?*
A No.

Addressing stress fractures we ask:

Q *Do you get impact pain?*
A Yes, it is painful when I land.
Q *Has the pain started gradually?*
A Yes, seems to have become worse recently.

Addressing Lisfranc injury we ask:

Q *Have you had any falls, or sprains of your ankle?*
A No, no other injuries for the last two years.
Q *Have you noticed any bruising of your foot?*
A No.

Differential diagnosis

More likely
> stress fracture metatarsals
> Lisfranc injury

Less likely
> hallux valgus
> hallux limitus
> Morton's neuroma
> Freiberg's osteochondritis
> Joplin's neuritis
> turf toe

This narrows our differential diagnosis somewhat, and we proceed to examination to narrow it further. By palpating painful structures, and recreating the pain through diagnostic maneuvers, we move toward a diagnosis, step 3.

Step 3: Palpate and re-create

We examine the foot, and see no signs of hallux valgus, with a normal first MTPJ. Range of movement of the first MTPJ is normal, and there is no pain on its movement. There is some pain on compression of the metatarsal heads, but no abnormal movement in disassociation testing. The palpation of the cuneiform/metatarsal joint reproduces the pain. On palpating the metatarsals, the patient is tender over the second metatarsal, and also in the second and third joint spaces. She is past the age for Freiberg's, and the history of no previous symptoms is likely to exclude this.

Given step 2 and the results of our palpation at step 3, it is likely that this is a stress fracture, or a Lisfranc ligament injury. We may now proceed to step 4 to confirm our clinical suspicion. It may be beneficial to consider a plain film, which is likely to be sensitive enough to detect a stress fracture if longstanding, but the Lisfranc injury, if mild (without large distraction on palpation), is unlikely to be demonstrated this way. In a female patient, rather than expose her to multiple films, we elect to order an MRI scan to look at the intertarsal ligaments and Lisfranc ligament, along with evidence from stress fracture.

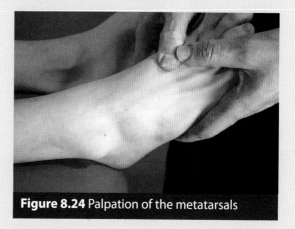

Figure 8.24 Palpation of the metatarsals

It is important to reiterate here the importance of a full clinical picture to the radiologist, in particular, the direct question regarding the differential clinical diagnosis. This will improve both the accuracy of reporting and the quality. An MRI scan will not demonstrate any dissociation of the mid-tarsal joints, although it would highlight the ligament injury or edema overlying it.

MRI confirms in this case a stress fracture of the second metatarsal.

Conclusion

While these case histories do not give typical examples for all conditions, they allow the reader to work through the process, and refresh the anatomy after reading the chapter. A familiarisation with the anatomy cannot fail to enhance your diagnostic skills, and you are encouraged to read widely among the reference material, to enhance knowledge in areas which are of particular interest. In the forefoot and midfoot, although we have divided the diagnoses based on the palpable anatomy, the reader should be aware of the possibility of structures in the ankle, in particular the nerve entrapments which occur around the ankle, of presenting as pain in the fore- and midfoot. We did not repeat ourselves by including these in the inferior and distal tables, but the reader should remain vigilant for the possibility, and always examine the foot and ankle as one structure.

References

1. Garrick JG. Epidemiologic perspective. Clin Sports Med 1982; 1(1):13–18.
2. Mangwani J, Gupta AK, Yadav CS, Rao KS. Unusual presentation of shoulder joint tuberculosis: A case report. J Orthop Surg (Hong Kong) 2001; 9(1):57–60.
3. Garrick JG. The frequency of injury, mechanism of injury, and epidemiology of ankle sprains. Am J Sports Med 1977; 5(6):241–42.
4. Ferran NA, Maffulli N. Epidemiology of sprains of the lateral ankle ligament complex. Foot Ankle Clin 2006; 11(3):659–62.
5. Hertel J, Braham RA, Hale SA, Olmsted-Kramer LC. Simplifying the star excursion balance test: analyses of subjects with and without chronic ankle instability. J Orthop Sports Phys Ther 2006; 36(3):131–37.
6. Malanga GA, Ramirez-Del Toro JA. Common injuries of the foot and ankle in the child and adolescent athlete. Phys Med Rehabil Clin N Am 2008; 19(2):347–71, ix.
7. Colville MR, Marder RA, Boyle JJ, Zarins B. Strain measurement in lateral ankle ligaments. Am J Sports Med 1990; 18(2):196–200.
8. van den Bekerom MP, Oostra RJ, Alvarez PG, van Dijk CN. The anatomy in relation to injury of the lateral collateral ligaments of the ankle: a current concepts review. Clin Anat 2008; 21(7):619–26.
9. Lohrer H, Nauck T, Arentz S, Vogl TJ. Dorsal calcaneocuboid ligament versus lateral ankle ligament repair: a case-control study. Br J Sports Med 2006; 40(10):839–43.
10. Harper MC. Deltoid ligament: an anatomical evaluation of function. Foot Ankle 1987; 8(1):19–22.
11. Kohls-Gatzoulis J, Angel JC, Singh D, Haddad F, Livingstone J, Berry G. Tibialis posterior dysfunction: a common and treatable cause of adult acquired flatfoot. BMJ 2004; 329(7478):1328–33.
12. Baxter DE, Thigpen CM. Heel pain – operative results. Foot Ankle 1984; 5(1):16–25.
13. Anderson IF, Crichton KJ, Grattan-Smith T, Cooper RA, Brazier D. Osteochondral fractures of the dome of the talus. J Bone Joint Surg Am 1989; 71(8):1143–52.
14. Berndt A, Harty M. Transchondral fractures (osteochondritis dissecans) of the talus. J Bone Joint Surg (Am) 1959; 41A:988–1020.
15. Anderson J, Read J. *Atlas of imaging in sports medicine.* 2nd ed. North Ryde: McGraw-Hill, 2008.
16. Verhagen RA, Struijs PA, Bossuyt PM, van Dijk CN. Systematic review of treatment strategies for osteochondral defects of the talar dome. Foot Ankle Clin 2003; 8(2):233–42, viii–ix.
17. Hayeri MR, Trudell DJ, Resnick D. Anterior ankle impingement and talar bony outgrowths: osteophyte or enthesophyte? Paleopathologic and cadaveric study with imaging correlation. AJR Am J Roentgenol 2009; 193(4):W334–38.
18. van Dijk CN, van Bergen CJ. Advancements in ankle arthroscopy. J Am Acad Orthop Surg 2008; 16(11):635–46.
19. Tol JL, van Dijk CN. Etiology of the anterior ankle impingement syndrome: a descriptive anatomical study. Foot Ankle Int 2004; 25(6):382–86.
20. Ivanenko YP, Poppele RE, Lacquaniti F. Five basic muscle activation patterns account for muscle activity during human locomotion. J Physiol 2004; 556(Pt 1):267–82.
21. Kennedy JG, Baxter DE. Nerve disorders in dancers. Clin Sports Med 2008; 27(2):329–34.
22. Fabre T, Piton C, Andre D, Lasseur E, Durandeau A. Peroneal nerve entrapment. J Bone Joint Surg Am 1998; 80(1):47–53.
23. Frost A, Roach R. Osteochondral injuries of the foot and ankle. Sports Med Arthrosc 2009; 17(2):87–93.
24. Verhagen RA, Maas M, Dijkgraaf MG, Tol JL, Krips R, van Dijk CN. Prospective study on diagnostic strategies in osteochondral lesions of the talus. Is MRI superior to helical CT? J Bone Joint Surg Br 2005; 87(1):41–46.
25. De Smet AA, Fisher DR, Burnstein MI, Graf BK, Lange RH. Value of MR imaging in staging osteochondral lesions of the talus (osteochondritis dissecans): results in 14 patients. AJR Am J Roentgenol 1990; 154(3):555–58.
26. O'Kane JW, Kadel N. Anterior impingement syndrome in dancers. Curr Rev Musculoskelet Med 2008; 1(1):12–16.
27. Robinson P. Impingement syndromes of the ankle. Eur Radiol 2007; 17(12):3056–65.
28. Bencardino JT, Rosenberg ZS, Serrano LF. MR imaging of tendon abnormalities of the foot and ankle. Magn Reson Imaging Clin N Am 2001; 9(3):475–92, x.
29. Beischer AD, Beamond BM, Jowett AJ, O'Sullivan R. Distal tendinosis of the tibialis anterior tendon. Foot Ankle Int 2009; 30(11):1053–59.

30. Alonso A, Khory L, Adams R. Clinical tests for ankle syndesmosis injury: reliability and prediction of return to function. J Orthop Sports Phys Ther 1998; 27(4):276–84.
31. Pneumaticos SG, Noble PC, Chatziioannou SN, Trevino SG. The effects of rotation on radiographic evaluation of the tibiofibular syndesmosis. Foot Ankle Int 2002; 23(2):107–11.
32. Milz P, Milz S, Steinborn M, Mittlmeier T, Reiser M. [13-MHc high frequency ultrasound of the lateral ligaments of the ankle joint and the anterior tibia-fibular ligament. Comparison and results of MRI in 64 patients]. Radiologe 1999; 39(1):34–40.
33. DiDomenico LA, Masternick EB. Anterior tarsal tunnel syndrome. Clin Podiatr Med Surg 2006; 23(3):611–20.
34. Shookster L, Falke GI, Ducic I, Maloney CT, Jr, Dellon AL. Fibromyalgia and Tinel's sign in the foot. J Am Podiatr Med Assoc 2004; 94(4):400–3.
35. Petrover D, Schweitzer ME, Laredo JD. Anterior process calcaneal fractures: a systematic evaluation of associated conditions. Skeletal Radiol 2007; 36(7):627–32.
36. Barei DP, Nork SE. Fractures of the tibial plafond. Foot Ankle Clin 2008; 13(4):571–91.
37. Conway JJ, Cowell HR. Tarsal coalition: clinical significance and roentgenographic demonstration. Radiology 1969; 92(4):799–811.
38. Hopkinson WJ, St Pierre P, Ryan JB, Wheeler JH. Syndesmosis sprains of the ankle. Foot Ankle 1990; 10(6):325–30.
39. Williams GN, Jones MH, Amendola A. Syndesmotic ankle sprains in athletes. Am J Sports Med 2007; 35(7):1197–207.
40. Nussbaum ED, Hosea TM, Sieler SD, Incremona BR, Kessler DE. Prospective evaluation of syndesmotic ankle sprains without diastasis. Am J Sports Med 2001; 29(1):31–35.
41. Bonar SK, Marsh JL. Tibial plafond fractures: changing principles of treatment. J Am Acad Orthop Surg 1994; 2(6):297–305.
42. Cook JL, Purdam CR. Is tendon pathology a continuum? A pathology model to explain the clinical presentation of load-induced tendinopathy. Br J Sports Med 2009; 43(6):409–16.
43. Rees JD, Maffulli N, Cook J. Management of tendinopathy. Am J Sports Med 2009.
44. Franklyn-Miller A, Falvey E, McCrory P. Fasciitis first before tendinopathy: does the anatomy hold the key? Br J Sports Med 2009; 43(12):887–89.
45. Tan SC, Chan O. Achilles and patellar tendinopathy: current understanding of pathophysiology and management. Disabil Rehabil 2008; 30(20–22):1608–15.
46. McGonagle D, Benjamin M. Towards a new clinico-immunopathological classification of juvenile inflammatory arthritis. J Rheumatol 2009; 36(8):1573–74.
47. Benjamin M, McGonagle D. The anatomical basis for disease localisation in seronegative spondyloarthropathy at entheses and related sites. J Anat 2001; 199(Pt 5):503–26.
48. Lee JC, Calder JD, Healy JC. Posterior impingement syndromes of the ankle. Semin Musculoskelet Radiol 2008; 12(2):154–69.
49. Bureau NJ, Cardinal E, Hobden R, Aubin B. Posterior ankle impingement syndrome: MR imaging findings in seven patients. Radiology 2000; 215(2):497–503.
50. Hendrix CL. Calcaneal apophysitis (Sever disease). Clin Podiatr Med Surg 2005; 22(1):55–62, vi.
51. Blankstein A, Cohen I, Diamant L, Heim M, Dudkiewicz I, Isreli A, et al. Achilles tendon pain and related pathologies: diagnosis by ultrasonography. Isr Med Assoc J 2001; 3(8):575–78.
52. Alfredson H, Masci L, Ohberg L. Partial midportion Achilles tendon ruptures: new sonographic findings helpful for diagnosis. Br J Sports ed 2009. Nov 27 epub ahead of print.
53. Khan RJ, Fick D, Keogh A, Crawford J, Brammar T, Parker M. Treatment of acute achilles tendon ruptures. A meta-analysis of randomized, controlled trials. J Bone Joint Surg Am 2005; 87(10):2202–10.
54. Kader D, Saxena A, Movin T, Maffulli N. Achilles tendinopathy: some aspects of basic science and clinical management. Br J Sports Med 2002; 36(4):239–49.
55. Sammarco GJ, Helfrey RB. Surgical treatment of recalcitrant plantar fasciitis. Foot Ankle Int 1996; 17(9):520–26.
56. Gehrmann RM, Renard RL. Current concepts review: Stress fractures of the foot. Foot Ankle Int 2006; 27(9): 750–57.
57. Subotnick SI. Achilles and peroneal tendon injuries in the athlete. An expert's perspective. Clin Podiatr Med Surg 1997; 14(3):447–58.

58. Khan KM, Forster BB, Robinson J, Cheong Y, Louis L, Maclean L, et al. Are ultrasound and magnetic resonance imaging of value in assessment of Achilles tendon disorders? A two year prospective study. Br J Sports Med 2003; 37(2):149–53.

59. Golano P, Mariani PP, Rodriguez-Niedenfuhr M, Mariani PF, Ruano–Gil D. Arthroscopic anatomy of the posterior ankle ligaments. Arthroscopy 2002; 18(4):353–58.

60. Schaffler GJ, Tirman PF, Stoller DW, Genant HK, Ceballos C, Dillingham MF. Impingement syndrome of the ankle following supination external rotation trauma: MR imaging findings with arthroscopic correlation. Eur Radiol 2003; 13(6):1357–62.

61. Linklater J. MR imaging of ankle impingement lesions. Magn Reson Imaging Clin N Am 2009; 17(4):775–800, vii–viii.

62. Schepsis AA, Jones H, Haas AL. Achilles tendon disorders in athletes. Am J Sports Med 2002; 30(2):287–305.

63. Fernandez-Palazzi F, Rivas S, Mujica P. Achilles tendinitis in ballet dancers. Clin Orthop Relat Res 1990; (257):257–61.

64. Peck DM. Apophyseal injuries in the young athlete. Am Fam Physician 1995; 51(8):1891–95, 1897–98.

65. Ogden JA, Ganey TM, Hill JD, Jaakkola JI. Sever's injury: a stress fracture of the immature calcaneal metaphysis. J Pediatr Orthop 2004; 24(5):488–92.

66. Simmonds FA. The diagnosis of the ruptured Achilles tendon. Practitioner 1957; 179(1069):56–58.

67. Matles AL. Rupture of the tendo achilles: another diagnostic sign. Bull Hosp Joint Dis 1975; 36(1):48–51.

68. O'Brien T. The needle test for complete rupture of the Achilles tendon. J Bone Joint Surg Am 1984; 66(7):1099–101.

69. Patel AT, Gaines K, Malamut R, Park TA, Toro DR, Holland N. Usefulness of electrodiagnostic techniques in the evaluation of suspected tarsal tunnel syndrome: an evidence-based review. Muscle & Nerve 2005; 32(2):236–40.

70. Diers DJ. Medial calcaneal nerve entrapment as a cause for chronic heel pain. Physiother Theory Pract 2008; 24(4):291–98.

71. Park TA, Del Toro DR. The medial calcaneal nerve: anatomy and nerve conduction technique. Muscle & Nerve 1995; 18(1):32–38.

72. Stankovic R, Johnell O, Maly P, Willner S. Use of lumbar extension, slump test, physical and neurological examination in the evaluation of patients with suspected herniated nucleus pulposus. A prospective clinical study. Man Ther 1999; 4(1):25–32.

73. Eizele SA, Sammarco GJ. Fatigue fractures of the foot and ankle in the athlete. Instr Course Lect 1993; 42: 175–83.

74. Weber JM, Vidt LG, Gehl RS, Montgomery T. Calcaneal stress fractures. Clin Podiatr Med Surg 2005; 22(1): 45–54.

75. Conti SF. Posterior tibial tendon problems in athletes. Orthop Clin North Am 1994; 25(1):109–21.

76. Premkumar A, Perry MB, Dwyer AJ, Gerber LH, Johnson D, Venzon D, et al. Sonography and MR imaging of posterior tibial tendinopathy. AJR Am J Roentgenol 2002; 178(1):223–32.

77. Hamilton WG. Stenosing tenosynovitis of the flexor hallucis longus tendon and posterior impingement upon the os trigonum in ballet dancers. Foot Ankle 1982; 3(2):74–80.

78. Schweitzer ME, Karasick D. MRI of the ankle and hindfoot. Semin Ultrasound CT MR 1994; 15(5):410–22.

79. Schweitzer ME, van Leersum M, Ehrlich SS, Wapner K. Fluid in normal and abnormal ankle joints: amount and distribution as seen on MR images. AJR Am J Roentgenol 1994; 162(1):111–14.

80. Lin CF, Gross ML, Weinhold P. Ankle syndesmosis injuries: anatomy, biomechanics, mechanism of injury, and clinical guidelines for diagnosis and intervention. J Orthop Sports Phys Ther 2006; 36(6):372–84.

81. Grath GB. Widening of the ankle mortise. A clinical and experimental study. Acta Chir Scand Suppl 1960; Suppl 263:1–88.

82. Khan KM, Brukner PD, Kearney C, Fuller PJ, Bradshaw CJ, Kiss ZS. Tarsal navicular stress fracture in athletes. Sports Med 1994; 17(1):65–76.

83. Lee S, Anderson RB. Stress fractures of the tarsal navicular. Foot Ankle Clin 2004; 9(1):85–104.

84. Kiss ZS, Khan KM, Fuller PJ. Stress fractures of the tarsal navicular bone: CT findings in 55 cases. AJR Am J Roentgenol 1993; 160(1):111–15.

85. Bradshaw C, Khan K, Brukner P. Stress fracture of the body of the talus in athletes demonstrated with computer tomography. Clin J Sport Med 1996; 6(1):48–51.

86. Rossi F, Dragoni S. Talar body fatigue stress fractures: three cases observed in elite female gymnasts. Skeletal Radiol 2005; 34(7):389–94.

87. Borges JL, Guille JT, Bowen JR. Kohler's bone disease of the tarsal navicular. J Pediatr Orthop 1995; 15(5):596–98.

88. Sammarco GJ, Cooper PS. Flexor hallucis longus tendon injury in dancers and nondancers. Foot Ankle Int 1998; 19(6):356–62.

89. Boruta PM, Beauperthuy GD. Partial tear of the flexor hallucis longus at the knot of Henry: presentation of three cases. Foot Ankle Int 1997; 18(4):243–46.

90. Yde J. The Lauge Hansen classification of malleolar fractures. Acta Orthop Scand 1980; 51(1):181–92.

91. Lauge-Hansen N. Fractures of the ankle. II. Combined experimental-surgical and experimental-roentgenologic investigations. Arch Surg 1950; 60(5):957–85.

92. Sangeorzan BJ, Benirschke SK, Mosca V, Mayo KA, Hansen ST, Jr. Displaced intra-articular fractures of the tarsal navicular. J Bone Joint Surg Am 1989; 71(10):1504–10.

93. Bennell KL, Malcolm SA, Thomas SA, Reid SJ, Brukner PD, Ebeling PR, et al. Risk factors for stress fractures in track and field athletes. A twelve-month prospective study. Am J Sports Med 1996; 24(6):810–18.

94. Torg JS, Pavlov H, Cooley LH, Bryant MH, Arnoczky SP, Bergfeld J, et al. Stress fractures of the tarsal navicular. A retrospective review of twenty-one cases. J Bone Joint Surg Am 1982; 64(5):700–12.

95. Saxena A, Fullem B. Navicular stress fractures: a prospective study on athletes. Foot Ankle Int 2006; 27(11): 917–21.

96. Balduini FC, Tetzlaff J. Historical perspectives on injuries of the ligaments of the ankle. Clin Sports Med 1982; 1(1):3–12.

97. Gebler C, Kukla C, Breitenseher MJ, Nellas ZJ, Mittlboeck M, Trattnig S, et al. Diagnosis of lateral ankle ligament injuries. Comparison between talar tilt, MRI and operative findings in 112 athletes. Acta Orthop Scand 1997; 68(3):286–90.

98. Sammarco GJ. Peroneal tendon injuries. Orthop Clin North Am 1994; 25(1):135–45.

99. Kijowski R, De Smet A, Mukharjee R. Magnetic resonance imaging findings in patients with peroneal tendinopathy and peroneal tenosynovitis. Skeletal Radiol 2007; 36(2):105–14.

100. Clarke HD, Kitaoka HB, Ehman RL. Peroneal tendon injuries. Foot Ankle Int 1998; 19(5):280–88.

101. Pisani G, Pisani PC, Parino E. Sinus tarsi syndrome and subtalar joint instability. Clin Podiatr Med Surg 2005; 22(1):63–77, vii.

102. Frey C, Feder KS, DiGiovanni C. Arthroscopic evaluation of the subtalar joint: does sinus tarsi syndrome exist? Foot Ankle Int 1999; 20(3):185–91.

103. Ferkel RD, Fasulo GJ. Arthroscopic treatment of ankle injuries. Orthop Clin North Am 1994; 25(1):17–32.

104. Robinson P, White LM, Salonen DC, Daniels TR, Ogilvie-Harris D. Anterolateral ankle impingement: MR arthrographic assessment of the anterolateral recess. Radiology 2001; 221(1):186–90.

105. Marshall P, Hamilton WG. Cuboid subluxation in ballet dancers. Am J Sports Med 1992; 20(2):169–75.

106. Klausner VB, McKeigue ME. The sinus tarsi syndrome: a cause of chronic ankle pain. Phys Sportsmed 2000; 28(5):75–80.

107. Breitenseher MJ, Haller J, Kukla C, Gebler C, Kaider A, Fleischmann D, et al. MRI of the sinus tarsi in acute ankle sprain injuries. J Comput Assist Tomogr 1997; 21(2):274–79.

108. Sanders TG, Rathur SK. Impingement syndromes of the ankle. Magn Reson Imaging Clin N Am 2008; 16(1): 29–38, v.

109. Jennings J, Davies GJ. Treatment of cuboid syndrome secondary to lateral ankle sprains: a case series. J Orthop Sports Phys Ther 2005; 35(7):409–15.

110. Mooney M, Maffey–Ward L. Cuboid plantar and dorsal subluxations: assessment and treatment. J Orthop Sports Phys Ther 1994; 20(4):220–26.

111. Subotnick SI. Peroneal cuboid syndrome. J Am Podiatr Med Assoc 1989; 79(8):413–14.

112. Ebraheim NA, Haman SP, Lu J, Padanilam TG. Radiographic evaluation of the calcaneocuboid joint: a cadaver study. Foot Ankle Int 1999; 20(3):178–81.

113. Styf J. Entrapment of the superficial peroneal nerve. Diagnosis and results of decompression. J Bone Joint Surg Br 1989; 71(1):131–35.

114. McCrory P. Exercise-related leg pain: neurological perspective. Med Sci Sports Exerc 2000; 32(3 Suppl):S11–14.

115. Riddle DL, Schappert SM. Volume of ambulatory care visits and patterns of care for patients diagnosed with plantar fasciitis: a national study of medical doctors. Foot Ankle Int 2004; 25(5):303–10.

116. Fredericson M, Misra AK. Epidemiology and etiology of marathon running injuries. Sports Med 2007; 37 (4–5):437–39.

117. Irving DB, Cook JL, Young MA, Menz HB. Obesity and pronated foot type may increase the risk of chronic plantar heel pain: a matched case-control study. BMC Musculoskelet Disord 2007; 8:41.

118. Wearing SC, Smeathers JE, Urry SR, Hennig EM, Hills AP. The pathomechanics of plantar fasciitis. Sports Med 2006; 36(7):585–611.

119. Falsetti P, Frediani B, Acciai C, Baldi F, Filippou G, Galeazzi M, et al. Ultrasonography and magnetic resonance imaging of heel fat pad inflammatory-oedematous lesions in rheumatoid arthritis. Scand J Rheumatol 2006; 35(6):454–58.

120. Falsetti P, Frediani B, Acciai C, Baldi F, Filippou G, Marcolongo R. Heel fat pad involvement in rheumatoid arthritis and in spondyloarthropathies: an ultrasonographic study. Scand J Rheumatol 2004; 33(5):327–31.

121. Kim DH, Hrutkay JM, Grant MP. Radiologic case study. Diagnosis: hypertrophic abductor hallucis muscle (causing tarsal tunnel syndrome). Orthopedics 1997; 20(4):376, 365–66.

122. Cameron AF, Rome K, Hing WA. Ultrasound evaluation of the abductor hallucis muscle: Reliability study. J Foot Ankle Res 2008; 1(1):12.

123. Glazer JL. An approach to the diagnosis and treatment of plantar fasciitis. Phys Sportsmed 2009; 37(2):74–79.

124. Sabir N, Demirlenk S, Yagci B, Karabulut N, Cubukcu S. Clinical utility of sonography in diagnosing plantar fasciitis. J Ultrasound Med 2005; 24(8):1041–48.

125. Jahss MH. The sesamoids of the hallux. Clin Orthop Relat Res 1981; (157):88–97.

126. Potter HG, Pavlov H, Abrahams TG. The hallux sesamoids revisited. Skeletal Radiol 1992; 21(7):437–44.

127. Cohen BE. Hallux sesamoid disorders. Foot Ankle Clin 2009; 14(1):91–104.

128. Dedmond BT, Cory JW, McBryde A, Jr. The hallucal sesamoid complex. J Am Acad Orthop Surg 2006; 14(13): 745–53.

129. Faciszewski T, Burks RT, Manaster BJ. Subtle injuries of the Lisfranc joint. J Bone Joint Surg Am 1990; 72(10):1519–22.

130. Donley BG, Tisdel CL, Sferra JJ, Hall JO. Diagnosing and treating hallux valgus: a conservative approach for a common problem. Cleve Clin J Med 1997; 64(9):469–74.

131. Hart ES, deAsla RJ, Grottkau BE. Current concepts in the treatment of hallux valgus. Orthop Nurs 2008; 27(5):274–80; quiz 81–82.

132. Durrant B, Chockalingam N. Functional hallux limitus: a review. J Am Podiatr Med Assoc 2009; 99(3):236–43.

133. Alexander IJ, Johnson KA, Parr JW. Morton's neuroma: a review of recent concepts. Orthopedics 1987; 10(1): 103–6.

134. Kinnard P, Lirette R. Freiberg's disease and dorsiflexion osteotomy. J Bone Joint Surg Br 1991; 73(5):864–65.

135. Rauh MJ, Macera CA, Trone DW, Shaffer RA, Brodine SK. Epidemiology of stress fracture and lower-extremity overuse injury in female recruits. Med Sci Sports Exerc 2006; 38(9):1571–77.

136. Milgrom C, Giladi M, Stein M, Kashtan H, Margulies JY, Chisin R, et al. Stress fractures in military recruits. A prospective study showing an unusually high incidence. J Bone Joint Surg Br 1985; 67(5):732–35.

137. Milgrom C, Giladi M, Chisin R, Dizian R. The long-term followup of soldiers with stress fractures. Am J Sports Med 1985; 13(6):398–400.

138. Curtis MJ, Myerson M, Szura B. Tarsometatarsal joint injuries in the athlete. Am J Sports Med 1993; 21(4): 497–502.

139. Still GP, Fowler MB. Joplin's neuroma or compression neuropathy of the plantar proper digital nerve to the hallux: clinicopathologic study of three cases. J Foot Ankle Surg 1998; 37(6):524–30.

140. McCrory P, Bell S, Bradshaw C. Nerve entrapments of the lower leg, ankle and foot in sport. Sports Med 2002; 32(6):371–91.

141. Fredericson M, Jennings F, Beaulieu C, Matheson GO. Stress fractures in athletes. Top Magn Reson Imaging 2006; 17(5):309–25.

142. Davidson G, Pizzari T, Mayes S. The influence of second toe and metatarsal length on stress fractures at the base of the second metatarsal in classical dancers. Foot Ankle Int 2007; 28(10):1082–86.

143. Paice E. Reflex sympathetic dystrophy. BMJ 1995; 310(6995):1645–48.

144. Hsu ES. Practical management of complex regional pain syndrome. Am J Ther 2009; 16(2):147–54.

145. Stiell IG, Greenberg GH, McKnight RD, Wells GA. Ottawa ankle rules for radiography of acute injuries. N Z Med J 1995; 108(996):111.

146. Shereff MJ, Cullivan WT, Johnson KA. Osteoid-osteoma of the foot. J Bone Joint Surg Am 1983; 65(5):638–41.

147. Davies M, Cassar-Pullicino VN, Davies AM, McCall IW, Tyrrell PN. The diagnostic accuracy of MR imaging in osteoid osteoma. Skeletal Radiol 2002; 31(10):559–69.

9

The spine triangle

Introduction

B ack pain is arguably the most prevalent and costly musculoskeletal condition in the western world.[1] About nine out of ten adults experience back pain at some point in their lives, and five out of ten working adults have back pain every year.[2] The vast majority (90%) improve over a three-month period, but nearly 50% have at least one recurrent episode. It is also the most common health condition causing individuals to be absent from the labor force, and healthcare costs are measured in billions of dollars.[3]

In sport, back pain is common, affecting up to 40% of participants in sports, especially running and rotation-based sports such as golf, tennis, and cricket.[4–6]

The anatomy of this area is complicated, and the authors believe a thorough knowledge of the anatomy of the area is necessary in order to correctly differentiate a diagnosis from within the possible pathologies. Even where it is not possible to make a precise anatomical and pathological diagnosis, this does not prevent management and treatment. In the majority of cases of low back pain, the principles of management depend on careful assessment to detect any abnormality, and then appropriate treatment to correct that abnormality.

The spine

The back consists of the posterior aspect of the trunk. The bony elements consist of the vertebrae, as well as the proximal ribs, superior aspect of the pelvis, and basal regions of the skull. The back muscles, which are distributed in three layers, connect the skeletal structures. The spinal canal runs through the spinal column, and provides nerves to the rest of the body.

There is a single triangle which is utilized in this chapter to enable the reader to fully appreciate the relationships between the structures in the back. These, as always, utilize bony landmarks to construct a relationship between various key tissues.

Functions of the back

The skeletal and muscular components of the back are designed to: (a) carry the head; (b) support the body's weight; (c) transmit forces through the pelvis to the lower limbs; (d) brace and help maneuver the upper limbs; (e) move the upper limbs, ribs, thorax, and neck; (f) maintain posture; and (g) protect the components of the nervous system, such as the spinal cord.[7, 8]

Key anatomical structures of the back

Bones

The skeletal components of the back consist mainly of the vertebral bones and associated intervertebral discs. The vertebral column is positioned posteriorly in the body at the midline. The base of the skull, scapulae, superior aspect of the pelvic bones, and proximal ribs also contribute to the bony framework and provide the base for muscle attachment. The vertebrae are divided into five groups, based on morphology and location. There are seven cervical, twelve thoracic, five lumbar, five sacral (usually fused into a single sacral bone), and up to four coccygeal vertebrae (also fused into the coccyx), making 33 vertebrae in total.

It is important for clinicians to know the key surface anatomical landmarks (Table 9.1). This aids in the examination of the back and localization of structures, and in the avoidance of injury with investigations and treatment. For example, certain investigations, such as a lumbar puncture, require specific anatomical knowledge that the needle must be inserted below the level of the spinal cord (which terminates at L1/L2 in adults) in order to avoid spinal cord injury, and above the level of S2 if the subarachnoid space is to be accessed.

Table 9.1 Key surface anatomical landmarks	
Spinal level	**Surface anatomical landmarks**
C7 spinous process	Easily located as a prominence at the lower part of the neck
T3 spinous process	At the level of the root or medial part of the spine of the scapula
T7 spinous process	At the level of the inferior angle of the scapula
L1/L2 intervertebral disc	In adults, the spinal cord terminates at this level
L4 spinous process	Highest point of the iliac crest
S2 spinous process	Level of the posterior superior iliac spine
T12 spinous process	Level with the mid-point of a vertical line between the inferior angle of the scapula and the iliac crest
S2 spinous process	The "sacral dimples", which mark the position of the posterior superior iliac spine, are level with this
S2	Subarachnoid space ends

Vertebral canal and spinal cord

The **spinal cord** lies within a bony vertebral canal and is surrounded by a series of three meningeal membranes (the pia mater, arachnoid mater, and dura mater). Between the walls of the vertebral canal and the dura is an extradural space, containing a plexus of veins emeshed in connective tissue. The spinal cord extends from the foramen magnum to approximately the level of the disc between L1 and L2 in adults. The distal end of the cord (the conus medullaris) is cone-shaped, with a thin tail (the filum terminale) which continues inferiorly from the apex of the conus medullaris. Below the end of the spinal cord, the cluster of lumbar, sacral, and coccygeal nerve roots is called the "cauda equina".

Joints

There are a number of different types of joints between the vertebrae, including the **intervertebral joints** between vertebral bodies, **zygapophyseal joints** between the superior and inferior articular processes of the adjacent vertebrae, and **uncovertebral joints** at the lateral margins of the upper surfaces of the cervical vertebrae (uncinate processes), which articulate with the body of the vertebrae above. Although the movement between any two vertebrae is small (each level contributes about 3% of the total spinal movement), the sum of movement among all vertebrae results in a large range of movement by the intact vertebral column.

Ligaments

The joints between the vertebrae are supported by a number of ligaments which connect the vertebral bodies, including the **interspinous ligaments** which pass between adjacent vertebral spinous processes, the **supraspinous ligaments** which pass along the tips of the vertebral spinous processes from C7 to the sacrum (above this level, the ligament becomes structurally distinct and forms a triangular structure termed the "ligamentum nuche"), the **anterior and posterior longitudinal ligaments** which lie on the anterior and posterior surfaces of the vertebrae, and the **ligamenta flava** which pass between the laminae of adjacent vertebrae and form part of the posterior surface of the vertebral canal.

Spinal nerves

The 31 pairs of spinal nerves emerge from the vertebral canal between the vertebrae; Figure 9.1. There are eight pairs of cervical nerves, twelve thoracic, five lumbar, five sacral and one coccygeal nerve. Each nerve is attached to the spinal cord by a posterior (sensory fibers) root and an anterior (motor fibers) root. A spinal segment is defined as the area of the spinal cord which gives rise to the posterior and anterior roots, which in turn form a single pair of spinal nerves. After leaving the vertebral canal, each spinal nerve branches into the anterior and posterior rami, which innervate most of the skeletal muscles of the body, and provide the cutaneous innervation of most regions of the body except the head, and in the case of the anterior rami form the major somatic plexi and visceral components of the sympathetic trunk and prevertebral plexus.

The major somatic plexi formed from the anterior rami of the spinal nerves are the cervical (C1 to C4), brachial (C5 to T1), lumbar (L1 to L4), sacral (L4 to S4), and coccygeal (S5 to Co) plexi. The most important of these clinically are the brachial and lumbosacral plexi, as these innervate the arm and leg respectively, and lesions of these relate to a number of important clinical problems. Figures 9.3 and 9.4.

Each spinal nerve exits the vertebral canal through the intervertebral foramen, which is formed by the vertebral arches of the adjacent vertebrae. Any pathology which reduces the size of an intervertebral foramen, such as intervertebral disc herniation or a degenerative zygapophyseal joint, can compress the associated spinal nerve. Once a spinal nerve is compressed or irritated, a variety of neurological signs may follow, including sensory loss, reduction in the deep tendon reflexes, and myotomal weakness. The patterns of the most common spinal nerve syndromes easily detected on clinical examination are illustrated in Table 9.2 and Figure 9.1 over page illustrates the relevant root sensory representation in more detail.

Muscles

The movement and clinical function of the back are largely generated by the muscles, which are arranged in three distinct anatomical layers; Figures 9.5 and 9.6. The superficial muscle layer is involved with movement of the upper limbs, shoulders and neck, the intermediate muscle layer acts on the ribs, and the deep muscle layer assists in moving and supporting

Figure 9.1 The spine

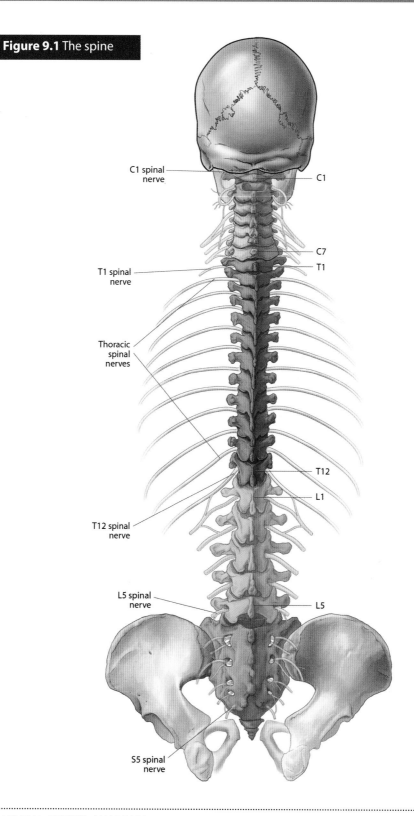

C1 spinal nerve

C1

C7

T1 spinal nerve

T1

Thoracic spinal nerves

T12

L1

T12 spinal nerve

L5 spinal nerve

L5

S5 spinal nerve

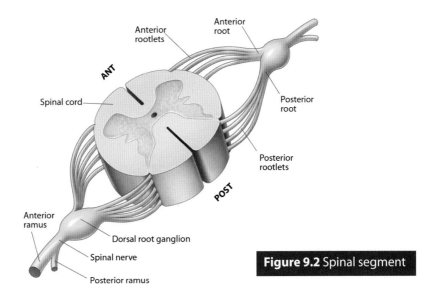

Figure 9.2 Spinal segment

Figure 9.3 Brachial plexus

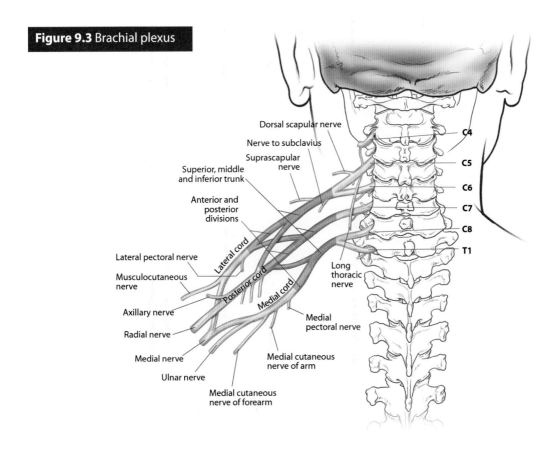

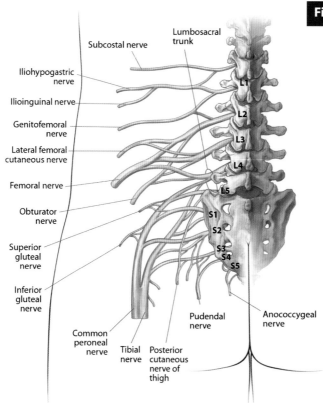

Figure 9.4 Lumbosacral plexus

Table 9.2 Most common spinal nerve syndromes			
Spinal nerve root	**Pattern of weakness**	**Pattern of sensory loss**	**Affected tendon reflex**
C5	Shoulder abduction	Lateral arm	Biceps
C5/C6	Elbow flexion, wrist extension, finger abduction	Lateral arm and forearm, thumb	Supinator
C6/C7	Elbow extension, wrist flexion, and hand abduction	Lateral forearm, digits 1–3	Triceps
T7–9	Abdominal	Lateral chest and upper abdomen to midline	Epigastric (abdominal)
T9–11	Abdominal	Lateral abdomen to midline	Upper abdominal
T11/T12	Abdominal	Lateral lower abdomen to midline	Lower abdominal
L1/L2	Hip flexion	Inguinal crease	Cremaster
L3/L4	Knee extension	Medial thigh, knee, and medial calf	Knee
S1	Knee flexion, foot plantar flexion, foot eversion	Lateral foot, heel, and distal mid-calf	Ankle
S4/S5	–	Perianal	Anal

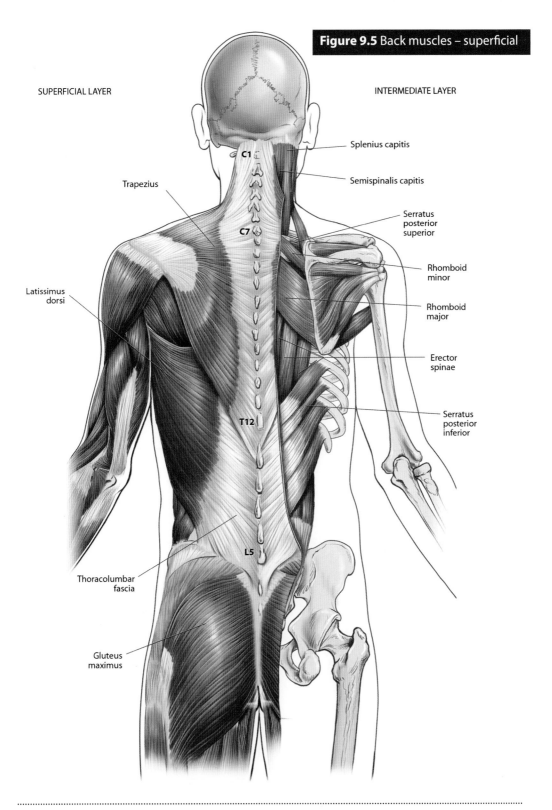

Figure 9.5 Back muscles – superficial

SUPERFICIAL LAYER

INTERMEDIATE LAYER

Splenius capitis

Semispinalis capitis

Trapezius

Serratus
posterior
superior

Rhomboid
minor

Rhomboid
major

Latissimus
dorsi

Erector
spinae

Serratus
posterior
inferior

Thoracolumbar
fascia

Gluteus
maximus

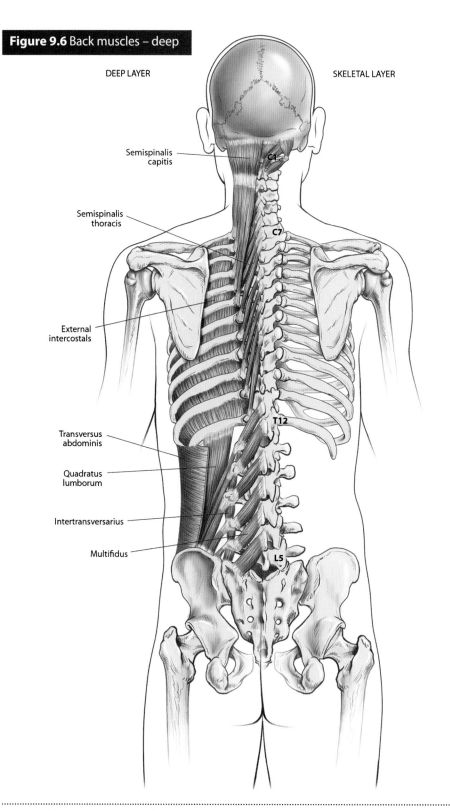

Figure 9.6 Back muscles – deep

DEEP LAYER

SKELETAL LAYER

Semispinalis
capitis

C1

Semispinalis
thoracis

C7

External
intercostals

T12

Transversus
abdominis

Quadratus
lumborum

Intertransversarius

Multifidus

L5

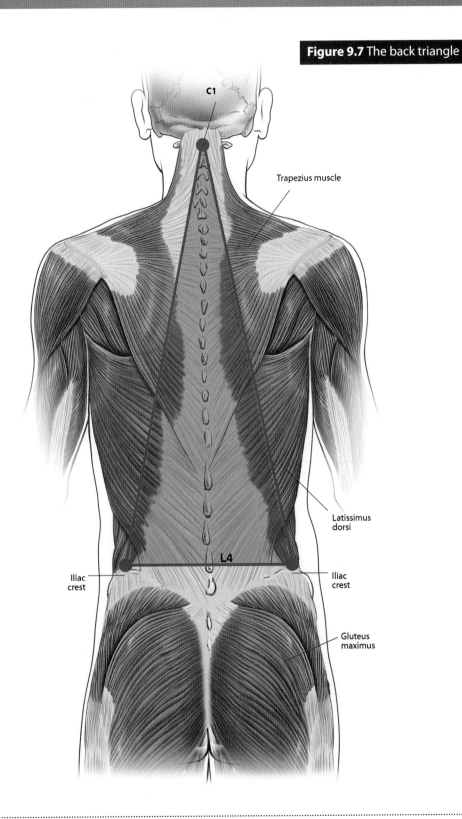

Figure 9.8 Back triangle—pathoanatomic approach

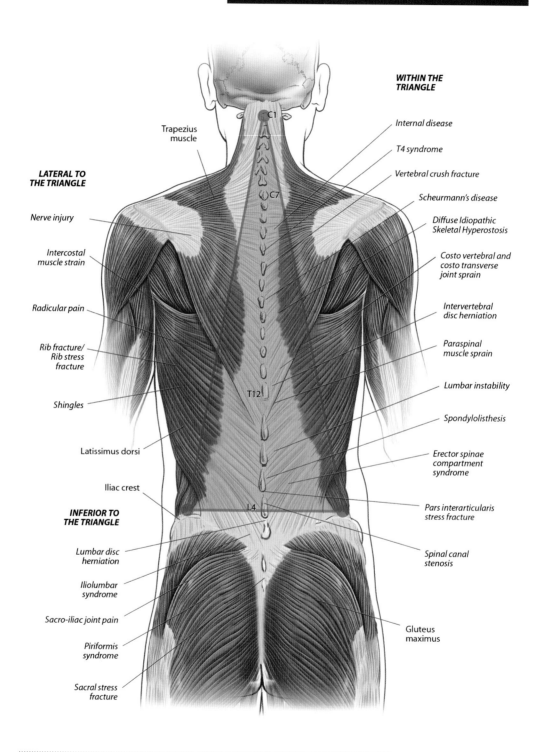

WITHIN THE TRIANGLE

Internal disease

T4 syndrome

Vertebral crush fracture

Scheurmann's disease

Diffuse Idiopathic Skeletal Hyperostosis

Costo vertebral and costo transverse joint sprain

Intervertebral disc herniation

Paraspinal muscle sprain

Lumbar instability

Spondylolisthesis

Erector spinae compartment syndrome

Pars interarticularis stress fracture

Spinal canal stenosis

Gluteus maximus

LATERAL TO THE TRIANGLE

Nerve injury

Intercostal muscle strain

Radicular pain

Rib fracture/ Rib stress fracture

Shingles

Latissimus dorsi

Iliac crest

INFERIOR TO THE TRIANGLE

Lumbar disc herniation

Iliolumbar syndrome

Sacro-iliac joint pain

Piriformis syndrome

Sacral stress fracture

Trapezius muscle

C1

C7

T12

L4

the spinal segments. This chapter will largely focus on the superficial and intermediate layers of muscles, given their importance clinically, and will present them in relation to the back triangle below.

Landmarks of the back triangle

There is one main triangle utilized in this chapter, to enable the reader to fully appreciate the relationships between structures; Figure 9.7. This, as always, utilizes bony landmarks to construct a relationship between various key tissues.

The landmarks of the back triangle are:

> the tip of the spinous process of C1

> the highest points of the iliac crest on both sides

Anatomical relationships of borders of the back triangle

The inferior border of the triangle runs in a straight line between the highest parts of the iliac crest. It is important to know the order in which the structures are palpable.

The structures palpable from lateral to medial along the inferior border are:

> iliac crest

> gluteus maximus (upper fibers)

> thoracolumbar fascia

> erector spine muscles (deep to TL fascia)

> spinous process of L4

The **iliac crest**: the bones of the pelvis consist of the right and left pelvic bones (called ilia), the sacrum, and the coccyx. The sacrum articulates superiorly with the vertebra L5 at the lumbosacral joint. The pelvic bones articulate posteriorly with the sacrum at the sacroiliac joints, and with each other anteriorly at the pubic symphysis. The iliac crest is the highest point of the ilia laterally.

The **gluteus maximus** is the largest muscle in the gluteal region, and lies on top of the other gluteal muscles. It has a broad origin, extending from the ilium behind the posterior gluteal line, and along the dorsal surface of the lower sacrum and the lateral surface of the coccyx, to the external surface of the sacrotuberous ligament. It is also attached to fascia overlying the gluteus medius muscle, and to fascia covering the erector spine muscle. The muscle inserts into the posterior aspect of the iliotibial tract. The function of the gluteus maximus is principally to extend the flexed thigh at the hip joint. In addition, it also plays a role in stabilizing the knee and hip joints. The muscle is innervated by the inferior gluteal nerve (L4, L5, S1).

The **thoracolumbar fascia** covers the deep muscles of the back and trunk, and is critical to the structural integrity of the region. Superiorly, it is continuous with the superficial lamina of the cervical fascia in the neck; in the thoracic region, it covers the deep muscles and separates them from the muscles in the superficial and intermediate groups; medially, it attaches to the spinous processes of the thoracic vertebrae; and laterally, to the angles of the ribs. The medial attachments of the latissimus dorsi and serratus posterior inferior muscles blend into the thoracolumbar fascia.

In the lumbar region, the thoracolumbar fascia consists of three distinct layers. The posterior layer is attached to the spinous processes of the lumbar vertebrae, sacral vertebrae, and supraspinous ligament – from these attachments, the middle layer is attached medially to the tips of the transverse processes of the lumbar vertebrae, and the anterior layer covers the anterior surface of the quadratus lumborum muscle, and is attached medially to the transverse processes of the lumbar vertebrae inferiorly. The anterior layer also forms the lateral arcuate ligament for the attachment of the diaphragm. At the lateral border of the quadratus lumborum, the anterior layer joins them and forms the aponeurotic origin for the transversus abdominis muscle of the abdominal wall.

The **erector spine** is the largest group of intrinsic back muscles, which lie posterolaterally to the vertebral column, between the spinous processes medially, and the angles of the ribs laterally. They are covered in the thoracic and lumbar regions by the thoracolumbar fascia, as well as the serratus posterior inferior, rhomboid, and splenius muscles. The muscle origin arises from a broad tendon attached to the sacrum, spinous processes of the lumbar and lower thoracic vertebrae, and iliac crest. This muscle mass divides in the upper lumbar region into three vertical columns of muscle, each of which is further subdivided regionally (lumborum, thoracis, cervicis, and capitis), depending on where the muscles attach superiorly. The muscle has three defined components – the most laterally placed column of the erector spine muscles is the **iliocostalis**, which passes from the common tendon of origin to multiple insertions into the angles of the ribs and the transverse processes of the lower cervical vertebrae; the middle column is the **longissimus**, which is the largest of the erector spine subdivisions, and extends from the common tendon of origin to the base of the skull; and the most medially placed column is the **spinalis**, which connects the spinous processes of the adjacent vertebrae.

The **L4 spinous process** projects posteriorly and inferiorly from the roof of the vertebral arch of the L4 vertebra.

The lateral borders of the triangle run from the lateral iliac crest to the spinous process of CI in the midline.

The structures palpable from lateral to midline are:

> iliac crest

> external oblique muscle

> internal oblique muscle

> latissimus dorsi muscle:
>   - serratus posterior inferior muscle (deep to latissimus dorsi)
>   - erector spine muscle (deep to latissimus dorsi)

> trapezius muscle:
>   - rhomboid major and minor muscles (deep to trapezius)

> thoracolumbar fascia:
> - splenius capitus (deep to thoracolumbar fascia)
> - semispinalis capitus (deep to thoracolumbar fascia)

> spinous process of C1

Iliac crest

The **external oblique** muscle, which lies immediately under the superficial fascia of the abdominal wall, is the most superficial of the abdominal wall muscles. Its fibers pass inferomedially, and it has an aponeurotic component which covers the anterior part of the abdominal wall to the midline. Approaching the midline, the aponeuroses form the linea alba, which extends from the xiphoid process to the pubic symphysis. The lower border of the external oblique aponeurosis forms the inguinal ligament on each side. The origin of the muscle is from muscular slips from the outer surfaces of the lower eight ribs (ribs 5 to 12), and it inserts into the lateral iliac crest, as well as the linea alba. The muscle derives its innervation from the anterior rami of the lower six thoracic spinal nerves (T7 to T12), and its function is to compress the abdominal contents, flex the trunk, and turn the anterior part of the abdomen to the opposite side.

Deep to the external oblique muscle is the **internal oblique** muscle. Its origin is from the thoracolumbar fascia, the iliac crest between the origins of the external and transversus muscles, and the lateral two-thirds of the inguinal ligament. It inserts into the inferior border of the lower three or four ribs, the linea alba, pubic crest, and pectineal line of the pelvis. It receives its innervation from the anterior rami of the lower six thoracic spinal nerves (T7 to T12) and L1. It has the same function as the external oblique muscle.

The **latissimus dorsi** is a triangular muscle which begins in the lower portion of the back, and tapers as it ascends to a narrow tendon which attaches to the humerus anteriorly. It arises from the spinous processes of T7 to L5 and the sacrum, iliac crest, and ribs 10 to 12, and inserts into the base of the intertubercular sulcus of the humerus. It is innervated by the thoracodorsal nerve (C6 to C8). Its role is to extend, adduct, and medially rotate the humerus.

The **serratus posterior inferior** is one of the intermediate muscle layers of the back, and is deep to the latissimus dorsi. The **serratus posterior superior** is deep to the rhomboid muscles. Both serratus posterior muscles arise from the spinous processes of T11 to L3 and the supraspinous ligaments, and insert into the lower border of ribs 9 to 12, just lateral to their angles. The muscles are innervated by the anterior rami of the lower thoracic nerves (T9 to T12) and have an important role in depressing ribs 9 to 12, which prevents the lower ribs from being elevated when the diaphragm contracts.

Erector spine muscle

The **trapezius** is a triangular muscle, with the base of the triangle (the muscle's origin) situated along the vertebral column, and the apex (the muscle's insertion) pointing toward the tip of the shoulder. It arises from the superior nuchal line, external occipital protuberance, ligamentum nuche, and spinous processes of C7 to T12, and inserts into the lateral one-third of the clavicle, acromion, and spine of the scapula. The innervation of this muscle arises from the accessory nerve (cranial nerve XI). In addition, there are proprioceptive fibers from the trapezius, which pass into the branches of the cervical plexus, and enter the spinal cord at spinal-cord levels C3 and C4. Contraction of the muscle elevates the scapula. In addition, the superior and inferior fibers work together to rotate the lateral aspect of the scapula upward, which needs to occur when raising the upper limb above the head.

The two **rhomboid muscles** are inferior to the levator scapulae. The rhomboid minor is superior to the rhomboid major, and is a small muscle which arises from the ligamentum nuche of the neck and the spinous processes of vertebrae C7 and T1, and attaches to the medial scapular border, opposite the root of the spine of the scapula. The rhomboid major originates from the spinous processes of the upper thoracic vertebrae, and inserts into the medial scapular border, inferior to the rhomboid minor. The dorsal scapular nerve, a branch of the brachial plexus, innervates both rhomboid muscles. The rhomboid muscles work to retract the scapula toward the vertebral column. With other muscles, they may also rotate the lateral aspect of the scapula inferiorly.

Thoracolumbar fascia

The **splenius capitis** arises from the lower half of the ligamentum nuche and spinous processes of C7 to T4, and inserts into the mastoid process and skull, below the lateral one-third of the superior nuchal line. It is innervated by the posterior rami middle cervical nerves. In conjunction with the other deep spinotransversales muscles, the splenius capitus draws the head backward, extending the neck, and each muscle individually draws and rotates the head to the ipsilateral side.

One muscle in the deep muscle layer, the **semispinalis capitis**, arises from the transverse processes of T1 to T6 (or T7) and C7 and articular processes of C4 to C6, and inserts into the area medially between the superior and inferior nuchal lines of the occipital bone. It is innervated by the posterior rami of the cervical nerves. The muscle works in conjunction with the other transversospinales muscles and, when contracting bilaterally, pulls the head posteriorly, whereas unilateral contraction pulls the head posteriorly and turns it, causing the chin to move superiorly and turn toward the side of the contracting muscle.

The **C1 spinous process** projects posteriorly from the vertebral arch of the axis vertebra.

Within the triangle lie:

> vertebral column (C1–L4)

> spinal cord and nerves

> trapezius muscles

> erector spine muscles

> latissimus dorsi muscle

> thoracolumbar fascia

> transversospinales and segmental muscles (deep to trapezius)

> rhomboid major muscle (deep to trapezius)

> serratus posterior superior muscle (deep to trapezius)

The anatomical details of all of these components, with the exception of the transverso-spinales and segmental muscles, have been discussed above.

The deep or intrinsic muscles of the back extend from the pelvis to the skull, and are innervated by the segmental branches of the posterior rami of the spinal nerves. They include the spinotransversales muscles (extensors and rotators of the head and neck), the erector spine and transversospinales (extensors and rotators of the vertebral column), and the interspinales and intertransversarii (the short segmental muscles of the spine).

The **transversospinales** muscles run obliquely upward and medially from the transverse processes to the spinous processes, filling the groove between these two vertebral projections, and are segmentally innervated by the posterior rami of the spinal nerves. They are deep to the erector spine, and consist of three major subgroups – the semispinalis, multifidus, and rotatores muscles. The **semispinalis** muscles are the most superficial group of muscles in the transversospinales group. These muscles arise from the transverse spinal processes in the lower thoracic region, and end by attaching to the vertebral spinous processes and nuchal line of the skull, crossing between four and six vertebrae from their point of origin to their point of attachment. Deep to the semispinalis is the **multifidus** group. Muscles in this group span the length of the vertebral column, arising from the sacrum, erector spine, posterior superior iliac spine, mammillary processes of the lumbar vertebrae, transverse processes of the thoracic vertebrae, and articular processes of the lower four cervical vertebrae. They insert into the base of the spinous processes of all vertebrae from L5 to C2. The small **rotatores** muscles are the deepest of the transversospinales group. They are present throughout the length of the vertebral column. Their fibers pass upward and medially from the transverse processes to the spinous processes, crossing two vertebrae (long rotators), or attaching to adjacent vertebrae (short rotators). When muscles in the transversospinales group contract bilaterally, they extend the vertebral column, an action similar to that of the erector spine group. However, when the muscles on only one side contract, they pull the spinous processes toward the transverse processes on that side, causing the trunk to turn or rotate in the opposite direction.

The two groups of **segmental** muscles are deeply placed in the back and innervated by the posterior rami of the spinal nerves. The first group of segmental muscles are the **levatores costarum** muscles, which arise from the transverse processes of vertebrae C7 to T11, and insert into the rib below the vertebra of origin in the area of the tubercle. The second group of segmental muscles are the true segmental muscles of the back – the **interspinales**, which pass between the adjacent spinous processes, and the **intertransversarii**, which pass between the adjacent transverse processes. Their innervation is segmental, and their function is to elevate the ribs and, most importantly, to stabilize the vertebrae during spinal movements.

Patho-anatomic approach

Back pain is an extremely common problem in sports, as well as in the general population. There are numerous causes, and in many cases it may not be possible to make a specific anatomical diagnosis. The back triangle system is designed to assist with the clinical presentations of these problems (see Figure 9.8).

Inferior to the triangle

Lumbar disc herniation occurs 15 times more often than cervical disc herniation, and it is one of the most common causes of lower back pain. Disc herniations can result from general wear and tear, or from acute events such as lifting. There is also a strong genetic component.

Table 9.3 A patho-anatomic approach; inferior to the spine triangle				
Define and align	**Pathology**	**Listen and localize**	**Palpate and recreate**	**Alleviate and investigate**
Inferior to the spine triangle	L5 disc herniation	Pain. Radicular symptoms (weakness, numbness) in L5 distribution	L5 weakness (toe extension, foot eversion), sensory loss in lateral calf and dorsum of foot, loss of ankle tenson reflex	MRI
	SIJ disorders	Upper buttock and low back pain. Spasm in hip external rotators. History of spondylo-arthropathy [9–15]	Localized tenderness over SIJ and attached ligaments. Positive SIJ stress tests, although reliability low [16, 17]	Plain x-ray and MRI may be helpful, although not specific.[18] Local anesthetic block is only reliable diagnostic method [19]
	Iliolumbar ligament syndrome	Upper buttock and low back pain. Difficult to differentiate from SIJ disorders [20]	Localized tenderness over iliolumbar ligaments	No reliable imaging modality. Local anesthetic diagnostic block may help localize [21, 22]
	Piriformis syndrome	Localized pain in buttock and posterior thigh	Tenderness in hip ER muscles. Reduced ROM in hip external rotators. Reduced straight leg raise. Freiberg's maneuver (forced internal rotation of extended thigh) may be useful [23–26]	Imaging not helpful. NCS/EMG occasionally positive [27, 23–26]
	Sacral stress fracture	Most common in female distance runners. Unilateral non-specific low back, buttock, or hip pain exacerbated by weight-bearing activity	Local bony tenderness [28, 29]	Bone scan, CT, or MRI [28, 29]

Mutation in genes coding for proteins involved in the regulation of the extracellular matrix, such as MMP2 and THBS2, has been demonstrated to contribute to lumbar disc herniation.[30] An L5 disc herniation presentation would be expected to result in radicular symptoms in L5 distribution, with weakness of the great toe/ankle dorsiflexion, and reduced sensation on the lateral calf and dorsum of the foot. Most disc herniations are self-limiting and simply require conservative treatment, with one study suggesting that 75% recover within three months.[31]

SIJ pain is usually due to inflammation of one of the sacroiliac joints, and this is a common cause of unilateral low back pain or buttock pain. In some individuals, this may be part of a generalized arthritis such as seronegative spondyloarthropathy.[9-15] Common problems of the sacroiliac joint are often called "sacroiliac joint dysfunction", and reflect either hypo- or hypermobility of this synovial joint. Mechanical SIJ dysfunction usually causes a dull, unilateral, low back pain ache.[32] The pain may become worse and sharp while doing activities such as standing up from a seated position, or lifting the knee up to the chest during stair climbing.[33] Occasionally there may be referred pain into the lower limb, which can be mistaken for sciatica from a herniated lumbar disc. This can be differentiated from radicular pain with a straight leg raise test. This test, when negative, rules out over 90% of patients with true radicular pain, or pain from a nerve root compression such as a disc herniation or protrusion.[34] Sacroiliac joint dysfunction is tested in many different ways, although the reliability of most individual clinical tests has been shown to be low.[16] Plain x-ray and MRI scan may be helpful, although they are not specific.[18] A local anesthetic block is often the only reliable diagnostic method.[19]

The **iliolumbar ligament** runs from the transverse process of the fifth lumbar vertebra to the posterior aspect of the iliac crest.[21] Damage to this ligament may cause pain in the sacroiliac joint area, and it can be virtually impossible to tell the difference between this injury and a sacroiliac joint injury.[20] There may be localized pain over the ligament, and there is no reliable imaging modality. A local anesthetic diagnostic block may help to localize it.[22]

Piriformis or deep gluteal syndrome[27] is often proposed in athletes as a cause of buttock and/or leg pain. Clinically, the findings are non-specific, with tenderness and reduced range of movement in the hip's external rotator muscles. If the sciatic nerve is involved, then the straight leg raise will be reduced. Imaging is generally not helpful; NCS and EMG are occasionally positive where longstanding nerve compression is present.[27, 23-26]

Sacral stress fractures are generally insufficiency fractures of the sacrum and pelvis, and may be confused with metastatic lesions, especially if bony resorption at the fracture is present on x-ray. These may be seen in individuals with osteoporosis, or in female long-distance runners with the so-called athletic triad. Generally there is a background of increasing exercise-related pain, and a sudden onset of severe pain at the site of the lesion with activity. An isotope bone scan is useful for localizing the lesion, and x-rays or CT scans through the lesion are usually necessary to confirm the diagnosis. Healing may take up to nine months, and patients need protected weight-bearing in order to avoid late displacement and possible malunion.[28, 29]

Lateral to the triangle

Intercostal muscle strain is an injury to the muscles between the ribs. It results in pain on coughing, chest wall movement, and breathing. Usually there is a history of trauma (e.g. a motor vehicle collision), a chronic cough or vomiting, and localized tenderness over the muscle. No imaging is required, although you may need to rule out rib stress fracture, depending on the clinical situation. Treatment is conservative.[35, 36]

Radicular pain from spinal nerve compression is similar to that discussed above. Clinically, there will be pain in the chest wall, with altered sensation corresponding to spinal dermatome,

Table 9.4 A patho-anatomic approach; lateral to the spine triangle				
Define and align	**Pathology**	**Listen and localize**	**Palpate and recreate**	**Alleviate and investigate**
Lateral to the spine triangle	Intercostal muscle strain	Pain on coughing, chest wall movement. History of chronic cough/vomiting. Common in rowers[35, 36]	Tenderness over muscle	No imaging required. May need to rule out rib stress fracture
	Radicular pain	Pain in chest wall corresponding to spinal dermatome[37–39]	Altered sensation in dermatomal distribution. Brachial plexus tension test (Elvey's test) may be useful[37–39]	No imaging required unless persistent > 6 weeks. CT or MRI may demonstrate cause. Nerve root infiltartion with local anesthetic occasionally useful[37]
	Rib fracture	History of blow to chest. Pain with inspiration and coughing[40, 41]	Local rib tenderness. Check for pneumothorax[40, 41]	Plain CXR, PA, and lateral film with rib views
	Rib stress fracture	Pain on coughing, chest wall movement. Seen in rowers, golfers, canoeists, baseball pitchers[42–44]	Tenderness over stress fracture. Pain on "springing" chest wall[42–44]	Ultrasound, plain film, bone scan, or MRI to exclude
	Nerve injury to localized back muscle	Pain. Localized weakness	Localized muscle weakness or abnormal movement	NCS or EMG
	Herpes zoster (shingles)	Localized dermatomal pain and vesicular rash. History of immunosuppression should be sought[45, 46]	Rash	No test required. Clinical diagnosis[45, 46]

and this is usually due to an intervertebral disc injury. Imaging modalities such as MRI will reveal the cause, and should be done if the pain is persistent (more than six weeks), systemic signs are present (e.g. loss of weight), there is a known history of malignancy, or if there are neurological signs to suggest spinal cord compression.[37-39]

Rib fracture is usually due to localized trauma, such as a blow to the chest wall while playing football. There is pain with inspiration, and coughing and localized tenderness on examination. Plain chest x-ray, including a lateral view with rib views, is important to rule out damage to underlying structures, in particular to exclude a pneumothorax.[40, 41]

By comparison, a rib stress fracture usually is seen in an individual with a chronic cough (e.g. a pertussis infection), and there will be localized pain on coughing, sneezing, and chest wall movement. Similar to the rib fracture above, there will be tenderness over the site of the stress fracture, and pain on "springing" the chest wall. Usually no imaging is required, as the causal history is clear, although plain film will reveal the fracture if required.[42-44]

Localized nerve injury to back muscles can occur after an illness such as neuritis, or trauma. For example, a particular complication of acute brachial neuritis, or Parsonage-Turner syndrome, is involvement of the suprascapular nerve, resulting in weakness of the spinati muscles, which in turn causes weakness of shoulder external rotation and abduction. The problem is usually apparent on neurological examination, and can be confirmed with nerve conduction studies and needle electromyography.

Herpes zoster (shingles) can present with involvement of a single spinal nerve, and presents with localized dermatomal pain, often very severe, associated with a pathognomonic vesicular rash. No investigative test is usually required, although the herpes infection can be confirmed with microbiological studies of the vesicular fluid. Treatment is usually pain relief and, if the infection is caught early, then antiviral therapy can minimize the symptomatic period.[45, 46]

Within the triangle

Intervertebral disc herniation has been discussed above. The critical clinical step is to exclude spinal cord compression, through a thorough neurological examination and imaging if required.[31, 47-54]

Intervertebral joint sprain is a common clinical problem, which may have either a sudden or gradual onset.[55] Clinical examination may reveal hypomobility in one or more segments, with reproduction of the pain with palpation of the involved joint. There is often associated spasm of the segmental paraspinal muscles. No imaging is required, unless it is persistent or not responding to conservative treatment.[56-64]

Paraspinal muscle sprain may occur following sudden movement, or where there is a history of trauma, coughing, or straining. Local muscular tenderness is present, and clinically it is important to differentiate the clinical findings from spinal or vertebral pathology, by accurate localization of the point of pain. No imaging is required and the treatment is conservative.

Costovertebral and costotransverse joint sprain presents with localized thoracic back pain, and may be seen in individuals with a chronic cough, or a history of inflammatory disease (e.g. ankylosing spondylitis), or degenerative osteoarthritis. Clinically, there is localized pain on inspiration and chest wall movement, with tenderness and hypo-mobility in one or more joints. No imaging is required, unless it is persistent or not responding to conservative modalities.[65]

Scheuermann's disease is a common osteochondritic condition affecting the thoracic spine, with acute pain presentation in adolescence, and late hypomobility/deformity in adulthood. Clinical presentations are thoracic spine pain, and stiffness of spinal movement. A thoracic spinal kyphosis is often present. A detailed training history is important, especially with extended periods in one posture (e.g. cycling), or loading into flexion.[66] Plain spine x-ray with a lateral view is diagnostic, with osteochrondritic change evident at the spinal endplates.[67, 68]

Vertebral crush fracture presents with localized spinal pain in the setting of a history of trauma, and/or risk factors for osteoporosis. Clinically, localized tenderness is present, and rarely is there radicular involvement. Imaging studies such as plain x-ray, CT, or MRI are diagnostic. The management of the pain is the main treatment, and addressing osteoporosis if present.

T4 syndrome[69] is an unusual condition seen in athletes. It presents with diffuse arm pain, and vague sensory symptoms.[70] Examination often demonstrates hypomobility of the upper to mid-thoracic spine segments, with poor cervical posture.[70] No imaging is required, and treatment is based around restoring normal mobility of the affected thoracic spinal segments.

Internal disease (e.g. peptic ulcer, aortic aneurysm, cardiac disease, pancreatitis) is an important differential in all patients with back pain, given the potentially catastrophic consequence of missed diagnoses. There should be an absent trauma history, and the presence of associated symptoms such as sweating, shortness of breath, hypotension, fever etc, which emphasizes the role of a complete and thorough physical exam in all cases of back pain. A back examination should be normal, and further investigations such as electrocardiography, blood tests, and imaging will be required, as appropriate to the underlying condition.[71]

Spondylolisthesis commonly presents as central low back pain aggravated by extension, in late childhood and adolescence. The most common age of onset is 9–14 years, but the condition may also be asymptomatic, and be noted as an incidental finding on a spinal x-ray in later life. Higher grades of spondylolisthesis result in a greater slip of one vertebra on another. Clinical examination is often unrevealing, and plain x-ray and/or CT scan is diagnostic.[72–77]

Spinal canal stenosis is due to degenerative osteoarthritic chanes in an ageing spine, with narrowing of the vertebral canal due to disc bulge, osteophytic formation, and thickening of the longitudinal ligaments. It results in chronic low back pain, radicular symptoms, and spinal claudication. Examination usually reveals little other than a hypomobile lumbar spine and possible radicular findings. CT and MRI imaging is usually diagnostic. If severe, then surgical treatment is often warranted.[78–82]

Lumbar instability is often proposed as a common cause of low back pain in the absence of structural pathology. There is a school of thought which suggests that the primary basis of this is impaired transversus abdominis function,[83–85] which may be associated with intrinsic back muscle wasting.[86] This is largely a clinical diagnosis, and imaging is usually unhelpful, other than to exclude other pathology. Isokinetic muscle testing has been proposed as a useful investigative modality,[87] and electromyography is reported as being abnormal in 75% of cases.[88] Treatment is usually with a program of core muscle strengthening such as Pilates.

Table 9.5 A patho-anatomic approach; within the spine triangle				
Define and align	**Pathology**	**Listen and localize**	**Palpate and recreate**	**Alleviate and investigate**
Within the spine triangle	Intervertebral disc herniation	Back pain, radicular symptoms (e.g. sciatica)	Localized tenderness. Neurological signs such as altered dermatomal sensation. Important to exclude spinal cord compression[10, 47–54]	No imaging required unless persistent > 6 weeks. CT or MRI may demonstrate cause[10, 47–54]
	Intervertebral joint sprain (disk, zygopophyseal joints)	Sudden or gradual onset[56–58]	Hypomobility in one or more segments[55] Local tenderness over spinous process, zygopophyseal joint Spasm of segmental paraspinal muscles[56–58]	No imaging required unless persistent[59–64]
	Paraspinal muscle sprain	Sudden onset. History of trauma, coughing, straining. Localized pain on movement	Local muscular tenderness	No imaging required
	Costovertebral and costotransverse joint sprain	Localized thoracic back pain. Pain on inspiration. History of inflammatory disease (e.g. ankylosing spondylitis), or degenerative OA	Hypomobility in one or more joints. Local tenderness over joints. Spasm of segmental paraspinal muscles[65]	No imaging required unless persistent[65]
	Scheuermann's disease	Adolescent. Thoracic pain. Training history important, especially with extended periods in one posture (e.g. cycling), or loading into flexion[66]	Thoracic kyphosis[67, 68]	Plain x-ray (lateral) is diagnostic[67, 68]
	Vertebral crush fracture	Localized pain. History of trauma and/or risk factors for osteoporosis	Local tenderness. Rarely radicular involvement	Plain x-ray, CT, or MRI
	T4 syndrome[69]	Diffuse arm pain and sensory symptoms[70]	Hypomobility of upper to mid thoracic spine segments. Poor cervical posture[70]	No imaging required
	Internal disease e.g. peptic ulcer, cardiac, pancreatitis	Absent trauma history. Associated symptoms e.g. sweating, SOB, hypotension, fever etc[71]	Exclude local pathology. No tenderness of back/chest wall. No hypomobility of spinal segments[71]	ECG, blood tests, imaging as appropriate

	Table 9.5 A patho-anatomic approach; within the spine triangle *(continued)*			
Define and align	**Pathology**	**Listen and localize**	**Palpate and recreate**	**Alleviate and Investigate**
	Spondylolisthesis	Most common age 9–14 yrs. Often asymptomatic. Higher grades cause low back pain aggravated by extension	Palpable dip at level of slip. Local soft tissue tenderness or spasm[72–77]	Plain x-ray with lateral views. CT scan[72–77]
	Spinal canal stenosis	Low back pain. Spinal claudication symptoms[78–82]	Hypomobile lumbar spine. Possible radicular findings[78–82]	CT, MRI
	Lumbar instability	Low back pain	Altered TA function.[83–85] Intrinsic back muscle wasting[86]	No imaging required. Isokinetic muscle testing.[87] EMG abnormal in 75%[88]
	Pars interarticularis stress fracture	Persistent, localized, unilateral back pain aggravated by movement involving lumbar extension. History of back rotation and hyperextension e.g. tennis player, pole vaulter, gymnast, cricket bowler[89]	Lumbar pain on extension and rotation. Tenderness over site of fracture. Excessive lordotic posture. Pain on stressing pars	Plain x-ray with 45° oblique view, isotope bone scan, reverse gantry CT or MRI[89]
	Spinal deformity e.g. scoliosis, spina bifida	Age of onset of deformity. Infantile forms may be associated with other developmental (e.g. genitourinary) abnormalities, or muscle disease. Back pain, limitation of movement[90]	Measurement of scoliosis in standing and flexion. Exclude other medical problems[90]	Plain x-ray, or CT scan
	Lumbar paraspinal compartment syndrome	Exercise-related low back pain and muscle spasm[94]	Tenderness and tenseness of erector spine muscles post exercise[91–94]	Compartment pressure test gives variable results[91–94]
	Diffuse idiopathic skeletal hyperostosis	Typically 6th and 7th decades of life. Stiffness and pain in back, dysphagia, often associated tendinitis	Stiffness of spine with reduced ROM. Possible myelopathy signs[95, 96]	Plain x-ray of spine, CT, and MRI[95, 96]

Pars interarticularis stress fracture results in persistent, localized, unilateral back pain, aggravated by movement involving lumbar extension. Typically, there is a history of back rotation and hyperextension, such as with tennis players, pole vaulters, gymnasts, and cricket bowlers.[89] Clinically, examination reveals lumbar pain on extension and rotation, with tenderness over the site of fracture, and reproduction of the pain on stressing the pars interarticularis at the affected level. There may be also an excessive lordotic posture. Plain x-ray with a 45° oblique view, isotope bone scan, reverse gantry CT, or MRI are diagnostic.[89]

Spinal deformity such as scoliosis, or spina bifida, may present with spinal pain. Infantile forms may be associated with other developmental (e.g. genitourinary) abnormalities or muscle disease. Later onset cases tend to present with pain and increasing deformity, particularly during the growth spurts in adolescence. Clinically, other than a deformity, there is usually restriction of spinal movement. It is important to measurement scoliosis in standing and flexion, to bring out the deformity more clearly. Plain x-ray or CT scan are usually diagnostic, and management is often in specialized clinics.[90]

Compartment syndromes of the erector spine muscles have been reported as an uncommon cause of chronic exercise-related back pain. Clinically, palpable rigidity without muscle spasm occurs in the affected muscles, and epaxial muscle contractions extend the spine, increasing lordosis.[91-94] Cadaveric dissections demonstrate fascial envelopment of these muscles, which may predispose some individuals to the developoment of this condition. Variable findings have been noted from compartment pressure testing studies in symptomatic patients, and the diagnosis may ultimately be a clinical one.[91-94] Fasciectomy may be curative.

Diffuse idiopathic skeletal hyperostosis is an uncommon but well recognized cause of spinal pain and dysfunction.[95, 96] The condition presents with anterior and lateral ossification of the spine, hyperostosis at sites of tendon and ligament insertion, ligamentous ossification, and periarticular osteophytes. The disease has about the same frequency in men (65%) and women (35%); it is most common in the thoracic spine, and occurs less frequently in the lumbar and cervical spine. The formal radiological diagnostic criteria require: (a) flowing ossification along the anterior and anterolateral aspects of at least four contiguous vertebrae; (b) preserved intervertebral disc height; (c) no bony ankylosis of the posterior spinal facet joints; and finally (d) no erosion, sclerosis, or bony ankylosis of the sacroiliac joints.[95, 96] Signs and symptoms include stiffness and pain in the back, dysphagia due to direct esophageal compression or distortion, pain related to associated tendinitis, myelopathy related to core compression associated with the ossification of the posterior longitudinal ligament, and pain related to vertebral complications such as fracture or subluxation. While conventional radiography clearly confirms the diagnosis of diffuse idiopathic skeletal hyperostosis, CT and MRI better detect associated findings (e.g. ossification of the posterior longitudinal ligament), and complications (e.g. spinal cord compressive myelomalacia). There is no treatment for this condition at present.[95, 96]

Systemic illness and malignancy

These conditions are beyond the scope of the diagnostic triangles, and care should always be taken to exclude systemic illness. The cardinal features of malignancy are unexplained weight loss, fever, nocturnal bone pain, and systemic illness, although of course these are commonly late-presenting signs. The clinician should always be aware of the potential for a musculoskeletal condition to mask an underlying systemic illness. Urgent imaging studies, such as plain x-ray, CT, MRI, or bone scans, are usually indicated if this is suspected.

Summary

Back problems are among the most common presentations seen in sports medicine. Although precise anatomical diagnoses are often difficult, the back triangle approach endeavors to simplify the diagnosis of pathology in this region in the active person. A complete, anatomically oriented differential diagnosis facilitates better initial diagnosis and, where a diagnosis is in doubt, allows an easy and complete review of potential pathologies.

Case histories

Case 1

A 30-year-old man presents with a six-week history of low back pain, associated with left lateral shin pain, numbness, and tingling. The numbness and tingling only began about 10 days ago, and these symptoms have gradually increased since that time.

Step 1: Define and align
Expose the patient properly; a pair of sports shorts will allow physical access and aid visibility.

Define the triangle: locate the high points of the iliac crest on both sides, and C1.

Align the patient's pain on the triangle. Here the pain is within the triangle, and localized to the central spinal region at the level of the iliac crest, which corresponds to the L4 vertebrae. From this point, we recommend that the reader attempt to exclude the potential pathologies. From Table 9.5, the potential causal structures in the lumbar region are:

Differential diagnosis

> intervertebral disc herniation

> intervertebral joint sprain (disk, zygopophyseal joints)

> paraspinal muscle sprain

> vertebral crush fracture

> spondylolisthesis

> spinal canal stenosis

> lumbar instability

> pars interarticularis stress fracture

> spinal deformity e.g. scoliosis, spina bifida

> tumor (e.g. secondary)

We proceed to differentiate between these structures, step 2.

Step 2: Listen and localize

Addressing intervertebral disc herniation we ask:

Q *What sort of work do you do, and do you do much activity in your job?*

A I work as an accountant, and sit at my desk throughout most days.

Q *Do you do much exercise, or other physical activity?*

A No, I do little physical activity.

Q *Is the pain worse on forward flexion?*

A Yes, I particularly find that driving in a car makes my back pain worse. The back pain and numbness are worse when sitting for prolonged periods of time, and tend not to be a problem when I am standing or walking.

Q *Where is the numbness and tingling?*

A Over the outside of my calf and top of my foot.

Q *Do you have any bowel or bladder dysfunction, or other symptoms in either leg?*

A No.

Addressing intervertebral joint sprain, or paraspinal muscle sprain we ask:

Q *Did the pain start suddenly, while lifting or straining?*

A No, there was no injury at the start. The pain just gradually increased.

Q *Is there any sharp pain in your back when moving?*

A No.

Addressing vertebral crush fracture we ask:

Q *Is there any problem with your bones, have you been on steroid therapy, or do you have an endocrine or hormonal problem?*

A No.

Addressing spondylolisthesis we ask:

Q *Is there any history of back pain as a child or adolescent?*

A No.

Q *Is there any pain on extension of the back?*

A No. Moving in that direction seems to reduce my pain.

Addressing spinal canal stenosis we ask:
Q *Is there any history of pain in your legs when you walk?*
A No.

Addressing lumbar instability we ask:
Q *Have you ever had an injury to your back in the past?*
A No.

Addressing pars interarticularis stress fracture we ask:
Q *Is the pain on one side of your back, or both sides?*
A It seems to be in the middle, and radiating to both sides.
Q *Do you do anything that may involve rotating and extending your back, such as tennis, or cricket bowling?*
A No.

Addressing spinal deformity we ask:
Q *Is there any history of spinal problems when you were a child, such as scoliosis or curvature of the spine?*
A No.

Addressing possible tumor we ask:
Q *Have you lost any weight recently, had pain in your back which wakes you at night, had a fever, or any other unusual symptoms?*
A No.
Q *Do you have any history of tumor, or malignancy?*
A No.

This narrows our differential diagnosis somewhat, and we proceed to examination to narrow it further. By palpating painful structures, and recreating the pain through diagnostic maneuvers, we move toward a diagnosis, step 3.

Step 3: Palpate and re-create
We palpate the spine and find tenderness over the L4 and L5 vertebrae. There is associated spasm in the paraspinal muscles at this level. The L4/5 and L5/S1 segments are hypomobile. Neurological examination of the lower limbs shows weakness on the left with ankle and toe dorsiflexion, a reduced ankle tendon reflex, decreased sensation over the lateral calf and dorsum of the foot (L5 dermatome), and a positive left straight leg raise test, with numbness reproduced below 40°.

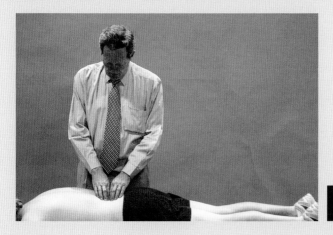

Figure 9.8 Palpation of vertebral levels

Differential diagnosis

More likely

> intervertebral disc herniation

Less likely

> intervertebral joint sprain (disk, zygopophyseal joints)

> spondylolisthesis

> lumbar instability

Unlikely but must not be forgotten

> tumor

Step 4: Alleviate and investigate

We may now proceed to step 4 to confirm our clinical suspicion via imaging. The most evidence-based test is MRI of the lumbar spine. The MRI confirms that there is a posterolateral disc prolapse at the L5/S1 level, with associated L5 nerve root compression.

Anatomical comment on symptoms

The numbness and tingling in the patient's left leg are likely to be due to a herniated disc, probably between the L5 and S1 vertebrae. The left leg symptoms are radicular in nature, from the compression of this nerve root. A herniated disc occurs when a tear exists in the outer portion of the disc (the anulus fibrosus), and the inner portion (the nucleus pulposus) seeps through the tear. If severe enough, the material compresses the nerve root, causing symptoms. Many people have a herniated nucleus pulposus, but do not report symptoms.

Case 2

A 20-year-old baseballer presents with a history of low back pain. He reports that the most severe pain occurs when sitting in class, standing for prolonged periods of time, and following baseball practise. The pain has been present since primary school, and gradually getting worse. Physiotherapy and massage seem to give temporary relief.

Step 1: Define and align

Expose the patient properly; a pair of sports shorts will allow physical access and aid visibility.

Define the triangle: locate the high points of the iliac crest on both sides, and C1.

Align the patient's pain on the triangle. Here the pain is within the triangle, and localized to the central spinal region, which corresponds to the lumbar vertebrae. From this point we recommend that the reader attempt to exclude the potential pathologies. From Table 9.5, the potential causal structures in the lumbar region are:

Differential diagnosis

> intervertebral disc herniation

> intervertebral joint sprain (disk, zygopophyseal joints)

> paraspinal muscle sprain

> vertebral crush fracture

> spondylolisthesis

> spinal canal stenosis

> lumbar instability

> pars interarticularis stress fracture

> spinal deformity (e.g. scoliosis, spina bifida)

> tumor (e.g. secondary)

We proceed to differentiate between these structures, step 2.

Step 2: Listen and localize

Addressing intervertebral disc herniation we ask:

Q *What sort of work do you do, and do you do much activity in your job?*

A I attend college, and sit at my desk for lectures throughout most days.

Q *Do you do much exercise, or other physical activity?*

A I do physical activity, playing for the college baseball team; otherwise I walk regularly.

Q *Is the pain worse on forward flexion?*

A Yes, I particularly find that sitting for prolonged periods of time tends to be a problem.

Q *Is there numbness and tingling in your legs?*

A No.

Q *Do you have any bowel or bladder dysfunction, or other symptoms in either leg?*

A No.

Addressing intervertebral joint sprain, or paraspinal muscle sprain we ask:

Q *Did the pain start suddenly, while lifting or straining?*

A No, there was no injury at the start. The pain just gradually increased over years.

Q *Is there any sharp pain in your back when moving?*

A No.

Addressing vertebral crush fracture we ask:

Q *Is there any problem with your bones, have you been on steroid therapy, or do you have an endocrine or hormonal problem?*

A No.

Addressing spondylolisthesis we ask:

Q *Is there any history of back pain as a child or adolescent?*

A No.

Q *Is there any pain on extension of the back?*

A No.

Addressing spinal canal stenosis we ask:

Q *Is there any history of pain in your legs when you walk?*

A No.

Addressing lumbar instability we ask:

Q *Have you ever had an injury to your back in the past?*

A No. The pain began in primary school, and has seemed to gradually get worse over my teenage years.

Addressing pars interarticularis stress fracture we ask:

Q *Is the pain on one side of your back, or both sides?*

A Both sides.

Q *Do you do anything which may involve rotating and extending your back, such as tennis, or cricket bowling?*

A Yes. I play baseball, but I don't get pain during practise, only afterwards.

Addressing spinal deformity we ask:

Q *Is there any history of spinal problems when you were a child, such as scoliosis or curvature of the spine?*

A No.

Addressing possible tumor we ask:

Q *Have you lost any weight recently, had pain in your back which wakes you at night, had a fever, or any other unusual symptoms?*

A No.

Q *Do you have any history of tumor, or malignancy?*

A No.

This narrows our differential diagnosis somewhat, and we proceed to examination to narrow it further. By palpating painful structures, and recreating the pain through diagnostic maneuvers, we move toward a diagnosis, step 3.

Step 3: Palpate and re-create

Examination shows no discrepancy in the patient's spinal and pelvic landmarks, and no neurological signs are present. During an active range of motion, the patient reports pain during flexion, and exhibits aberrant movements (thigh climbing) when returning to neutral from flexion. His passive straight leg raise is normal. Spring testing on the patient's spinous processes (by placing the patient in a prone position and applying an anterior force on each spinous process) results in pain when pressure is applied to L2–L4. Also, the patient shows hypermobility in each lumbar segment. A prone instability test is done, to determine whether a diagnosis of instability is indicated. The patient is placed in a prone position, with his hips on the edge of the table and his legs hanging off the table. Spring testing is again performed in this position, and again the patient reports pain at L2–4. The patient is then instructed to extend his hips, so that his body is in a straight position, and his erector spine muscles are activated. Again spring testing

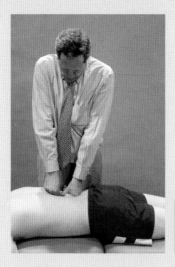

Figure 9.9 Spring testing for lumbar instability

is performed while he holds this position. If he does not report pain during this, the test is positive for instability. In this case, he does not report pain, which is consistent with a lumbar instability.

Differential diagnosis

More likely
> lumbar instability

Less likely
> intervertebral joint sprain (disk, zygopophyseal joints)
> spondylolisthesis

Unlikely but must not be forgotten
> tumor

Step 4: Alleviate and investigate

We may now proceed to step 4 to confirm our clinical suspicion. In this case, no imaging is required, and the patient can be treated clinically. It has been reported that isokinetic muscle testing may be useful diagnostically,[87] as well as needle electromyography, although only 75% of patients will demonstrate abnormalities.[88]

Case 3

A 51-year-old doctor presents with a recent history of left lateral thoracic pain. He reports that the pain has come on over the past 3–4 weeks, associated with a chronic cough, recently diagnosed by his general practitioner as pertussis. Other than a past history of hypertension and hypercholesterolemia, he is well.

Step 1: Define and align

Expose the patient properly; a pair of sports shorts will allow physical access and aid visibility.

Define the triangle: locate the high points of the iliac crest on both sides, and C1.

Align the patient's pain on the triangle. Here the pain is lateral to the triangle, and localized to the lateral chest wall. From this point we recommend that the reader attempt to exclude the potential pathologies. From Table 9.4, the potential causal structures in this region are:

Differential diagnosis

> intercostal muscle strain
> radicular pain
> rib fracture

> rib stress fracture

> nerve injury to localized back muscle

> herpes zoster (shingles)

> tumor (e.g. secondary)

We proceed to differentiate between these structures, step 2.

Step 2: Listen and localize

Addressing intercostal muscle strain we ask:

Q *What sort of work do you do, and do you do much activity in your job?*

A I work as a doctor, and mostly sit at my desk seeing patients, or at my computer throughout most days.

Q *Do you do much exercise, or other physical activity?*

A I walk the dog regularly and, before I was sick, I used to go to the gym three times per week.

Q *Is the pain worse on movement?*

A Yes, I particularly find that moving in any direction causes pain. Also coughing, sneezing, and straining.

Q *Is there numbness and tingling in your legs?*

A No.

Q *Did the pain start suddenly, while lifting or straining?*

A No, there was no obvious injury at the start.

Q *Do you have any bowel or bladder dysfunction, or other symptoms in either leg?*

A No.

Addressing radicular pain or nerve injury to localized back muscles we ask:

Q *Does the pain radiate around your chest at all?*

A No, it seems to be in one spot.

Q *Is there any numbness, or tingling in your chest?*

A No.

Q *Is there any weakness of any muscle in your chest or back?*

A No.

Addressing rib fracture or stress fracture we ask:

Q *Is there any problem with your bones, have you been on steroid therapy, or do you have an endocrine or hormonal problem?*

A Yes, I had a single course of steroids early on, for the treatment of the severe pertussis-related cough.

Q *Was there any trauma to your chest?*

A No.

Addressing herpes zoster (shingles) we ask:

Q *Is there any rash?*

A No.

Q *Have you ever had chicken pox?*

A Yes, as a child.

Addressing possible tumor we ask:

Q *Have you lost any weight recently, had pain in your back which wakes you at night, had a fever, or any other unusual symptoms?*

A No.

Q *Do you have any history of tumor, or malignancy?*

A No.

This narrows our differential diagnosis somewhat, and we proceed to examination to narrow it further. By palpating painful structures, and recreating the pain through diagnostic maneuvers, we move toward a diagnosis, step 3.

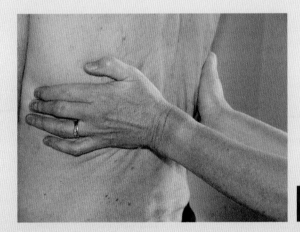

Figure 9.10 Rib tenderness on springing of ribs

Step 3: Palpate and re-create

Examination shows a localized area of tenderness over the sixth rib laterally. The patient's pain is reproduced when springing the chest wall. The tenderness is localized to the rib, with no muscle tenderness in relation to the rib. Auscultation of the lung is normal.

Differential diagnosis

More likely

> rib (stress) fracture

> intercostal muscle strain

Less likely
> herpes zoster
> localized nerve injury

Unlikely but must not be forgotten
> tumor

Step 4: Alleviate and investigate

We may now proceed to step 4 to confirm our clinical suspicion. In this case, plain chest x-ray, including a lateral view with rib views, demonstrates an undisplaced sixth rib fracture, and there is no evidence of any underlying chest disease (e.g. infection or pneumothorax).

References

1. Andersson GB. Epidemiology of low back pain. Acta Orthop Scand Suppl. 1998 Jun; 281:28–31.
2. Patel AT, Ogle AA. Diagnosis and management of acute low back pain. Am Fam Physician. 2000 Mar 15; 61(6):1779–86, 89–90.
3. Walker BF, Muller R, Grant WD. Low back pain in Australian adults: the economic burden. Asia Pac J Public Health. 2003; 15(2):79–87.
4. Harris-Hayes M, Sahrmann S, Van Dillen L. Relationship between the hip and low back pain in athletes who participate in rotation-related sports. J Sports Rehabiliation. 2009; 18(1):60–75.
5. Fritz J, Clifford S. Low back pain in adolescents: a comparison of clinical outcomes in sports participants and nonparticipants. J Athl Train 2010; 45(1):61–66.
6. Woolf S, Glaser J. Low back pain in running-based sports. South Med J. 2004; 97(9):847–51.
7. Hansen L, de Zee M, Rasmussen J, Andersen TB, Wong C, Simonsen EB. Anatomy and biomechanics of the back muscles in the lumbar spine with reference to biomechanical modeling. Spine (Phila Pa 1976). 2006 Aug 1; 31(17):1888–99.
8. Hoskisson JB. Posture and comparative anatomy as guiding principles in the treatment of back disorders. Br J Phys Med. 1957 Jun; 20(6):121–26.
9. Dreyfuss P, Michelsen M, Pauza K, McLarty J, Bogduk N. The value of medical history and physical examination in diagnosing sacroiliac joint pain. Spine (Philadelphia PA 1976). 1996 Nov 15; 21(22):2594–602.
10. Olivieri I, van Tubergen A, Salvarani C, van der Linden S. Seronegative spondyloarthritides. Best Pract Res Clin Rheumatol. 2002 Dec; 16(5):723–39.
11. Onsel C, Collier BD, Kir KM, Larson SJ, Meyer GA, Krasnow AZ, et al. Increased sacroiliac joint uptake after lumbar fusion and/or laminaectomy. Clin Nucl Med. 1992 Apr; 17(4):283–87.
12. Puhakka KB, Jurik AG, Schiottz-Christensen B, Hansen GV, Egund N, Christiansen JV, et al. MRI abnormalities of sacroiliac joints in early spondylarthropathy: a 1-year follow-up study. Scand J Rheumatol. 2004; 33(5):332–38.
13. Puhakka KB, Jurik AG, Schiottz-Christensen B, Hansen GV, Egund N, Christiansen JV, et al. Magnetic resonance imaging of sacroiliitis in early seronegative spondylarthropathy. Abnormalities correlated to clinical and laboratory findings. Rheumatology (Oxford). 2004 Feb; 43(2):234–37.
14. Puhakka KB, Melsen F, Jurik AG, Boel LW, Vesterby A, Egund N. MR imaging of the normal sacroiliac joint with correlation to histology. Skeletal Radiol. 2004 Jan; 33(1):15–28.
15. Slipman CW, Sterenfeld EB, Chou LH, Herzog R, Vresilovic E. The value of radionuclide imaging in the diagnosis of sacroiliac joint syndrome. Spine (Philadelphia PA 1976). 1996 Oct 1; 21(19):2251–54.
16. Freburger J, Riddle D. Measurement of sacroiliac joint dysfunction: a multicenter intertester reliability study. Phys Ther. 1999; 79:1134–41.
17. Broadhurst NA. Sacroiliac dysfunction as a cause of low back pain. Aust Fam Physician. 1989 Jun; 18(6):623–24, 26–27, 29.
18. Brolinson PG, Kozar AJ, Cibor G. Sacroiliac joint dysfunction in athletes. Curr Sports Med Rep. 2003 Feb; 2(1):47–56.

19. Bogduk N. *Clinical anatomy of the lumbar spine and sacrum.* 4th ed. Edinburgh: Churchill–Livingstone; 2004.
20. Broadhurst N. The iliolumbar ligament syndrome. Aust Fam Physician. 1989 May; 18(5):522.
21. Rucco V, Basadonna P, Gasparini D. The anatomy of the iliolumbar ligament. Am J Phys Med Rehab. 1996; 75(6):451–55.
22. Neim F, Froetscher L, Hirschberg G. Treatment of the chronic iliolumbar syndrome by infiltration of the iliolumbar ligament. West J Med. 1982; 136(4):372–74.
23. Beatty RA. The piriformis muscle syndrome: a simple diagnostic maneuver. Neurosurgery. 1994 Mar; 34(3):512–14; discussion 14.
24. Fishman LM, Anderson C, Rosner B. BOTOX and physical therapy in the treatment of piriformis syndrome. Am J Phys Med Rehabil. 2002 Dec; 81(12):936–42.
25. Fishman LM, Dombi GW, Michelsen C, Ringel S, Rozbruch J, Rosner B, et al. Piriformis syndrome: diagnosis, treatment, and outcome – a 10-year study. Arch Phys Med Rehabil. 2002 Mar; 83(3):295–301.
26. Fishman LM, Zybert PA. Electrophysiologic evidence of piriformis syndrome. Arch Phys Med Rehabil. 1992 Apr; 73(4):359–64.
27. McCrory P, Bell S. Nerve entrapment syndromes as a cause of pain in the hip, groin and buttock. Sports Med. 1999 Apr; 27(4):261–74.
28. Lin J, Lane J. Sacral stress fracture. J Women's Health. 2004; 12(9):879–88.
29. Zaman F, Frey M, Slipman C. Sacral stress fractures. Current Sports Medicine Reports. 2006; 5(1):37–43.
30. Hirose Y. A functional polymorphism in THBS2 that affects alternative splicing and MMP binding is associated with lumbar-disc herniation. American Journal of Human Genetics. 2008; 82(5):1122–29.
31. Vroomen P, de Krom M, Knottnerus J. Predicting the outcome of sciatica at short-term follow-up. Br J Gen Pract 2002; 52:119–23.
32. Cibulka M, Delitto A, Erhard R. Pain patterns in patients with and without sacroiliac joint dysfunction. In: Vleeming A, Mooney V, Snijders C, Dorman T, eds., *Low back pain and its relation to the sacroiliac joint.* San Diego; 1992. p. 363–70.
33. Fortin J, Falco F. The Fortin finger test: an indicator of sacroiliac pain. Am J Orthop. 1997; 26:477–80.
34. Andersson G, Deyo R. History and physical examination in patients with herniated lumbar discs. Spine (Philadelphia PA 1976). 1996; 21:10S–18S.
35. Hickey GJ, Fricker PA, McDonald WA. Injuries to elite rowers over a 10-year period. Med Sci Sports Exerc. 1997 Dec; 29(12):1567–72.
36. Hickey GJ, Fricker PA, McDonald WA. Injuries of young elite female basketball players over a six-year period. Clin J Sport Med. 1997 Oct; 7(4):252–56.
37. Dooley JF, McBroom RJ, Taguchi T, Macnab I. Nerve root infiltration in the diagnosis of radicular pain. Spine (Philadelphia PA 1976). 1988 Jan; 13(1):79–83.
38. Quintner JL. A study of upper limb pain and paresthesie following neck injury in motor vehicle accidents: assessment of the brachial plexus tension test of Elvey. Br J Rheumatol. 1989 Dec; 28(6):528–33.
39. Viikari-Juntura E. Interexaminer reliability of observations in physical examinations of the neck. Phys Ther. 1987 Oct; 67(10):1526–32.
40. Griffith J, Rainer T, Ching A, Law K, Cocks R, Metreweli C. Sonography compared with radiography in revealing acute rib fracture. American Journal of Roentgenology.173:1603–9.
41. Schurink GW, Bode PJ, van Luijt PA, van Vugt AB. The value of physical examination in the diagnosis of patients with blunt abdominal trauma: a retrospective study. Injury. 1997 May; 28(4):261–65.
42. Connolly LP, Connolly SA. Rib stress fractures. Clin Nucl Med. 2004 Oct; 29(10):614–16.
43. Iwamoto J, Takeda T. Stress fractures in athletes: review of 196 cases. J Orthop Sci. 2003; 8(3):273–78.
44. Karlson KA. Rib stress fractures in elite rowers. A case series and proposed mechanism. Am J Sports Med. 1998 Jul–Aug; 26(4):516–19.
45. Ragozzino MW, Melton LJ, 3rd, Kurland LT, Chu CP, Perry HO. Population-based study of herpes zoster and its sequele. Medicine (Baltimore). 1982 Sep; 61(5):310–16.
46. Ragozzino MW, Melton LJ, 3rd, Kurland LT, Chu CP, Perry HO. Risk of cancer after herpes zoster: a population-based study. N Engl J Med. 1982 Aug 12; 307(7):393–97.
47. Atlas SJ, Deyo RA. Evaluating and managing acute low back pain in the primary care setting. J Gen Intern Med. 2001 Feb; 16(2):120–31.

48. Atlas SJ, Deyo RA, van den Ancker M, Singer DE, Keller RB, Patrick DL. The Maine–Seattle back questionnaire: a 12-item disability questionnaire for evaluating patients with lumbar sciatica or stenosis: results of a derivation and validation cohort analysis. Spine (Philadelphia PA 1976). 2003 Aug 15; 28(16):1869–76.

49. Atlas SJ, Nardin RA. Evaluation and treatment of low back pain: an evidence-based approach to clinical care Muscle & Nerve. 2003 Mar; 27(3):265–84.

50. Atlas SJ, Volinn E. Classics from the spine literature revisited: a randomized trial of 2 versus 7 days of recommended bed rest for acute low back pain. Spine (Philadelphia PA 1976). 1997 Oct 15; 22(20):2331–37.

51. Maigne R. Low back pain of thoracolumbar origin. Arch Phys Med Rehabil. 1980 Sep; 61(9):389–95.

52. Vroomen PC, de Krom MC, Knottnerus JA. Diagnostic value of history and physical examination in patients suspected of sciatica due to disc herniation: a systematic review. J Neurol. 1999 Oct; 246(10):899–906.

53. Vroomen PC, de Krom MC, Wilmink JT, Kester AD, Knottnerus JA. Lack of effectiveness of bed rest for sciatica. N Engl J Med. 1999 Feb 11; 340(6):418–23.

54. Weinstein JN, Lurie JD, Tosteson TD, Skinner JS, Hanscom B, Tosteson AN, et al. Surgical vs nonoperative treatment for lumbar disk herniation: the Spine Patient Outcomes Research Trial (SPORT) observational cohort. JAMA. 2006 Nov 22; 296(20):2451–59.

55. Dreyer SJ, Dreyfuss PH. Low back pain and the zygapophyseal (facet) joints. Arch Phys Med Rehabil. 1996 Mar; 77(3):290–300.

56. Bogduk N, Long DM. The anatomy of the so-called "articular nerves" and their relationship to facet denervation in the treatment of low back pain. J Neurosurg. 1979 Aug; 51(2):172–77.

57. Boswell MV, Colson JD, Sehgal N, Dunbar EE, Epter R. A systematic review of therapeutic facet joint interventions in chronic spinal pain. Pain Physician. 2007 Jan; 10(1):229–53.

58. Dreyfuss P, Tibiletti C, Dreyer SJ. Thoracic zygapophyseal joint pain patterns. A study in normal volunteers. Spine (Philadelphia PA 1976). 1994 Apr 1; 19(7):807–11.

59. Carrera GF. Lumbar facet arthrography and injection in low back pain. Wis Med J. 1979 Dec; 78(12):35–37.

60. Carrera GF. Lumbar facet joint injection in low back pain and sciatica: description of technique. Radiology. 1980 Dec; 137(3):661–64.

61. Carrera GF, Haughton VM, Syvertsen A, Williams AL. Computed tomography of the lumbar facet joints. Radiology. 1980 Jan; 134(1):145–48.

62. Carrera GF, Williams AL. Current concepts in evaluation of the lumbar facet joints. Crit Rev Diagn Imaging. 1984; 21(2):85–104.

63. Lilius G, Laasonen EM, Myllynen P, Harilainen A, Gronlund G. Lumbar facet joint syndrome. A randomized clinical trial. J Bone Joint Surg Br. 1989 Aug; 71(4):681–84.

64. Lilius G, Laasonen EM, Myllynen P, Harilainen A, Salo L. [Lumbar facet joint syndrome. Significance of non-organic signs. A randomized placebo-controlled clinical study]. Rev Chir Orthop Reparatrice Appar Mot. 1989; 75(7):493–500.

65. Young BA, Gill HE, Wainner RS, Flynn TW. Thoracic costotransverse joint pain patterns: a study in normal volunteers. BMC Musculoskelet Disord. 2008; 9:140.

66. Ashton–Miller JA. Thoracic hyperkyphosis in the young athlete: a review of the biomechanical issues. Curr Sports Med Rep. 2004 Feb; 3(1):47–52.

67. Alexander C. Scheuermann's disease. Skeletal Radiology. 1977; 1(4):209–21.

68. Aufdermaur M. Juvenile kyphosis (Scheuermann's disease): radiography, histology, and pathogenesis. Clin Orthop Relat Res. 1981 Jan–Feb; (154):166–74.

69. Brukner P, Khan K. Clinical sports medicine. 3rd ed. Sydney, Australia: McGraw–Hill; 2007.

70. Defranca G, Levine L. The T4 syndrome. J Manipulative Physiol Ther. 1995; 18(1):34–37.

71. Smith MD, Russell A, Hodges PW. How common is back pain in women with gastrointestinal problems? Clin J Pain. 2008 Mar–Apr; 24(3):199–203.

72. Capener N. Skiagrams of a very early case of spondylolisthesis. Proc R Soc Med. 1935 Aug; 28(10):1369–70.

73. Capener N. Spondylolisthesis. Brit J Surg. 2005; 17(75):374–86.

74. Fredrickson BE, Baker D, McHolick WJ, Yuan HA, Lubicky JP. The natural history of spondylolysis and spondylolisthesis. J Bone Joint Surg Am. 1984 Jun; 66(5):699–707.

75. Middleton K, Fish DE. Lumbar spondylosis: clinical presentation and treatment approaches. Curr Rev Musculoskelet Med. 2009 Jun; 2(2):94–104.

76. Standert CJ, Herring SA. Spondylolysis: a critical review. Br J Sports Med. 2000 Dec; 34(6):415–22.

77. Standert CJ, Herring SA, Halpern B, King O. Spondylolysis. Phys Med Rehabil Clin N Am. 2000 Nov; 11(4): 785–803.
78. Amundsen T. Why are female birds ornamented? Trends Ecol Evol. 2000 Apr; 15(4):149–55.
79. Amundsen T, Weber H, Lilleas F, Nordal HJ, Abdelnoor M, Magnes B. Lumbar spinal stenosis. Clinical and radiologic features. Spine (Philadelphia PA 1976). 1995 May 15; 20(10):1178–86.
80. Amundsen T, Weber H, Nordal HJ, Magnes B, Abdelnoor M, Lilleas F. Lumbar spinal stenosis: conservative or surgical management?: A prospective 10-year study. Spine (Philadelphia PA 1976). 2000 Jun 1; 25(11):1424–35; discussion 35–36.
81. Tan S. Spinal canal stenosis. Singapore Med J. 2003; 44(4):168–69.
82. Teh J, Imam A, Watts C. Imaging of back pain. Imaging. 2005; 17:171–207.
83. Hodges PW. Core stability exercise in chronic low back pain. Orthop Clin North Am. 2003 Apr; 34(2):245–54.
84. Hodges PW, Richardson CA. Delayed postural contraction of transversus abdominis in low back pain associated with movement of the lower limb. J Spinal Disord. 1998 Feb; 11(1):46–56.
85. Hodges PW, Richardson CA. Inefficient muscular stabilization of the lumbar spine associated with low back pain. A motor control evaluation of transversus abdominis. Spine (Philadelphia PA 1976). 1996 Nov 15; 21(22): 2640–50.
86. Hides JA, Stokes MJ, Saide M, Jull GA, Cooper DH. Evidence of lumbar multifidus muscle wasting ipsilateral to symptoms in patients with acute/subacute low back pain. Spine (Philadelphia PA 1976). 1994 Jan 15; 19(2): 165–72.
87. McGill S. *Low back disorders: Evidence based prevention and rehabilitation.* Champaign, IL: Human Kinetics; 2002.
88. Sihvonen T, Lindgren KA, Airaksinen O, Manninen H. Movement disturbances of the lumbar spine and abnormal back muscle electromyographic findings in recurrent low back pain. Spine (Philadelphia PA 1976). 1997 Feb 1; 22(3):289–95.
89. Brukner P, Bennell K, Matheson G. *Stress fractures.* Melbourne: Blackwell Scientific; 1999.
90. Rogala EJ, Drummond DS, Gurr J. Scoliosis: incidence and natural history. A prospective epidemiological study. J Bone Joint Surg Am. 1978 Mar; 60(2):173–76.
91. Styf J, Lysell E. Chronic compartment syndrome in the erector spine muscle. Spine (Philadelphia PA 1976). 1987 Sep; 12(7):680–82.
92. Styf J, Korner L, Suurkula M. Intramuscular pressure and muscle blood flow during exercise in chronic compartment syndrome. J Bone Joint Surg Br. 1987 Mar; 69(2):301–05.
93. Styf J. Pressure in the erector spine muscle during exercise. Spine (Philadelphia PA 1976). 1987 Sep; 12(7): 675–79.
94. Carr D, Gilbertson L, Frymoyer J, Krag M, Pope M. Lumbar paraspinal compartment syndrome. A case report with physiologic and anatomic studies. Spine (Philadelphia PA 1976). 1985 Nov; 10(9):816–20.
95. Cammisa M, de Serio A, Gugliemi G. Diffuse idiopathic skeletal hyperostosis. Eur J Radiol. 1998; 27(Suppl 1):S7–11.
96. Mata S, Fortin P, Fitcharles M, Starr M, Lawrence M, Watts C, et al. A controlled study of diffuse idiopathic skeletal hyperostosis: clinical features and functional status. Medicine. 1997; 76(2):104–17.

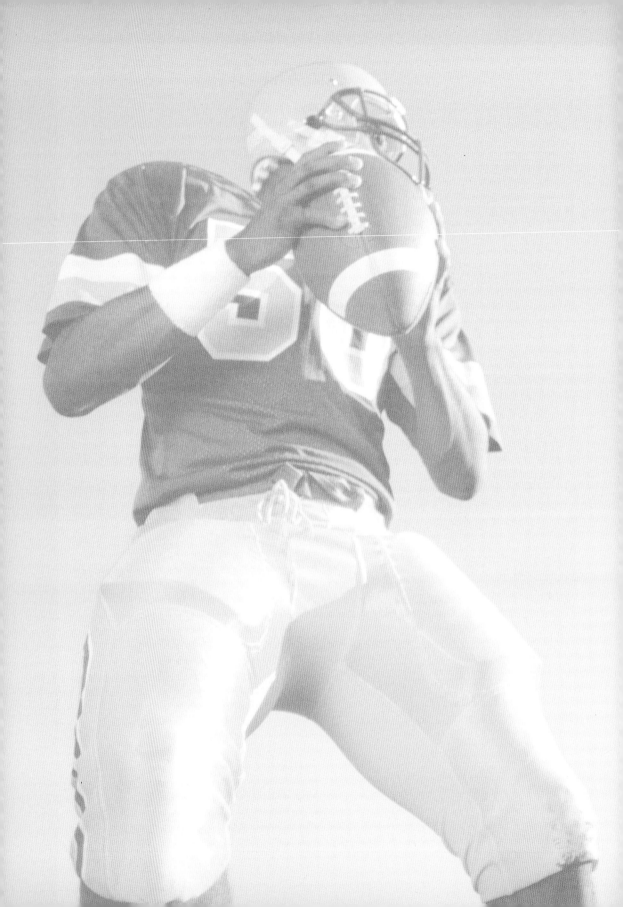

Index

Page numbers in *italics* indicate tables or figures.

adductor pollicis (AP)
  injury, *126*
  origin, insertion, nerve supply, *115*
  at radial border, 104–105
  in thumb, *109*
  on volar clockface, 110, *110*
adhesive capsulitis, *24*, 25
  diagnosis, *28*, 42–48
  stages of, *26*
ADM. *See* abductor digiti minimi
adolescents
  back pain in, *388*, 389
  hamstring injury in, *239*, 241
  hip pain in, 198–200, *200*
  Sever's disease in, *333*, *334*
AIIS. *See* anterior inferior iliac spine
AL. *See* adductor longus
ALCL. *See* anterolateral collateral ligament
Alcmaeon of Croton, *1*
align, *5*
American Society for Surgery of the Hand, *101*
anatomical clock, *9*, *9*
anatomical illustrations, 9–10, *10*
anatomical landmarks, *5*. *See also specific landmark*
"anatomical snuffbox," *102*, *106*, *125*
anatomical triangles, *8*, 8–9. *See also specific triangle*
anatomy teaching
  history of, 1–2
  trends in, 2–5, 7
anconaeus, *70*, *73*
ankle, 307–365
  anterior border, *318*, 318–319
  joint, 308–309, 308–312, *312*
  landmarks, 312, 316
  lateral border, *316*, 317–318
  medial border, 312–316, *314*
  movements, 308–309, *327*
  muscles, *325*–326
  nerves, *325*–326
  palpation, *328*, *348*, *351*, *353*, *353*, *355*
  posterior border, 319–320, *320*
ankle pathology. *See also specific disorder*
  anterior, 328–331, *329*–*331*, 347–349
  case histories, 347–360
  complex regional pain syndrome, 345–346
  lateral, *338*–*340*, 338–341, 354–356
  malignancy, 346

medial, 335–336, *336*–*337*, 352–354
Ottawa ankle rules, 346
posterior, 331–335, *332*–*334*, 349–352
referred pain, *332*, *334*, 335, 349–352
annular ligament, 64, *64*, 80
anterior band
  elbow, 63
  shoulder, 15, 21, 30
anterior capsule (shoulder), 15
anterior circumflex humeral artery, *19*
anterior cruciate ligament (ACL), *261*–262, 263–264
  at medial border, *270*
  pathology, 260, 280, 283
    diagnosis, 282, 299–302
anterior impingement syndrome, 328, *329*–*330*, 347–349
anterior inferior iliac spine (AIIS), 150, 154, 189, 198
anterior interosseus nerve, *73*, *82*, *115*
anterior joint line (knee), 267–268
anterior ligament (pubic symphysis), 147
anterior longitudinal ligaments, 369
anterior primary rami, 156–157, 196
anterior sacroiliac ligament, 220
anterior superior iliac spine (ASIS)
  in gluteal triangle, 229
  in greater trochanter triangle, *188*, *189*, *191*, *198*
  in groin triangle, *148*, *149*, *150*
    at lateral border, 153–154
    neuropathy and, *158*
    at superior border, *151*
anterior talofibular ligament (ATFL), 310, *310*, *316*
  pathology, *338*, *338*–*339*, 354–356
anterior tarsal tunnel syndrome, 328, *329*–*330*
anterior tibiofibular ligament, *265*, 310, 311
anterior tibiotalar ligament, 311, *312*
anterolateral collateral ligament (ALCL), *81*
anterolateral impingement (ankle), *316*, *338*, 339
  diagnosis, *340*, 354–356
aorta, 147
AP. *See* adductor pollicis
APB. *See* abductor pollicis brevis
APL. *See* abductor pollicis longus
Apley scarf test, 48
aponeuroses
  ankle, 315
  back, 379
  foot, 321

osteoid osteoma, 346
osteolysis, clavicular, *39, 40, 41*
osteoporosis, hip, *199,* 207–209
osteosarcoma, 242
os trigonum, *308*
Ottawa rules
   ankle, 346
   knee, 289

P
"Paget-Schroetter syndrome," 35
pain. *See also specific site or type of pain*
   alleviation of, 7
   radicular (*See* radicular pain)
   referred (*See* referred pain)
pain provocation test, 45, 56
palmar digital artery, *102*
palmar digital nerve, *102*
palmar interossei, *111, 115*
palmaris longus (PL)
   at elbow, 68, 69, *71, 72*
   origin, insertion, nerve supply, *114*
   at wrist, 101, *102–103*
palmar metacarpal ligament, *99*
palpation, 6. *See also specific site or technique*
   anatomical clock for, *9, 9*
Panner's disease, 73, *74, 75, 76*
paraspinal muscle sprain, *376,* 385
   diagnosis, *387,* 390–397
parasthesia, groin, *158*
pars interarticularis fracture, 232, *376,* 389
   diagnosis, *388,* 394–397
patella, 262, 263, 269, 271
   pathology, *277,* 284, *284–286*
      diagnosis, 285–286, 299–302
patellar ligament, 263
patellar retinaculum, *284*
   lateral, *279, 279, 281,* 293–296
   medial, *268, 277*
patellar tendon, 267–268
   pathology, *277,* 283, 285, 299–302
patellofemoral joint, 261–262, *261–262*
   pathology, 284, *284*
      diagnosis, 285, 293–296, 299–302
Patte's test, 47, *47,* 55
PCL. *See* posterior cruciate ligament
pectineal line, *152*
pectineus, *148, 149, 150, 152*
   origin, insertion, nerve supply, *157, 197*

pathology, *158, 205*
pectoralis major, 18, *20*
   origin, insertion, nerve supply, *22*
   pathology, *24, 27, 35, 39*
      diagnosis, *28, 38,* 42–51
pectoralis minor, 20, *22*
Pellegrini-Stieda syndrome, 277, *277, 278,* 291–293
pelvic bones, 219–221, *367, 377. See also* sacroiliac joint; *specific bone*
pelvic floor dysfunction, *238, 239,* 250–253
pelvic viscera, *150,* 168–169
peroneal nerve
   common (*See* common peroneal nerve)
   deep (*See* deep peroneal nerve)
   pathology, *338,* 354–356
   superficial, 274, 317, 318, *319, 324, 325, 326*
peroneal tendons, *318*
   pathology, *316, 339,* 354–356
peroneus brevis, *316, 317, 320, 324*
   origin, insertion, nerve supply, *326*
   pathology, *332, 338, 339,* 354–356
peroneus longus, 274, *316, 317, 320, 324*
   origin, insertion, nerve supply, *326*
   pathology, *332, 338, 339,* 354–356
Perthes' disease, 186, 199, *200*
   diagnosis, *201,* 210–212
pes anserinus, 268–270, *270*
   pathology, 277, *277*
      diagnosis, *278,* 291–293
phalanges
   foot, *309,* 322
   hand, 96–97
Phalen's test, 122–123, *140*
phrenic nerve, 35
pincer deformity, *198*
PIPJ. *See* proximal interphalangeal joint
piriformis, 190, *191–192*
   in gluteal triangle, 225, 227, *228,* 229–230
      pathology, *236, 238,* 250–253
   origin, insertion, nerve supply, *196, 223*
   tendinopathy, *204, 204*
piriformis nerve, *223*
piriformis syndrome, 236, *376,* 382, 383
pisiform bone, 96, 97, 98, *100, 113*
   fracture, 123, *123, 125, 126*
      diagnosis, 124, 137–140
   on volar clockface, *110,* 110–111
pisometacarpal ligament, *99*